THE PHYSICAL PRINCIPLES
of
ELECTRON PARAMAGNETIC RESONANCE

SECOND EDITION

FRONTIERS IN PHYSICS

David Pines, Editor

S. L. Adler and R. F. Dashen
    Current Algebras and Applications to Particle Physics, 1968

P. W. Anderson   *Concepts in Solids: Lectures on the Theory of Solids, 1965 (2nd printing, 1971)*

V. Barger and D. Cline
    Phenomenological Theories of High Energy Scattering: An Experimental Evaluation, 1967

N. Bloembergen   *Nonlinear Optics: A Lecture Note and Reprint Volume, 1965*

N. Bloembergen   *Nuclear Magnetic Relaxation: A Reprint Volume, 1961*

R. Brout   *Phase Transitions, 1965*

G. F. Chew   *S-Matrix Theory of Strong Interactions: A Lecture Note and Reprint Volume, 1961*

P. Choquard   *The Anharmonic Crystal, 1967*

P. G. de Gennes   *Superconductivity of Metals and Alloys, 1966*

R. P. Feynman   *Quantum Electrodynamics: A Lecture Note and Reprint Volume, 1961 (2nd printing, with corrections, 1962)*

R. P. Feynman   *The Theory of Fundamental Processes: A Lecture Note Volume, 1961*

R. P. Feynman   *Statistical Mechanics: A Set of Lectures, 1972*

R. P. Feynman   *Photon-Hadron Interactions, 1972*

H. Frauenfelder   *The Mössbauer Effect: A Review—with a Collection of Reprints, 1966*

S. C. Frautschi   *Regge Poles and S-Matrix Theory, 1963*

H. L. Frisch and J. L. Lebowitz
    The Equilibrium Theory of Classical Fluids: A Lecture Note and Reprint Volume, 1964

M. Gell-Mann and Y. Ne'eman
    The Eightfold Way: (A Review—with a Collection of Reprints), 1964

W. A. Harrison   *Pseudopotentials in the Theory of Metals, 1966 (2nd printing 1971)*

R. Hofstadter   *Electron Scattering and Nuclear and Nucleon Structure: A Collection of Reprints with an Introduction, 1963*

D. Horn and F. Zachariasen
   Hadron Physics at Very High Energies, 1973

M. Jacob and G. F. Chew
   Strong-Interaction Physics: A Lecture Note Volume, 1964

L. P. Kadanoff and G. Baym
   Quantum Statistical Mechanics: Green's Function Methods in Equilibrium and Nonequilibrium Problems, 1962 (2nd printing, 1971)

I. M. Khalatnikov
   An Introduction to the Theory of Superfluidity, 1965

J. J. J. Kokkedee
   The Quark Model, 1969

A. M. Lane   *Nuclear Theory: Pairing Force Correlations to Collective Motion, 1963*

T. Loucks   *Augmented Plane Wave Method: A Guide to Performing Electronic Structure Calculations—A Lecture Note and Reprint Volume, 1967*

A. B. Migdal and V. Krainov
   Approximation Methods in Quantum Mechanics, 1969

A. B. Migdal   *Nuclear Theory: The Quasiparticle Method, 1968*

Y. Ne'eman   *Algebraic Theory of Particle Physics: Hadron Dynamics in Terms of Unitary Spin Currents, 1967*

P. Nozières   *Theory of Interacting Fermi Systems, 1964*

R. Omnès and M. Froissart
   Mandelstam Theory and Regge Poles: An Introduction for Experimentalists, 1963

FRONTIERS IN PHYSICS *(continued)*

David Pines, Editor

G. E. Pake and T. L. Estle
> *The Physical Principles of Electron Paramagnetic Resonance, 2nd edition, completely revised, enlarged, and reset, 1973*

D. Pines
> *The Many-Body Problem: A Lecture Note and Reprint Volume, 1961*

R. Z. Sagdeev and A. A. Galeev
> *Nonlinear Plasma Theory, 1969*

J. R. Schrieffer   *Theory of Superconductivity, 1964 (2nd printing, 1971)*

J. Schwinger   *Quantum Kinematics and Dynamics, 1970*

E. J. Squires   *Complex Angular Momenta and Particle Physics: A Lecture Note and Reprint Volume, 1963*

L. Van Hove, N. M. Hugenholtz, and L. P. Howland
> *Problems in Quantum Theory of Many-Particle Systems: A Lecture Note and Reprint Volume, 1961*

IN PREPARATION

E. R. Caianiello   *Combinatorics and Renormalization in Quantum Field Theory*

S. Doniach and E. H. Sondheimer
> *Green's Functions for Solid State Physicists*

S. Ichimaru   *Basic Principles of Plasma Physics: A Statistical Approach*

THE PHYSICAL PRINCIPLES
of
ELECTRON PARAMAGNETIC
RESONANCE

SECOND EDITION

COMPLETELY REVISED, ENLARGED, AND RESET

G. E. Pake   *Xerox Palo Alto Research Center, Palo Alto, California*

T. L. Estle   *Rice University, Houston, Texas*

1973

W. A. Benjamin, Inc.

ADVANCED BOOK PROGRAM

Reading, Massachusetts

London · Amsterdam · Don Mills, Ontario · Sydney · Tokyo

Library of Congress Cataloging in Publication Data

Pake, George Edward.
    The physical principles of electron paramagnetic resonance.

    (Frontiers in physics)
    First ed. published in 1962 under title:
Paramagnetic resonance.
    Includes bibliographical references.
    1. Electron paramagnetic resonance.
I. Estle, Thomas Leo, 1931-   joint author.
II. Title. III. Series.

QC762.P3 1973   538'.3   73-15842
ISBN 0-8053-7702-6
ISBN 0-8053-7703-4 (pbk.)

CONTENTS

EDITOR'S FOREWORD

The problem of communicating in a coherent fashion the recent developments in the most exciting and active fields of physics seems particularly pressing today. The enormous growth in the number of physicists has tended to make the familiar channels of communication considerably less effective. It has become increasingly difficult for experts in a given field to keep up with the current literature; the novice can only be confused. What is needed is both a consistent account of a field and the presentation of a definite "point of view" concerning it. Formal monographs cannot meet such a need in a rapidly developing field, and, perhaps more important, the review article seems to have fallen into disfavor. Indeed, it would seem that the people most actively engaged in developing a given field are the people least likely to write at length about it.

FRONTIERS IN PHYSICS has been conceived in an effort to improve the situation in several ways: first, to take advantage of the fact that the leading physicists today frequently give a series of lectures, a graduate seminar, or a graduate course in their special fields of interest. Such lectures serve to summarize the present status of a rapidly developing field and may well constitute the only coherent account available at the time. Often, notes on lectures exist (prepared by the lecturer himself, by graduate students, or by postdoctoral fellows) and have been distributed in mimeographed form on a limited basis. One of the principal purposes of the FRONTIERS IN PHYSICS Series is to make such notes available to a wider audience of physicists.

It should be emphasized that lecture notes are necessarily rough and informal, both in style and content, and those in the series will prove no exception. This is as it should be. The point of the series is to offer new, rapid, more informal, and it is hoped, more effective ways for physicists to teach one another. The point is lost if only elegant notes qualify.

The second way to improve communication in very active fields of physics is by the publication of collections of reprints of recent articles. Such collections are themselves useful to people working in the field. The value of the reprints would, however, seem much enhanced if the collection would be accompanied by an introduction of moderate length which would serve to tie the collection together and, necessarily, constitute a brief survey of the present status of the field. Again, it is appropriate that such an introduction be informal, in keeping with the active character of the field.

A third possibility for the series might be called an informal monograph, to connote the fact that it represents an intermediate step between lecture notes and formal monographs. It would offer the author an opportunity to present his views of a field that has developed to the point at which a summation might prove extraordinarily fruitful, but for which a formal monograph might not be feasible or desirable.

Fourth, there are the contemporary classics—papers or lectures which constitute a particularly valuable approach to the teaching and learning of physics today. Here one thinks of fields that lie at the heart of much of present-day research, but whose essentials are by now well understood, such as quantum electrodynamics or magnetic resonance. In such fields some of the best pedagogical material is not readily available, either because it consists of papers long out of print or lectures that have never been published.

———————

The above words, written in August, 1961, seem equally applicable today (which may tell us something about developments in communication in physics during the past decade). It was our hope that as a field matured authors who had published a lecture note volume in FRONTIERS IN PHYSICS would choose to review their notes and cast them into a somewhat more polished text or monograph. This has not happened with any great frequency—I suspect, because as a field matures, scientists who have been working at the frontier prefer to go on to another field rather than tidying up some of the remaining unresolved questions. It is therefore a special pleasure to welcome this revision, after ten years, by George Pake and Thomas Estle, of George Pake's lecture notes on paramagnetic resonance. Those notes represent one of the "classics" of modern physics; they have served to introduce thousands of students into the field, which has itself undergone a substantial expansion as part of its maturing process. It is our hope and expectation that the present volume will continue this important educational contribution, addressed as it is both to the student seeking an introduction to magnetic resonance, and especially paramagnetic resonance, and to the scientist who wishes to obtain a better understanding of the fundamental principles of the subject.

DAVID PINES

Fall 1973

PREFACE

During the decade since the appearance of the first edition of this book, the study and use of electron paramagnetic resonance have grown enormously. It has become a fairly standard tool in many fields of science and technology. At the same time the basic concepts have been more thoroughly investigated and are better understood. The goal of this new edition is similar to that of the first, to present the essential ideas and concepts needed to understand electron paramagnetic resonance. In the second edition, we hope to retain many features of the original version while including material which seems appropriate in view of another decade of thought and research.

This book is addressed to the student seeking an introduction to magnetic resonance, especially electron paramagnetic resonance, and to the scientist who wishes to better understand the fundamental principles of this subject. The minimum preparation needed would be roughly a one-year course on quantum mechanics. Since this is now frequently taught at the undergraduate level, the book should be of interest to upper-level undergraduates as well as to graduate students. Many of the changes are in fact an outgrowth of the way in which one of the authors (TLE) has attempted to explain this subject to students and to apply it in his own research.

Over the years of development of the subject of electron paramagnetic resonance it has become commonplace to bridge the gap between fundamental theory and the experimentalist's spectra by the use of an intermediate description, the spin Hamiltonian. The spin Hamiltonian is an effective Hamiltonian which, in its most general form, can describe exactly a group of states which are close in energy to each other but far from all others. The terms in the spin Hamiltonian do not always have an easy physical interpretation, however. These properties make it an extremely useful meeting ground for experiment and theory. It is also possible to develop a considerable amount of physical insight in terms of the spin Hamiltonian. For example anisotropic g factors and zero-field splittings are meaningful and convenient concepts in considering paramagnets. In a general discussion of electron paramagnetic resonance there is another important advantage of the spin Hamiltonian. A common description of quite diverse paramagnets, such as free radicals, transition group ions, donors and acceptors in semiconductors, or color centers in ionic crystals, can be given even though a theoretical description of these paramagnets can differ considerably from one type to another.

Believing that extensive use of the spin Hamiltonian is an effective way of approaching the subject and in particular in giving it a cohesiveness that it sometimes seems to lack, we have utilized this approach at every opportunity. This has meant some selection of topics but more it has meant selection of methods of presentation. A general form for the spin Hamiltonian is often most conveniently obtained using symmetry arguments. These, of course, are most efficiently and elegantly handled by group theory. For those readers conversant with group theory it should be relatively easy to establish most of the results using group theory and to extend them where desired. It is our hope that the major features and many of the results will be understandable without a knowledge of group theory, although some knowledge of point symmetry would certainly be valuable.

In keeping with the view that the spin Hamiltonian approach is the simplest general approach to the subject, we have tried, where possible, to simplify the treatment in other ways without damaging the physical content. For example the solutions of the spin Hamiltonian eigenvalue problems are usually discussed using first order perturbation theory, whereas quantitative analysis of spectra usually requires higher order terms or exact solutions (numerical in most cases). Most of the concepts of importance appear in first order. In these solutions we have used tensor relationships which give general results quickly and without tedious coordinate transformations. In some ways a more serious approximation is made in discussing dynamic properties. These are discussed using rate equations for the most part. This method is simple and leads to a great deal of insight. More refined treatments often can be difficult to understand and apply.

No attempt has been made to survey the experimental results in this field. The last such attempt was in the 1950's with the articles in *Reports on Progress in Physics* from the Oxford group. The book by Abragam and Bleaney (see bibliography at the end of Chapter 1) is the closest approach to a recent attempt and they only consider transition group ions. It is unlikely that any extensive survey will ever be attempted again. We have therefore chosen examples for illustrative purposes. We have attempted to make choices which did not follow traditional patterns (i.e., we use few examples of iron group impurities, F-centers, or donors in semiconductors).

We should like to express our appreciation to the many colleagues and students who have contributed in various ways to this book. A particular debt is owed to R. K. Watts and T. G. Castner, Jr., for reading and commenting on the manuscript during its development. We should also like to acknowledge the cheerful and skillful help of Mary Comerford who typed the majority of the manuscript.

One of the authors (T.L.E.) would like to take this opportunity to acknowledge the encouragement and the sacrifices of his wife, Arlene. His contribution to this book is dedicated to her.   T. L. Estle

G. E. Pake

CHAPTER 1

Introduction

1–1 Magnetic Resonance

Paramagnetic resonance is a form of spectroscopy in which an oscillating magnetic field* induces magnetic dipole transitions between the energy levels of a system of paramagnets. We shall be concerned with paramagnets at the atomic or molecular level, each paramagnet possessing a permanent magnetic dipole moment associated with the motion of its charged particles. Paramagnetic resonance usually is confined to the radio-frequency (10^6 to 10^9 Hz) or microwave-frequency (10^9 to 10^{11} Hz) range; this means that the initial and final states must lie within a few reciprocal centimeters of each other.

Electron paramagnetic resonance (or EPR[†]) is restricted to the study of magnetic dipoles of electronic origin and is usually studied at microwave frequencies [nuclear magnetic resonance (or NMR) by contrast is paramagnetic resonance using nuclear magnetic dipoles]. In addition to the transitions induced by the oscillating magnetic field there are transitions produced by the thermal excitation of other degrees of freedom of the system such as vibration or translation. These processes constitute spin-lattice relaxation. If the system of paramagnets is at thermal equilibrium, the lower energy levels of the magnetic system are more heavily populated and there is net absorption of energy from the oscillating field. In steady state the rate at which energy is absorbed from the oscillating magnetic field is equal to the rate at which energy leaves paramagnetic degrees of freedom and enters other degrees of freedom. The paramagnetic degrees

---

* We will follow the most common convention and use magnetic field, **H**, and gauss as the name, symbol, and unit to describe magnetic fields. What may appear to the reader as a confusing or arbitrary choice is discussed in detail starting on p. 389 of E. M. Purcell, *Electricity and Magnetism*, Berkeley Physics Course, Vol. 2, McGraw-Hill, New York, 1965.

[†] The term electron spin resonance (or ESR) is a commonly used synonym but will not be employed here, in order to avoid any possible implication that only electron spin angular momentum is involved. Also paramagnets are frequently called spins or, collectively, a spin system. This does not necessarily imply that only spin angular momentum is involved.

of freedom are frequently called the spin system and the other degrees of freedom are termed the lattice.

Occasionally we will consider closely related phenomena which do not fit our definition, and yet we will refer to them loosely as electron paramagnetic resonance also. Examples of these are transitions between close-lying levels of a paramagnetic entity which are excited by oscillating electric fields or stresses. Also we will recognize superficially such related subjects as ferromagnetic resonance, ferrimagnetic resonance, and antiferromagnetic resonance when strongly interacting permanent magnetic dipoles are involved.

In paramagnetic resonance a second magnetic field is usually employed. It is essentially static, being varied only slowly for purposes of tuning the desired energy differences to resonance with the energy of the oscillating field quanta. This tuning arises via the Zeeman interaction. Observing the magnetic field or fields at which resonance occurs may allow one to determine the magnetic dipole moment, the local magnetic field or fields, and any nonmagnetic energy splittings. In the simplest case tuning to resonance establishes the condition

$$h\nu = g\beta H, \qquad (1\text{-}1)$$

where H is the local magnetic field (thus including hyperfine fields), β is the Bohr magneton, and g is a dimensionless constant that determines the magnetic dipole moment. The nonmagnetic energy splittings (zero-field splittings) yield more complicated resonance conditions which we will discuss in Chapter 5. For frequencies near 10^{10} Hz the resonance condition of Eq. (1-1) is satisfied for fields near 3500 G for most paramagnets (i.e., those with g about 2).

The first experimental observations of electron paramagnetic resonance were reported in 1945 by Zavoisky [1]. The initial experiments observed the power absorbed from a 12 MHz radio-frequency magnetic field as a function of the magnetic field in substances with lines roughly 50 G wide or larger. At such low frequencies the approximate field for resonance is 4 G, and the resonance was scarcely discernible. A second series of experiments found a resonance maximum for Cu^{2+} ions at 47.6 G, using a frequency of 133 MHz. Subsequently Zavoisky [2] pushed the frequency of his equipment into the microwave region and observed well-defined resonances with widths of 200 to 300 G at fields of about 1000 G. Cummerow and Halliday [3] also published in 1946 an account of EPR measurements in the microwave region. An example of such a resonance is shown in Fig. 1-1. The paramagnets were Mn^{2+} ions in $MnSO_4 \cdot 4H_2O$, and the data were taken by Cummerow and Halliday [3]. Then in 1947 Bagguley and Griffiths [4] performed an experiment at 9.4 GHz (or approximately 3 cm wavelength) in the x-band of microwave frequencies, a frequency region which remained the one most commonly used during the following two decades. There followed, primarily

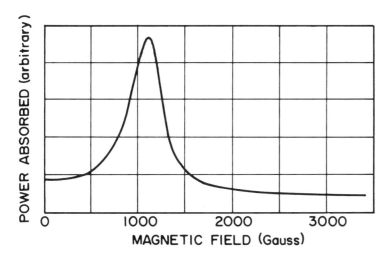

FIG. 1-1 The electron paramagnetic resonance of Mn^{2+} ions in $MnSO_4 \cdot 4H_2O$, observed at 2930 MHz by Cummerow and Halliday [3] in early experiments. The large line width resulted from the high concentration of paramagnetic ions.

at the Clarendon Laboratory in Oxford, an important and fruitful period of EPR researches in which the subject was extensively explored and much of our present-day understanding was established [5].

The magnetic resonance principle had first been applied by Rabi and his coworkers [6] in their classic experiments on molecular beams. Unsuccessful attempts to detect magnetic dipole transitions in bulk samples of matter were first made by Gorter [7], in whose laboratory early nonresonance experiments on paramagnetism in oscillating fields helped to develop some of the basic concepts. This work included extensive studies of paramagnetic relaxation, a topic closely related to EPR. The first experimental observations of magnetic resonance in bulk matter were the early EPR results of Zavoisky [1]. Very shortly thereafter, nuclear magnetic resonance in solids and liquids was observed independently by two groups [8]. Both EPR and NMR observations in condensed matter were greatly facilitated by microwave- and radio-frequency techniques developed during World War II.

1–2 Electronic Paramagnetism

Paramagnetism arises from the circulation of charge on an atomic scale. The circulation of mass represented by angular momentum has associated with it a circulation of charge, thus leading to permanent magnetic dipoles. If the angular momentum arises from electronic motion only, then, for a given angular momentum, the angular frequency will be much greater than for nuclear motion because of the ratio of 10^3 to 10^5 in the masses of nuclei and electrons. Thus, although nuclei may affect and indeed do influence many EPR spectra, we can drop from primary consideration nuclear spin or nuclear motion associated with rotation of molecules. We can include nuclear paramagnetism simply by adding the appropriate term to our definition of the magnetic dipole moment given below, and we can then develop many of the essential concepts of NMR.

It suffices therefore to consider electronic spin and orbital angular momentum which, in units of $\hbar$, are denoted by $\mathbf{S}$ and $\mathbf{L}$. These quantities are operators in quantum mechanics (some useful properties of angular momentum operators for this section and later ones are given in Appendix A). In terms of $\mathbf{L}$ and $\mathbf{S}$ the magnetic dipole moment operator, $\boldsymbol{\mu}$, is given by

$$\boldsymbol{\mu} = -\beta(\mathbf{L} + g_e\mathbf{S}), \tag{1-2}$$

where β is the Bohr magneton, $|e|\hbar/2mc$, which in convenient units is approximately 1.4 MHz/G. This applies rigorously only to spherical symmetry, for which angular momentum is well defined. For a rigorous treatment of nonspherical environments such as those in a solid, $\mathbf{L}$ must be replaced by $\Sigma_i\mathbf{r}_i \times \mathbf{p}_i/\hbar$, where $\mathbf{r}_i$ and $\mathbf{p}_i$ are the position and the linear momentum, respectively, of the ith electron. For electrons localized primarily on a single atom this is not usually necessary (see Section 7.4 in Slichter [9] for a case where the more general form is used). Note that β is positive and that the negative charge of the electron produces the minus sign in Eq. (1-2). When corresponding equations for nuclei are written, the minus sign of Eq. (1-2) is missing. The factor g_e is the spectroscopic splitting factor for electrons, a value which is nearly 2 (actually 2.0023). As we will see, it is customary to define a g factor to relate the magnetic dipole moment to the angular momentum in general. Equation (1-2) equates the magnetic dipole moment to the sum of a magnetic dipole moment proportional to $\mathbf{L}$ and another proportional to $\mathbf{S}$, with a different constant of proportionality. This is the most general form the vector $\boldsymbol{\mu}$ can have for spherical symmetry, provided that orbital motion and spin are the only two physically different circulations present. The constants of proportionality and the form follow directly from the Dirac equation [10]. The orbital magnetic moment can be obtained classically as well*. The magnetic dipole moment resulting from spin is g_e times the classical value.

---

* If an electron with velocity v has a circular orbit of radius r, the orbital angular momentum is

$$\hbar L = mvr$$

and the magnetic dipole moment of the current loop (writing charge in electromagnetic

The energy of a magnetic dipole, $\boldsymbol{\mu}$, in a magnetic field, $\mathbf{H}$, is given classically by

$$E = -\boldsymbol{\mu}\cdot\mathbf{H}, \tag{1-3}$$

or in quantum-mechanical language the Hamiltonian for spherical symmetry is

$$\mathcal{H} = -\boldsymbol{\mu}\cdot\mathbf{H} = \beta(\mathbf{L}+g_e\mathbf{S})\cdot\mathbf{H}. \tag{1-4}$$

Equations (1-3) and (1-4) lead to the Zeeman effect, well known in optical spectroscopy. It is more convenient in dealing with free atoms or ions to use an expression which explicitly recognizes that electronic states can be described by their total angular momentum, $\mathbf{J} = \mathbf{L}+\mathbf{S}$. We want to find the matrix elements of $\boldsymbol{\mu} = -\beta(\mathbf{L}+g_e\mathbf{S})$, or equivalently $\mathcal{H}$, among states of a system corresponding to a given value of J. They can be written as

$$\langle J, M_J|\boldsymbol{\mu}|J, M_J'\rangle = \frac{\langle J|\mathbf{J}\cdot\boldsymbol{\mu}|J\rangle}{J(J+1)}\langle J, M_J|\mathbf{J}|J, M_J'\rangle, \tag{1-5}$$

where the Wigner-Eckart theorem [11] can be used to show that the matrix elements of the two first-rank irreducible tensor operators, $\boldsymbol{\mu}$ and $\mathbf{J}$, are proportional and the constant of proportionality is evaluated following Condon and Shortley [12]. Assuming Russell-Saunders coupling so that L, S, and J are all good quantum numbers, we may then evaluate the constant of proportionality, the Landé g-factor [13]:

$$g_L = \frac{-1}{\beta J(J+1)}\langle J|\mathbf{J}\cdot\boldsymbol{\mu}|J\rangle. \tag{1-6}$$

We see that explicit recognition has been given to the fact that the scalar $\mathbf{J}\cdot\boldsymbol{\mu}$ has matrix elements independent of M_J:

$$\mathbf{J}\cdot\boldsymbol{\mu} = -\beta[\mathbf{L}^2+\mathbf{S}\cdot\mathbf{L}+g_e(\mathbf{L}\cdot\mathbf{S}+\mathbf{S}^2)],$$

$$\mathbf{L}\cdot\mathbf{S} = \tfrac{1}{2}(\mathbf{J}^2-\mathbf{L}^2-\mathbf{S}^2), \tag{1-7}$$

$$\mathbf{J}\cdot\boldsymbol{\mu} = -\tfrac{1}{2}\beta[\mathbf{J}^2+\mathbf{L}^2-\mathbf{S}^2 + g_e(\mathbf{J}^2-\mathbf{L}^2+\mathbf{S}^2)].$$

Thus

$$g_L = 1 + \frac{J(J+1)+S(S+1)-L(L+1)}{2J(J+1)}(g_e-1), \tag{1-8}$$

where g_e-1 is normally given its approximate value of 1. Thus we may write for a free atom or ion

$$\boldsymbol{\mu} = -g\beta\mathbf{J}, \tag{1-9}$$

---

units) is

$$\mu = IA = \left(\frac{e/c}{2\pi r/v}\right)\pi r^2 = \frac{evr}{2c} = \frac{eh}{2mc}L.$$

This is, of course, the Bohr magneton times the orbital angular momentum.

where it is understood that the operator $\mathbf{\mu}$ is to operate only within the $2J+1$ states having a given value of J. The g factor appearing in this expression will be the Landé g factor if L-S coupling is a good approximation. The g factor will be approximately 2 if $J = S$, that is, for an S state. Therefore, even though the magnetic moment arises from the circulation of charge caused by the two angular momenta $\mathbf{L}$ and $\mathbf{S}$, it can be regarded as arising from $\mathbf{J}$ since $\mathbf{J}$ is strictly the only defined angular momentum vector for such spherically symmetric systems. Chapter 2 will describe magnetic resonance entirely in terms of Eq. (1-9), that is, only a vaguely defined spherically symmetric paramagnetic entity will be assumed. Then in Chapter 3 and later chapters we will take up the question of defining the paramagnetic entities and their properties more precisely. At that point we will drop the simplifying assumption of spherical symmetry.

Using Eq. (1-9) or its equivalent,

$$\mathbf{\mu} = -\gamma\hbar\mathbf{J}, \qquad (1\text{-}10)$$

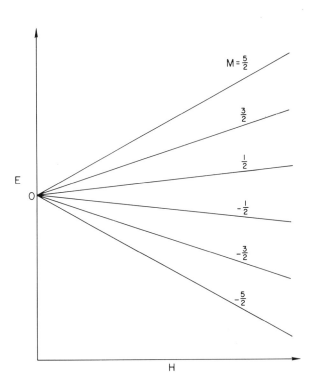

FIG. 1-2   The energy levels for a spherically symmetric paramagnet with $J = \frac{5}{2}$ as a function of the magnetic field.

which defines the "magnetogyric" or gyromagnetic ratio, γ, let us calculate some of the properties of paramagnetic systems. The Hamiltonian for one magnetic dipole in an assembly of identical dipoles that are noninteracting (this represents an immense simplification, as we see in Chapter 6) is

$$\mathcal{H} = -\boldsymbol{\mu} \cdot \mathbf{H} = g\beta \mathbf{H} \cdot \mathbf{J} = g\beta H J_z, \tag{1-11}$$

where the z axis is chosen to be the direction of the applied static field $\mathbf{H}$ (we here exclude hyperfine or other internal fields for simplicity). The solutions for the energy are then

$$E = g\beta H M \qquad (M = -J, -J+1, \cdots, J-1, J), \tag{1-12}$$

a set of $2J+1$ evenly spaced levels each of which corresponds to one value of M and whose spacing is directly proportional to H (see Fig. 1-2).

The probability that a dipole within the assembly at temperature T has the energy E_j is, according to Maxwell-Boltzmann statistics*,

$$p_j = \frac{\exp(-E_j/kT)}{\sum_i \exp(-E_i/kT)}, \tag{1-13}$$

where the sum over i extends over all levels, E_i, which are populated. In the present case inserting Eq. (1-12) into (1-13) gives

$$p_M = \frac{\exp(-g\beta H M/kT)}{\sum_{M'=-J}^{J} \exp(-g\beta H M'/kT)}. \tag{1-14}$$

The magnetization $\mathbf{M}$, defined as the magnetic moment per unit volume, is one of the most frequently studied observables of the system. The only nonzero component of $\mathbf{M}$ is along z and is given by

$$M_z = N \sum_{M=-J}^{J} \langle M|\mu_z|M\rangle p_M, \tag{1-15}$$

where N is the number of dipoles per unit volume. Substituting the values of p_M and $\langle M|\mu_z|M\rangle$ into Eq. (1-15), we obtain

$$M_z = N \frac{\sum_{M=-J}^{J} -g\beta M \exp(-g\beta H M/kT)}{\sum_{M'=-J}^{J} \exp(-g\beta H M'/kT)} = kT \frac{\partial}{\partial H} \log Z, \tag{1-16}$$

---

* Electrons obey Fermi-Dirac statistics, and the use of Boltzmann statistics here should not be thoughtlessly accepted. We suppose that the electrons on a Cu^{2+} ion, for example, definitely obey the Pauli exclusion principle insofar as they compete with each other for quantum states within the ion. Once the paramagnetic properties of the ion are so determined, however, our assumption of independent, noninteracting Cu^{2+} ions implies a spatial separation and, in effect, a spatial distinguishability of particles. This spatial distinguishability means that Boltzmann statistics are appropriate.

where the partition function, Z, is

$$Z = \sum_{M=-J}^{J} \exp\left(-g\beta HM/kT\right). \qquad (1\text{-}17)$$

By summing the geometric series one obtains

$$Z = \frac{\sinh\left(J+\tfrac{1}{2}\right)g\beta H/kT}{\sinh g\beta H/2kT} \qquad (1\text{-}18)$$

and

$$M_z = Ng\beta J B_J\left(\frac{g\beta H}{kT}\right), \qquad (1\text{-}19)$$

where

$$B_J\left(\frac{g\beta H}{kT}\right) = \frac{1}{J}\left[\left(J+\tfrac{1}{2}\right)\coth\left(J+\tfrac{1}{2}\right)\frac{g\beta H}{kT} - \tfrac{1}{2}\coth\frac{g\beta H}{2kT}\right]. \qquad (1\text{-}20)$$

For $g\beta H/kT \ll 1$, as would be obtained at low fields or high temperatures, we find that

$$M_z = NJ(J+1)\frac{g^2\beta^2 H}{3kT}, \qquad (1\text{-}21)$$

the usual form for Curie's law. By contrast, saturation of the magnetization results from the complete alignment of the dipoles, that is, all dipoles are in the state with $M = -J$. That limit results if $g\beta H/kT \gg 1$, which gives for Eqs. (1-19) and (1-20)

$$M_z = Ng\beta J. \qquad (1\text{-}22)$$

Typically temperatures below $1\,°\mathrm{K}$ and fields well in excess of $10\,\mathrm{kG}$ are required for saturation. The magnetizations of several paramagnetic crystals are shown in Fig. 1-3 (note both the linear dependence on H at low fields and the subsequent saturation). More information on non-resonant aspects of electronic paramagnetism can be found in reference 14.

1-3 Paramagnetic Entities

As stated in Section 1-2, we will not discuss the actual nature of the paramagnetic entities until Chapter 3 and subsequent chapters. However, at this point a brief listing of some of the more common types of paramagnets will help to clarify the early discussions.

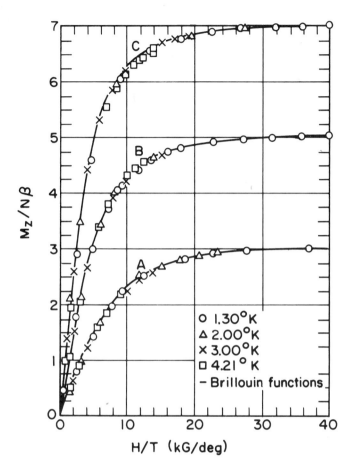

FIG. 1-3   The magnetization of three paramagnetic crystals as a function of H and T (actually H/T) [15]. Note the linear region described by Curie's law for low values of H/T and the saturation for large H/T. The solid curves are the appropriate Brillouin functions given in Eq. (1-20). Crystal A is potassium chrome alum, in which Cr^{3+} is paramagnetic with $J = S = \frac{3}{2}$. Crystal B is iron ammonium alum with Fe^{3+} having $J = S = \frac{5}{2}$. Crystal C contains Gd^{3+} $(J = S = \frac{7}{2})$ in gadolinium sulfate octahydrate.

The most commonly encountered forms of matter are not electronically paramagnetic in their pure and perfect forms (although they usually exhibit nuclear paramagnetism). In a perfect crystal of silicon all of the electrons are in completely filled inner atomic shells or they occupy the covalent bonds in such a way that no resultant angular momentum exists. A pure silicon crystal is not electronically paramagnetic. Similarly an ionic crystal such as sodium chloride consists of ions; hence all electrons are in closed-shell configurations. Thus perfect NaCl crystals are not electronically paramagnetic. Similarly many molecular species which may exist in gaseous or liquid form are, like silicon, such that all covalent bonds are filled and they are not electronically paramagnetic. Carbon dioxide and methane are molecules of this sort.

How then does electronic paramagnetism arise?

1. Atoms and ions. All electronic configurations with an odd number of electrons must possess spin angular momentum and therefore must be paramagnetic. This applies generally but in particular also to atoms or ions. In addition, for atoms or ions with an even number of electrons, many configurations will correspond to unfilled shells and hence usually a nonzero angular momentum. Thus most configurations for atoms and ions will be paramagnetic. However, these usually correspond to chemically unstable charge states so that in practice they are not easily observed. Atomic sodium, chlorine, and silicon are examples.

2. Molecules and molecule ions. Stable molecules usually have filled atomic shells and saturated bonds, and this leads only to diamagnetism. Exceptions occur, however, such as the molecules NO and NO_2, which have odd numbers of electrons and are therefore paramagnetic. Also O_2, although having an even number of electrons, has a ground state with only a partially filled molecular shell and is thus paramagnetic. Similarly many large molecules can exist stably with an odd number of electrons and are therefore paramagnetic. Triphenyl methyl, DPPH, naphthalene negative ion, and many other free radicals, as they are usually called, are well known. These paramagnetic molecules and molecule ions (and to a lesser extent the atoms and ions discussed above) can exist in several ways in matter—as gases, as liquids, in solution, as solids, or rather undisturbed in solid matrices. The stability of the paramagnetic species in these several forms will vary.

3. Excited states. Although the ground states of most molecules are nonmagnetic singlets, one can occasionally observe paramagnetism from excited triplet states. For example, the excited triplet state of naphthalene can be populated by irradiating with ultraviolet light. Other types of interesting excited-state paramagnetism also exist.

4. Point imperfections in solids. Point imperfections in crystalline solids may be visualized as molecule-like complexes embedded in the crystalline matrix. Therefore the considerations applied to molecules and molecule ions in paragraph 2 apply also here. Two important distinctions, however, should be made. First, a wider variety of stable charge states can occur in nonmetallic solids than is usually encountered for molecules. In addition, the neutral charge state, that is, the one with the same net charge

as the perfect crystal, is commonly paramagnetic, as can easily be seen if the point imperfection is an impurity with one more or one less nuclear charge than the crystalline constituent it replaces. Numerous examples exist, including the following:

(a) donors and acceptors in semiconductors, such as phosphorus donor impurities in silicon;

(b) activators and coactivators in phosphors, such as self-activated ZnS;

(c) electron or hole traps in photoconductors, such as Fe^{3+} in CdS;

(d) color centers in insulators, such as the F center in KCl;

(e) radiation-damage centers, such as the Si vacancy in silicon crystals;

(f) transition-group impurities such as Mn^{2+} in MgO. These are atoms or ions with incomplete $3d$, $4d$, $5d$, $4f$, or $5f$ shells; they will be discussed more thoroughly in Chapter 3. Those with incomplete $3d$ shells are termed the iron group; those with the $4d$ shell unfilled, the palladium group; those with the $5d$ shell incomplete, the platinum group. The incomplete $4f$ shell characterizes the rare-earth group, and for the actinide group the $6d$ and $5f$ shells are unfilled.

5. Highly delocalized electrons in solids. This includes conduction electrons in metals, that is, solids with unfilled energy bands. Metallic sodium is a good example. Somewhere between the descriptions of paragraphs 4 and 5 are the impurity bands in semiconductors. A somewhat similar behavior can occur for solid molecular free radicals. Finally, although not examples of paramagnetism, the ferromagnetic, ferrimagnetic, and antiferromagnetic solids fall within this category.

1–4 Supplemental Bibliography

Electron paramagnetic resonance has been the subject of an immense number of research papers, many fine reviews of selected aspects, and a few general reviews or introductions. As a guide to the reader we include here a list of some generally useful publications. More specialized references appear at appropriate places in the text. References to books or reviews published before 1960 can be found in many of the books in this list.

1. A. Abragam and B. Bleaney, *Electron Paramagnetic Resonance of Transition Ions*, Oxford, New York, 1970. This book is almost encyclopedic in the treatment of its subject matter. Although EPR is broader than the study of transition-group ions, the latter represent the topic most thoroughly investigated by the use of this phenomenon. For this reason this book will undoubtedly become a requirement for any serious student of EPR.

2. A. Abragam, *The Principles of Nuclear Magnetism*, Oxford, New York, 1961. Although, strictly speaking, this is a book on nuclear magnetic resonance,

the similarity of NMR and EPR and the extensive and elegant coverage that Abragam gives to NMR makes this book of great importance to anyone studying magnetic resonance.

3. C. P. Slichter, *Principles of Magnetic Resonance, with Examples from Solid State Physics*, Harper and Row, New York, 1963. An introduction to magnetic resonance with applications to both nuclear and electronic paramagnetism. Very clear and readable with excellent treatments of many important topics.

4. J. W. Orton, *Electron Paramagnetic Resonance: An Introduction to Transition Group Ions in Crystals*, Gordon and Breach, New York, 1968. An effective introduction to EPR with emphasis on transition-group ions.

5. A. Carrington and A. D. McLachlan, *Introduction to Magnetic Resonance*, Harper and Row, New York, 1967. An introduction to both NMR and EPR such that each adds to the other. The treatment of many aspects of magnetic resonance of chemical interest is particularly noteworthy.

6. M. Bersohn and J. C. Baird, *An Introduction to Electron Paramagnetic Resonance*, Benjamin, New York, 1966. An elementary introduction to EPR that is particularly appropriate for the chemical aspects of the subject.

7. G. E. Pake, *Paramagnetic Resonance*, Benjamin, New York, 1962. Although the present volume is a revision of this book, the changes have been so extensive that reference to the earlier version may be useful.

8. H. G. Hecht, *Magnetic Resonance Spectroscopy*, Wiley, New York, 1967. Covers all forms of magnetic resonance. An introductory text oriented primarily toward chemistry.

9. H. M. Assenheim, *Introduction to Electron Spin Resonance*, Hilger and Watts, London, 1966. This book, the first of several in a series dealing with EPR, provides a general introduction.

10. J. Dieleman, "Electron Spin Resonance in Luminescent Solids," Chapter 6 of *Luminescence of Inorganic Solids* (P. Goldberg, ed.), Academic, New York, 1966. Not as specialized as the title may sound, this is actually a compact description of EPR with selected illustrations from luminescent solids.

11. S. A. Al'tshuler and B. M. Kozyrev, *Electron Paramagnetic Resonance*, Academic, New York, 1964. An English translation of the Russian text published in 1961.

12. W. Low, *Paramagnetic Resonance in Solids*, Academic, New York, 1960, Suppl. 2 of *Solid State Physics*.

13. J. A. McMillan, *Electron Paramagnetism*, Reinhold, New York, 1968.

References Cited in Chapter 1

[1] E. Zavoisky, *J. Phys. USSR* **9**, 211, 245 (1945).
[2] E. Zavoisky, *J. Phys. USSR* **10**, 197 (1946).
[3] R. L. Cummerow and D. Halliday, *Phys. Rev.* **70**, 433 (1946).
[4] D. M. S. Bagguley and J. H. E. Griffiths, Nature **160**, 532 (1947).
[5] For references to this early work consult the following sequence of review articles: B. Bleaney and K. W. H. Stevens, *Rept. Progr. Phys.* **16**, 108

(1953); K. D. Bowers and J. Owen, *Rept. Progr. Phys.* **18**, 304 (1955); D. M. S. Bagguley and J. Owen, *Rept. Progr. Phys.* **20**, 304 (1957); J. W. Orton, *Rept. Progr. Phys.* **22**, 204 (1959).

[6] I. I. Rabi, J. R. Zacharias, S. Millman, and P. Kusch, *Phys. Rev.* **53**, 318 (1938).

[7] C. J. Gorter, *Physica* **3**, 995 (1936).

[8] F. Bloch, W. W. Hansen, and M. Packard, *Phys. Rev.* **69**, 127 (1946); E. M. Purcell, H. C. Torrey, and R. V. Pound, *Phys. Rev.* **69**, 37 (1946).

[9] C. P. Slichter, *Principles of Magnetic Resonance*, Harper and Row, New York, 1963.

[10] See, for example, Section 17.3 of A. Abragam and B. Bleaney, *Electron Paramagnetic Resonance of Transition Ions*, Oxford, New York, 1970.

[11] A. R. Edmonds, *Angular Momentum in Quantum Mechanics*, Princeton University Press, Princeton, N.J., 1957, p. 73; H. Watanabe, *Operator Methods in Ligand Field Theory*, Prentice-Hall, Englewood Cliffs, N.J., 1966, p. 15; A. Messiah, *Quantum Mechanics*, North Holland, Amsterdam, 1962, Vol. II, p. 573; reference 9, p. 164.

[12] E. U. Condon and G. H. Shortley, *The Theory of Atomic Spectra*, Cambridge, 1953, p. 59; E. Feenberg and G. E. Pake, *Notes on the Quantum Theory of Angular Momentum*, Addison-Wesley, Reading, Mass., 1953, p. 33.

[13] A vector model derivation is given on pp. 109–111 of G. Herzberg, *Atomic Spectra and Atomic Structure*, Dover, New York, 1944, and on pp. 249–251 of J. C. Slater, *Quantum Theory of Atomic Structure*, McGraw-Hill, New York, 1960, Vol. I.

[14] J. A. McMillan, *Electron Paramagnetism*, Reinhold, New York, 1968; D. H. Martin, *Magnetism in Solids*, Iliffe, London, 1967; C. Kittel, *Introduction to Solid State Physics*, 3rd ed., Wiley, New York, 1967, p. 427; R. A. Levy, *Principles of Solid State Physics*, Academic, New York, 1968, p. 198.

[15] W. E. Henry, *Phys. Rev.* **88**, 559 (1952).

CHAPTER 2

The Phenomenon
of Magnetic Resonance

We have yet to develop a detailed concept of the paramagnetic entities in nature. More definite ideas will be presented in Chapters 3, 4, and 5. However, in order to discuss magnetic resonance in a simple context, we will use a paramagnet that has the dominant feature of all paramagnets: the direct association of the magnetic dipole moment with the angular momentum. We choose a system with spherical symmetry described by its total angular momentum and use the following [in this chapter it is more convenient to employ Eq. (1-10), repeated below as Eq. (2-1), than Eq. (1-9)]:

$$\boldsymbol{\mu} = -\gamma \hbar \mathbf{J}. \qquad (2\text{-}1)$$

We also assume noninteracting dipoles. This chapter applies also to nuclear magnetic resonance by a proper choice for γ and $\mathbf{J}$, although our main concern is with electron paramagnetic resonance.

2–1 The Description of Magnetic Resonance by Precession

Classically a magnetic dipole experiences a torque in a uniform magnetic field. If it also possesses angular momentum about the dipolar axis, it will precess about the magnetic field. A similar behavior is observed quantum mechanically for the expectation value of the magnet dipole moment operator. The expectation value is the quantum-mechanical average value, given by

$$\langle \boldsymbol{\mu} \rangle = \int \psi^* \boldsymbol{\mu} \psi \, d\tau, \qquad (2\text{-}2)$$

where ψ is the time-dependent wave function describing the state of the dipole, and the integration extends over all coordinates, including summation over spin coordinates. This average should not be confused with the statistical averaging, which amounts to considering a random set of initial conditions for ψ. Equation (2-1) shows that $\boldsymbol{\mu}$ is proportional to $\mathbf{J}$ and is not explicitly a function of time. A theorem of quantum mechanics [1] gives the following equation for the time derivative of the expectation value of a time-independent operator:

$$\frac{d}{dt}\langle\boldsymbol{\mu}\rangle = \frac{i}{\hbar}\langle[\mathcal{H}, \boldsymbol{\mu}]\rangle, \tag{2-3}$$

where an explicit time dependence appears because

$$\mathcal{H} = -\boldsymbol{\mu}\cdot\mathbf{H} = \gamma\hbar\mathbf{H}\cdot\mathbf{J} \tag{2-4}$$

and **H** will generally depend on time. Substituting Eqs. (2-1) and (2-4) into (2-3) and defining the z axis as parallel to **H**, we find

$$\frac{d}{dt}\langle\boldsymbol{\mu}\rangle = -i\gamma^2\hbar H\langle[J_z, \mathbf{J}]\rangle. \tag{2-5}$$

Applying the commutation relations for angular momenta (given in Appendix A), we obtain

$$\frac{d}{dt}\langle\boldsymbol{\mu}\rangle = \gamma^2\hbar H\langle J_y\mathbf{i} - J_x\mathbf{j}\rangle. \tag{2-6}$$

If we expand the cross product $\mathbf{H}\times\mathbf{J}$, we see that Eq. (2-6) can be written in the desired form,

$$\frac{d}{dt}\langle\boldsymbol{\mu}\rangle = \gamma\mathbf{H}\times\langle\boldsymbol{\mu}\rangle. \tag{2-7}$$

If we have a large number of noninteracting dipoles and if N is the number of dipoles per unit volume, then the magnetization, which is the magnetic dipole moment per unit volume, is given by

$$\mathbf{M} = N\langle\boldsymbol{\mu}\rangle_{avg}, \tag{2-8}$$

where $\langle\boldsymbol{\mu}\rangle_{avg}$ indicates that the statistical average over the initial conditions is also taken. Although Eq. (2-7) is frequently written as

$$\frac{d}{dt}\boldsymbol{\mu} = \gamma\mathbf{H}\times\boldsymbol{\mu}, \tag{2-9}$$

we should remember that $\boldsymbol{\mu}$ can be **M**, $\langle\boldsymbol{\mu}\rangle$, or $\langle\boldsymbol{\mu}\rangle_{avg}$, each having its appropriate quantum-statistical meaning. Also $\boldsymbol{\mu}$ is frequently regarded as a magnetic dipole behaving classically, since a classical dipole would have the same equation of motion. To show this, we start with the equation for the energy: $E = -\boldsymbol{\mu}\cdot\mathbf{H} = -\mu H\cos\theta$. The only generalized force on the dipole (arising because E depends on θ) is a torque equal to $-\partial E/\partial\theta$, tending to align μ along H. Setting the time derivative of the angular momentum, $-\mu/\gamma$, equal to the torque gives

$$\frac{d}{dt}\mu = \gamma H \times \mu, \tag{2-10}$$

which is identical to Eq. (2-9).

Let us consider the simplest solution of this equation, the case in which H is independent of time. Although it may be unnecessary to do so for this simple case, we will employ a rotating reference system (coordinate system) for this problem. This technique will be very useful in analyzing more complicated cases. In Fig. 2-1 we show the fixed

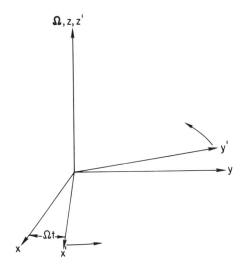

FIG. 2-1   Fixed laboratory coordinates, x, y, and z, and rotating coordinates, x', y', and z', for the angular velocity, Ω, along the z axis, the primed and unprimed axes being the same at $t = 0$.

laboratory system (unprimed) and the rotating coordinate system (primed), which has an angular frequency of Ω. For simplicity we show the case in which Ω is along the z axis. The general case can be obtained by a coordinate transformation in the laboratory frame of reference. We wish to describe an infinitesimal change in μ measured in the fixed coordinate system, $d\mu$, in terms of an infinitesimal change measured in the rotating coordinate system, $d'\mu$, and in terms of the rotation of the two coordinate systems. This relationship is [2]

$$d\mathbf{\mu} = d'\mathbf{\mu} + \mathbf{\Omega}\,dt \times \mathbf{\mu}, \tag{2-11}$$

where the last term is simply the change in $\mathbf{\mu}$ observed in the fixed system if $\mathbf{\mu}$ is constant in the rotating system. This becomes

$$\frac{d\mathbf{\mu}}{dt} = \frac{d'\mathbf{\mu}}{dt} + \mathbf{\Omega} \times \mathbf{\mu}, \tag{2-12}$$

where the terms have obvious meanings. Returning to the solution of Eq. (2-9) for constant $\mathbf{H}$, we obtain

$$\frac{d'\mathbf{\mu}}{dt} = (\gamma\mathbf{H} - \mathbf{\Omega}) \times \mathbf{\mu}. \tag{2-13}$$

If we now choose $\mathbf{\Omega} = \gamma\mathbf{H}$, we find that $\mathbf{\mu}$ is a constant in the rotating system. Transforming back to the fixed coordinate system, we find that $\mathbf{\mu}$ precesses about $\mathbf{H}$ at the Larmor frequency, γH. This behavior is shown in Fig. 2-2. Precession, with $\mathbf{\mu}$ fixed in magnitude and at a constant angle with $\mathbf{H}$, is the simplest possible behavior for a dipole in a magnetic field. The sense of the precession is consistent with the negative charge of the electron and opposite to the convention employed for nuclear dipoles.

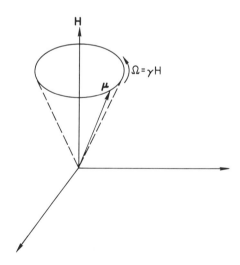

FIG. 2-2 The Larmor precession of $\mathbf{\mu}$ about a constant magnetic field, $\mathbf{H}$. The vector $\mathbf{\mu}$ may represent the magnetization or the expectation value of the operator $\mathbf{\mu}$. The sense of precession is that which occurs when the magnetic dipole moment and the angular momentum are antiparallel, as for individual electrons.

Returning to Eq. (2-13), we note that we chose the value of Ω as γH purely as a matter of convenience. More generally we define an effective field in the rotating coordinate system by

$$\mathbf{H}_e \equiv \mathbf{H} - \frac{\Omega}{\gamma}. \qquad (2\text{-}14)$$

For more complicated problems it is usual to choose $\mathbf{H}_e$ or Ω so as to obtain some desired simplification in the equation of motion. The two most common choices are for Ω to equal the Larmor frequency in some magnetic field, as above, or to equal the frequency of an oscillating component of the field. In the next paragraph we will make the latter choice.

Magnetic resonance experiments do not use a constant $\mathbf{H}$ but rather employ time-dependent components which are usually small compared to the constant component. The geometry most frequently encountered is that of a constant component, $\mathbf{H}_0$, along what we will call the z axis and an oscillating component along the x axis and with a peak-to-peak amplitude of $4H_1$. Although this is the most convenient geometry experimentally, it is less convenient theoretically than one in which the time-dependent field rotates.

To see the relationship let us write the usual experimental time-dependent field as follows:

$$\mathbf{H}_1 = \mathbf{i}2H_1 \cos \omega t = H_1(\mathbf{i} \cos \omega t + \mathbf{j} \sin \omega t) + H_1(\mathbf{i} \cos \omega t - \mathbf{j} \sin \omega t). \quad (2\text{-}15)$$

The first term is a field of constant amplitude H_1 rotating about $\mathbf{H}_0$ at frequency ω in the same sense as electronic Larmor precession. The second term is a similar field but with the opposite sense of rotation. Expressing the time-dependent field as two oppositely rotating fields allows us to examine the effect of each of these on magnetic resonance. The component rotating opposite to the sense of the Larmor precession does not cause magnetic resonance and will result in only minor modifications of the effects of the other component provided that $H_1 \ll H_0$. Henceforth, we will usually consider the total field to be

$$\mathbf{H} = \mathbf{i}H_1 \cos \omega t + \mathbf{j}H_1 \sin \omega t + \mathbf{k}H_0 \qquad (2\text{-}16)$$

as illustrated in Fig. 2-3. Now by transformation to a coordinate system rotating about $\mathbf{H}_0$ at a frequency ω (shown in Fig. 2-3) we find that the magnetic field is constant in this rotating frame. The equation of motion [Eq. (2-9)] is

$$\frac{d\boldsymbol{\mu}}{dt} = \gamma \mathbf{H} \times \boldsymbol{\mu} \qquad (2\text{-}17)$$

where **H** is given by Eq. (2-16). Transformed to the rotating system, this becomes

$$\frac{d'\mathbf{\mu}}{dt} = (\gamma\mathbf{H} - \omega\mathbf{k}) \times \mathbf{\mu} = \gamma\mathbf{H}_e \times \mathbf{\mu}. \qquad (2\text{-}18)$$

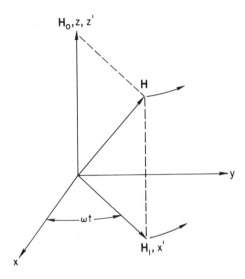

FIG. 2-3   The magnetic field, **H**, usually considered in magnetic resonance experiments. This field consists of a static component, **H₀**, and a component, **H₁**, rotating in the *xy* plane at the angular velocity ω in the same sense as the Larmor precession. Normally $H_0 \gg H_1$, and thus the relative sizes of **H₀** and **H₁** are not as shown in the figure. The magnetic field, **H**, is constant in the primed coordinate system rotating at the same angular velocity, ω, as **H₁**.

The effective field in the rotating coordinate system is shown in Fig. 2-4 and is given by

$$\mathbf{H}_e = H_1\mathbf{i}' + \left(H_0 - \frac{\omega}{\gamma}\right)\mathbf{k}'. \qquad (2\text{-}19)$$

The condition known as magnetic resonance occurs when $H_0 = \omega/\gamma$ and hence $\mathbf{H}_e = \mathbf{H}_1$. Far away from magnetic resonance, $\mathbf{H}_e$ is either nearly parallel or antiparallel to **H₀** and is much larger than H_1.

Returning to the solution of the equation of motion, we see that $\mathbf{H}_e$ in the rotating system is a time-independent field. Thus, as we have shown

above, μ will precess about $\mathbf{H}_e$ in the rotating frame at the angular frequency γH_e. If we wish, we can demonstrate this by going to a third
coordinate system rotating at $\Omega = \gamma \mathbf{H}_e$ relative to the rotating coordinate
system already introduced. The equation of motion in the new system
(double primed) becomes

$$\frac{d''\mu}{dt} = 0. \qquad (2\text{-}20)$$

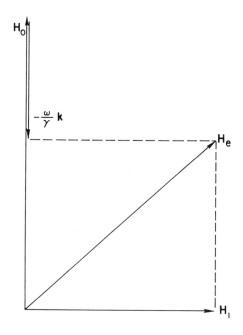

FIG. 2-4   The effective magnetic field, $\mathbf{H}_e$, in the coordinate system rotating
with $\mathbf{H}_1$. Normally $H_0 \gg H_1$ so that the relative magnitudes differ from those
in the figure. Magnetic resonance occurs when $\mathbf{H}_e = \mathbf{H}_1$.

.Thus the motion in the fixed frame consists of μ precessing around $\mathbf{H}_e$ at
the frequency γH_e while $\mathbf{H}_e$ precesses about $\mathbf{H}_0$ at the angular frequency ω.
This is illustrated in Fig. 2-5. The resultant motion depends on the initial
conditions for μ as well as on the quantities ω and $\mathbf{H}_e$. Figure 2-5 does not
employ a thermal equilibrium value for μ initially, but rather uses an
initial large inclination of μ relative to $\mathbf{H}_0$ so as to increase the clarity of
the diagram. We can gain a clearer impression of the motion of μ if we

draw the locus of the end point of **μ** on a spherical surface in the laboratory, as was done for gravitational tops by Goldstein [3]. In our case the frequency γH_e is much less than ω if we are near magnetic resonance. This leads to the behavior shown in Fig. 2-6. Goldstein [3] has other, similar diagrams that represent cases for which $\gamma H_e \gtrsim \omega$ and that are therefore of little interest for magnetic resonance.

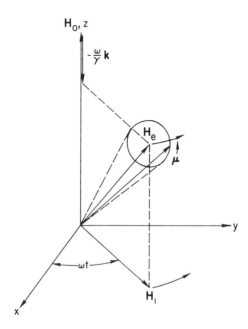

FIG. 2-5   The motion of **μ** close to magnetic resonance for a rotating component of the magnetic field. The vector **μ** precesses about H_e in the rotating coordinate system. The complete motion is then obtained by rotating H_e about H_0 at the angular velocity ω. The figure exaggerates the length of H_1 relative to H_0 and assumes that **μ** does not have its thermal equilibrium orientation initially.

   Let us examine in somewhat more detail a very useful case. It occurs when $\omega = \gamma H_0$ and **μ** is initially parallel to H_0 (assuming $H_1 \ll H_0$), as occurs if H_1 at the Larmor frequency is quickly applied. In this case $H_e = H_1$ and is perpendicular to H_0. Thus **μ** will precess about H_1 going from parallel to antiparallel and back. The locus of the end point of **μ** is shown in Fig. 2-7. Thus **μ** spirals down and back up repetitiously with a period $2\pi/\gamma H_1$. For a better picture of this behavior let us plot some of the components of **μ**. In Fig. 2-8 we show the component of **μ** along H_0 plotted as a function of time. In a similar fashion we plot the y' component of μ (note that $\mu_{x'} = 0$) in Fig. 2-9. This component in the rotating coordinate system gives very similar figures for both the x and the y components when transformed back to a fixed coordinate system. The x component is plotted in Fig. 2-10.

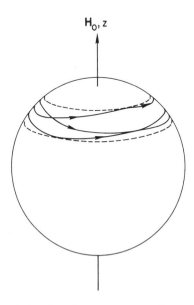

FIG. 2-6   The path of the tip of μ near magnetic resonance. The vector μ rotates about H_0 at the angular frequency ω because of the rotation of H_1 and wobbles at the frequency γH_e because of the precession of μ about H_e in the rotating coordinate system. The initial value of μ and the relationship between γH_0 and ω determine the region of the sphere which will be covered. This region lies between the dashed lines in the figure.

Let us recall our earlier statement that μ represents M, $\langle \mu \rangle$, or $\langle \mu \rangle_{avg}$. If we consider the case of M, then Fig. 2-10 shows that a transverse component of M will oscillate at the Larmor frequency, although with varying amplitude. A transverse coil or its microwave cavity equivalent will pick up a signal at the Larmor frequency, a process referred to as induction. These signals fall off rapidly in intensity as one moves away from resonance.

Next let us consider $\langle \mu \rangle$ (refer to Fig. 2-8). We see that, if the system starts out in the lowest-energy stationary state, after a time $\pi/\gamma H_1$ it is in the highest-energy stationary state, and then at $2\pi/\gamma H_1$ it is back in the lowest-energy stationary state [4].

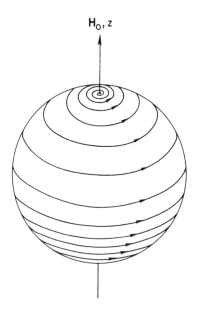

FIG. 2-7   The path of the tip of **μ** at magnetic resonance with **μ** initially along
H$_0$ as it would be in thermal equilibrium.

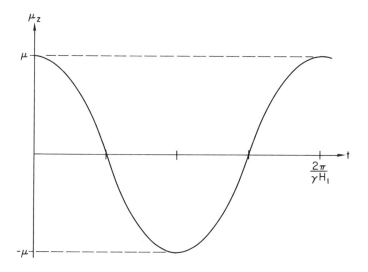

FIG. 2-8   The component of **μ** along **H**$_0$ versus time at magnetic resonance.
At $t = 0$ it is assumed that **μ** is along **H**$_0$.

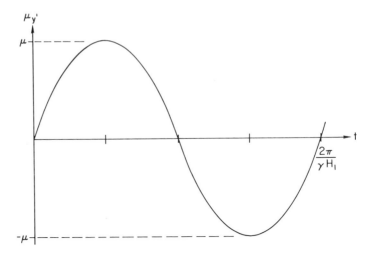

FIG. 2-9   The component of **μ** at magnetic resonance transverse to **H₀** in the coordinate system rotating at the Larmor frequency. This component is 90° out of phase with **H₁**. The component in phase with **H₁** is zero.

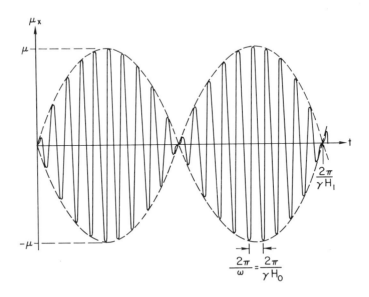

FIG. 2-10   A component of **μ** at magnetic resonance transverse to **H₀** in the laboratory coordinate system. A transverse pickup coil will have a voltage induced at the Larmor frequency, providing one way to detect magnetic resonance.

We have not yet discussed any of the techniques for observing magnetic resonance; rather we have discussed two very simple solutions to the equation of motion, that for a constant field and that for a rotating transverse component of an otherwise constant field. Resonance experiments require a way of sweeping the field or frequency through magnetic resonance or a similar way of comparing the behavior of the system on and off resonance. We can see one practical way of doing this by using the two solutions already obtained. Let us assume initially that $\mathbf{M}$ has its thermal equilibrium value, $\mathbf{M}_0 = \chi_0 \mathbf{H}_0$, where χ_0 is the static magnetic susceptibility. If we now allow $\mathbf{H}_1$ to be turned on for a time $\pi/2\gamma H_1$, and if $\omega = \gamma H_0$, then after the 90° pulse, as it is called, the magnetization will have the same magnitude but will be precessing at the Larmor frequency in the xy plane. Since now the magnetic field is constant, our solutions suggest that it would precess indefinitely and an induction signal could be observed. Actually this free precession will eventually decay, usually because different parts of the sample experience slightly different fields, and thus the precession is not coherent over the whole sample. The subsequent decay of the induction signal, called free induction decay, may be studied both to observe the resonance and to investigate the mechanisms for the decay.

2–2 A Phenomenological Description of Relaxation; the Bloch Equations

If inhomogeneity of the magnetic field is not the cause of free induction decay, then relaxation usually is responsible. For an understanding of most observations of magnetic resonance we must include relaxation in our description. In this section we will give a phenomenological discussion based on Bloch's [5] early description of nuclear magnetic resonance.

With the introduction of relaxation we find ourselves dealing with a statistical problem; therefore Eq. (2-9) will be used to describe the magnetization:

$$\frac{d\mathbf{M}}{dt} = \gamma \mathbf{H} \times \mathbf{M}. \tag{2-21}$$

If $\mathbf{M}$ does not have its thermal equilibrium value at a given time, not only will it precess about $\mathbf{H}$ but also for small H_1 it will approach its thermal equilibrium value, $\mathbf{M}_0 = \chi_0 \mathbf{H}_0$. For example, a nonequilibrium value of $\mathbf{M}$ (a different orientation) could be obtained by the 90° pulse described in Section 2–1.

We will consider the nature of relaxation for a constant magnetic field. We then make the assumption that, if the time-varying components are much smaller than the constant component, the form of the equations is unchanged. Taking the z axis to be the direction of $\mathbf{H}_0$, the constant field, we note that the energy density, U, depends only on the z components of $\mathbf{M}$:

$$U = N\langle \mathcal{H} \rangle_{\text{avg}} = N\langle -\mathbf{\mu} \cdot \mathbf{H} \rangle_{\text{avg}} = -N\langle \mathbf{\mu} \rangle_{\text{avg}} \cdot \mathbf{H} = -M_z H_0 . \quad (2\text{-}22)$$

By means of processes in which energy flows from the spin system (the degrees of freedom determining $\mathbf{M}$, i.e., the dipoles) to the lattice (all other degrees of freedom coupled to the spin system) or the reverse, the z component of the magnetization will approach its thermal equilibrium value, M_0. This is called longitudinal or spin-lattice relaxation. If this process is assumed to lead to an exponential approach to equilibrium, the equation for M_z can be written as

$$\frac{d}{dt} M_z = \frac{M_0 - M_z}{T_1} , \quad (2\text{-}23)$$

where T_1 is the spin-lattice relaxation time.

In contrast the transverse components of the magnetization do not influence the energy, and so they can change without coupling to the lattice. This often makes the transverse or spin-spin relaxation, as it is called, faster than spin-lattice relaxation. One spin-spin relaxation mechanism involves dipoles close enough so that they experience various local fields resulting from the dipolar fields of their neighbors. These local field variations lead to different precessional frequencies and an eventual incoherence in the precessing component of $\mathbf{M}$. If this loss of the transverse components is also assumed to occur exponentially, we have

$$\frac{d'M_{x'}}{dt} = -\frac{M_{x'}}{T_2} , \qquad \frac{d'M_{y'}}{dt} = -\frac{M_{y'}}{T_2} \quad (2\text{-}24)$$

in a coordinate system rotating with the transverse magnetization at the Larmor frequency, γH_0. The quantity T_2 is called the spin-spin relaxation time and is at least as small as T_1. Transforming back to the laboratory system and allowing a small time-varying component of $\mathbf{H}$ (z is still the direction of $\mathbf{H}_0$), we have the Bloch equations for electrons (negative magnetic moments):

$$\frac{dM_x}{dt} = \gamma(\mathbf{H} \times \mathbf{M})_x - \frac{M_x}{T_2} ,$$

$$\frac{dM_y}{dt} = \gamma(\mathbf{H} \times \mathbf{M})_y - \frac{M_y}{T_2} , \quad (2\text{-}25)$$

$$\frac{dM_z}{dt} = \gamma(\mathbf{H} \times \mathbf{M})_z + \frac{M_0 - M_z}{T_1} .$$

The Bloch equations represent about the simplest mathematical description possible for magnetic resonance when relaxation is included.

It is important to realize, however, that many paramagnetic samples will not obey the Bloch equations, although frequently these equations are still of qualitative or even semiquantitative value in suggesting the behavior of such samples. This may be the situation for interacting dipoles, for dipoles corresponding to $J > \frac{1}{2}$ at low temperatures, for cases of low static field, or for saturation.

We will now examine a few types of magnetic resonance experiments using the Bloch equations. First let us briefly mention again the free induction decay following a 90° pulse, as described in Section 2–1. We may choose $t = 0$ as the time when the 90° pulse is removed. Then the initial value of **M** is given by

$$\mathbf{M}(0) = M_0 \mathbf{i}, \tag{2-26}$$

where the z axis is along $\mathbf{H}_0$, the x axis is chosen as the transverse direction along $\mathbf{M}(0)$, and the fact that $M(0) = M_0$ indicates that the pulse was short relative to T_1 or T_2. The Bloch equations in a coordinate system rotating at the Larmor frequency, $\omega = \gamma H_0$, are as follows:

$$\frac{d'M_{x'}}{dt} = -\frac{M_{x'}}{T_2},$$

$$\frac{d'M_{y'}}{dt} = -\frac{M_{y'}}{T_2}, \tag{2-27}$$

$$\frac{d'M_{z'}}{dt} = \frac{dM_z}{dt} = \frac{M_0 - M_z}{T_1}.$$

The solution of these equations for $t > 0$ is

$$M_{x'} = M_0 \exp\left(-\frac{t}{T_2}\right),$$

$$M_{y'} = 0, \tag{2-28}$$

$$M_z = M_0\left[1 - \exp\left(-\frac{t}{T_1}\right)\right].$$

Transformed to the fixed laboratory frame, this becomes

$$M_x = M_0 \exp\left(-\frac{t}{T_2}\right)\cos\omega t,$$

$$M_y = M_0 \exp\left(-\frac{t}{T_2}\right)\sin\omega t, \tag{2-29}$$

$$M_z = M_0\left[1 - \exp\left(-\frac{t}{T_1}\right)\right].$$

As shown in Fig. 2-11, M_z approaches M_0 with a characteristic time T_1. Figure 2-12 shows M_x (M_y would look similar) approaching zero with a characteristic time T_2; M_x also oscillates at the Larmor frequency. The

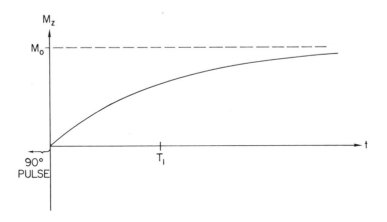

FIG. 2-11   The growth of the component of the magnetization **M** along **H**$_0$ following a 90° pulse. At $t = T_1$, the spin-lattice relaxation time, M_z has reached a value of $(1 - 1/e)M_0$, where M_0 is the thermal equilibrium value.

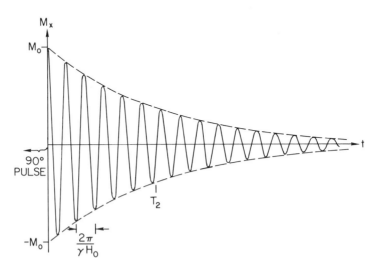

FIG. 2-12   A component of **M** transverse to **H**$_0$ following a 90° pulse. This free induction decay has a characteristic time, T_2, the spin-spin relaxation time.

damped oscillation shown in Fig. 2-12 is the form of the signal observed for a free induction decay experiment.

The magnetic resonance condition is sought by varying parameters in the Hamiltonian, such as the magnetic field or the frequency, and observing the effect on the magnetization. These changes may be made suddenly or adiabatically, rapidly or slowly. In addition to these limiting cases, changes can be made which are neither sudden nor adiabatic. Also, changes which are neither rapid nor slow occur. A sudden change is one made so fast that the time-dependent wave function of an individual dipole does not change during the time in which the change in parameters is taking place. This means that $\langle \mu \rangle$ cannot change and therefore the magnetization remains unchanged. In other words, the change occurs in a time short compared to a Larmor period and hence no precessional motion of **M** can occur. An adiabatic change, in contrast, is one which is so slow that no additional transitions between the stationary states are induced, but the stationary states change as the parameters change. Thus the wave function is always the same combination of stationary eigenfunctions, which are, however, at any instant always the correct instantaneous stationary eigenfunctions of the system. This means that **M** makes many precessional circuits during the time in which a significant change in the Hamiltonian occurs. In consequence, as we will show later, **M** makes a constant angle with **H**. Note that we are using "adiabatic" not in the thermodynamic sense of isentropic (no heat flow) but in the Ehrenfest sense [6]. The question of whether a change in field or frequency is adiabatic, sudden, or neither depends on the coordinate system (fixed or rotating), since this can greatly influence the rate of change of the magnetic field.

Another important feature is the relationship of the rates of the changes to the relaxation times. A change is rapid if it occurs in a time short compared to the relaxation times, and it is slow if it occurs in a time long compared to the relaxation times. Hence for a rapid process no relaxation can occur, while for a slow process relaxation occurs so fast that thermal equilibrium exists at all times.

From these two classifications we can obtain three types of changes for a system with a clearly resolved magnetic resonance: sudden, adiabatic rapid, and slow. (By introducing another time-varying field, a modulation of the swept nearly constant field, Weger [7] obtains many more cases. These three are adequate, however, for the simple situations that we wish to consider.) To illustrate a sudden process we might consider an alternative to the 90° pulse as preparation for the observation of free induction decay. Consider a very fast rotation of the magnetic field by 90°, so fast that no precession occurs until the change has been made. The subsequent decay occurs just as for the 90° pulse (assuming that no $\mathbf{H}_1$ is present).

An important type of magnetic resonance process is referred to as adiabatic rapid passage. Before discussing this we will consider adiabatic rapid processes in general [8]. If a process is rapid, we may ignore the relaxation terms in the Bloch equations during the time of the rapid change. Thus we have

$$\frac{d\mathbf{M}}{dt} = \gamma\mathbf{H} \times \mathbf{M}, \qquad (2\text{-}30)$$

the same as Eq. (2-9). We note that

$$\frac{d(M^2)}{dt} = \frac{d}{dt}(\mathbf{M} \cdot \mathbf{M}) = 2\mathbf{M} \cdot \frac{d\mathbf{M}}{dt} = 2\gamma\mathbf{M} \cdot \mathbf{H} \times \mathbf{M} = 0, \qquad (2\text{-}31)$$

that is, $\mathbf{M}$ is constant in magnitude and changes only in direction. This arises because without relaxation we have only a torque acting on $\mathbf{M}$. The same behavior occurred throughout Section 2–1.

In general the time derivative of $\mathbf{H}$ can be written as

$$\frac{d\mathbf{H}}{dt} = \boldsymbol{\Omega} \times \mathbf{H} + \Omega'\mathbf{H} \qquad (2\text{-}32)$$

the first term being an arbitrary component transverse to $\mathbf{H}$, and the second being an arbitrary longitudinal component. The quantities $\boldsymbol{\Omega}$ and Ω' are a general time-dependent vector (which we will take perpendicular to $\mathbf{H}$)

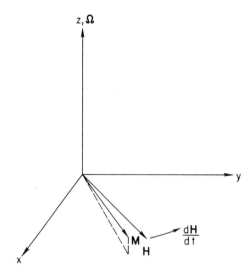

FIG. 2-13 The magnetization and the magnetic field in the laboratory coordinate system. The magnetic field rotates in the xy plane as shown. This geometry is used to discuss an adiabatic rapid rotation of the magnetic field.

and scalar, respectively, both having the dimensions of frequency. Since **M** is constant, we are interested only in the rotation of **H** (provided Ω' is so small that H changes very little). To simplify the problem further, let us consider that Ω is constant and $\Omega' = 0$. If we now transform to a (primed) coordinate system rotating with respect to the laboratory system at the angular frequency Ω (it is for this reason that we used Ω for the frequency of rotation of **H**), we obtain the equation of motion:

$$\frac{d'\mathbf{M}}{dt} = (\gamma\mathbf{H} - \mathbf{\Omega}) \times \mathbf{M} = \gamma\mathbf{H}_e \times \mathbf{M}. \qquad (2\text{-}33)$$

But in this coordinate system the magnetic field is constant; hence $\mathbf{H}_e$ is time independent. From our experience in Section 2-1 we know that in the rotating frame **M** simply precesses around $\mathbf{H}_e$ at the frequency γH_e, the angle of **M** with respect to $\mathbf{H}_e$ remaining fixed. This is illustrated in Figs. 2-13, 2-14, and 2-15, which show the fields and the magnetization for the fixed and the rotating coordinate system, respectively, and the motion of **M** in the fixed system.

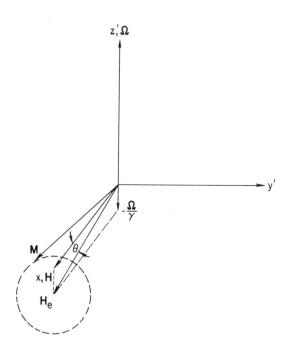

FIG. 2-14   The magnetization and the magnetic fields in the rotating coordinate system for the geometry shown in Fig. 2-13. The magnetization precesses about the effective magnetic field resulting from rotation of **H**.

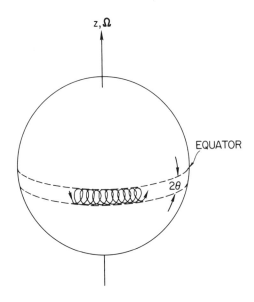

FIG. 2-15   The path of the tip of **M** during an adiabatic rapid rotation of the magnetic field with **M** initially along **H**. Refer to Figs. 2-13 and 2-14 for the geometry employed. The angle θ is $\tan^{-1} \Omega/\gamma H$, which is usually a very small quantity. Thus **M** roughly follows **H**.

The angular separation, θ, of **H** and $\mathbf{H}_e$ is given by

$$\tan \theta = \frac{\Omega}{\gamma H}. \qquad (2\text{-}34)$$

Thus we see that, if $\Omega \ll \gamma H$, then $\theta \simeq \Omega/\gamma H \ll 1$ and **H** and $\mathbf{H}_e$ differ by a very small amount. Hence our conclusion that **M** will remain at a fixed angle with respect to $\mathbf{H}_e$ can now be used to argue that **M** makes a fixed angle with respect to **H**. In particular, if **M** is originally along **H**, it will follow **H**.

The condition $\Omega \ll \gamma H$ states that the rate of angular change of **H** is slow compared to the Larmor frequency and hence the process is adiabatic. We have shown that, if Ω is a constant, **M** remains at a fixed angle with **H**. In general, however, Ω will be time dependent. The argument above can still be applied at any instant of time. But in order not to be troubled by being near magnetic resonance in the rotating reference system we must also require that Ω not have any time variations with frequencies near γH, the Larmor frequency. Since we now have the restrictions imposed by adiabaticity for a general motion of **H** (except for the effect of Ω', which is not important for a rapid change), let us express them in a somewhat more useful fashion in terms of $d\mathbf{H}/dt$ rather than $\mathbf{\Omega}$:

$$\frac{d\mathbf{H}}{dt} = \mathbf{\Omega} \times \mathbf{H} + \Omega'\mathbf{H}, \tag{2-35}$$

$$\mathbf{H} \times \frac{d\mathbf{H}}{dt} = \mathbf{H} \times (\mathbf{\Omega} \times \mathbf{H}) = H^2\mathbf{\Omega} - (\mathbf{H} \cdot \mathbf{\Omega})\mathbf{H}. \tag{2-36}$$

Since $\mathbf{\Omega}$ is perpendicular to $\mathbf{H}$,

$$\left| \mathbf{H} \times \frac{d\mathbf{H}}{dt} \right| = H^2\Omega \tag{2-37}$$

or the adiabatic condition becomes

$$\frac{1}{H^2} \left| \mathbf{H} \times \frac{d\mathbf{H}}{dt} \right| \ll \gamma H. \tag{2-38}$$

This is occasionally replaced by the more severe restriction on $\mathbf{H}$,

$$\frac{1}{H} \left| \frac{d\mathbf{H}}{dt} \right| \ll \gamma H. \tag{2-39}$$

In either case we also must have no time variations of $H^{-2}\mathbf{H} \times d\mathbf{H}/dt$ with frequencies near the Larmor frequency.

It may seem that an angular difference between $\mathbf{M}$ and $\mathbf{H}$ (assuming they were initially parallel) could be accumulated after a large number of Larmor periods by a properly chosen time dependence for $\mathbf{\Omega}$. This could happen only if variations of $\mathbf{\Omega}$ with a frequency near γH were allowed. In other cases incremental increases and decreases will cancel, as was shown in a clear pictorial fashion for adiabatic rapid passage by Powles [9].

We will now apply our conclusions concerning processes which are adiabatic and rapid to the type of magnetic resonance experiment called adiabatic rapid passage. In order to have magnetic resonance we must have a time-varying component of the magnetic field. Let us take the geometry used previously: a small rotating field perpendicular to a larger, nearly constant field. Because the total field now has time variations at the frequency ω, which is near the Larmor frequency, we cannot have any adiabatic processes in the laboratory frame of reference. However, if we transform to a coordinate system rotating with $\mathbf{H}_1$ at the frequency ω, then the field is nearly constant. It varies only because of the relatively slow changes in H_0. The behavior upon passing through magnetic resonance by varying H_0 adiabatically in this rotating system is called adiabatic rapid passage.

The effective field in the rotating system $\mathbf{H}_e$ is given by [see Fig. 2-4 and Eq. (2-19)]

$$\mathbf{H}_e = H_1 \mathbf{i}' + \left(H_0 - \frac{\omega}{\gamma} \right) \mathbf{k}'. \tag{2-40}$$

This field is nearly constant. It varies because we sweep H_0 or ω to pass through magnetic resonance. In order for this sweep of H_0 or ω to result in an adiabatic process in the coordinate system rotating at ω, we must apply Eq. (2-38) in the rotating system:

$$\frac{1}{H_e^2} \left| \mathbf{H}_e \times \frac{d'\mathbf{H}_e}{dt} \right| \ll \gamma H_e. \tag{2-41}$$

Using Eq. (2-40) for $\mathbf{H}_e$, we obtain

$$\frac{H_1}{H_e^2} \left| \frac{d}{dt} \left(H_0 - \frac{\omega}{\gamma} \right) \right| \ll \gamma H_e. \tag{2-42}$$

This is usually replaced by the more restrictive condition required near resonance:

$$\frac{1}{H_1} \left| \frac{d}{dt} \left(H_0 - \frac{\omega}{\gamma} \right) \right| \ll \gamma H_1. \tag{2-43}$$

The restriction on the time dependence of $\mathbf{\Omega}$ becomes in this case that $H_e^{-2}(d/dt)(H_0 - \omega/\gamma)$ have no frequency components near γH_e. Since the processes are rapid, we have the additional restriction that

$$\frac{1}{H_1} \left| \frac{d}{dt} \left(H_0 - \frac{\omega}{\gamma} \right) \right| \gg \frac{1}{T_1}, \frac{1}{T_2}. \tag{2-44}$$

If these conditions are satisfied, the sweep is adiabatic in the rotating coordinate system and the magnetization will follow the effective field of Eq. (2-40) (or maintain a constant angle of precession about it). Two initial conditions are commonly encountered; in both, the magnetization is equal to its thermal equilibrium value $\mathbf{M}_0$ along $\mathbf{H}_0$, but in one case H_0 is above ω/γ, the value of the field at which magnetic resonance occurs, whereas in the second it is below this value. The effective fields for these two cases are shown together with the value at resonance in Fig. 2-16 (where the frequency is varying). We see that for the first initial condition, with $H_0 > \omega/\gamma$, both the magnetization and the effective field start nearly along $\mathbf{H}_0$. The magnetization follows $\mathbf{H}_e$, so that at $H_0 = \omega/\gamma$ it is along $\mathbf{H}_1$ and finally it ends up for $H_0 < \omega/\gamma$ in the opposite direction from $\mathbf{H}_0$. This process is termed adiabatic inversion. If the second initial condition were

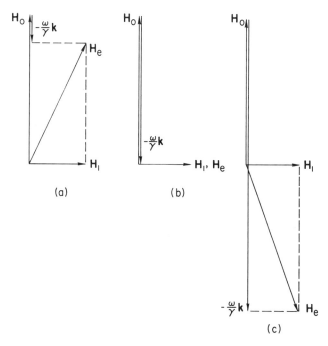

FIG. 2-16   The magnetic fields of importance in adiabatic rapid passage shown in the coordinate system rotating with $\mathbf{H}_1$. Case (b) is for magnetic resonance; the frequency for case (a) is well below the Larmor frequency; for case (c) it is well above.

employed, a similar behavior of the magnetization would occur although there would be a constant angle of 180° with $\mathbf{H}_e$. The path of the magnetization vector is shown in the rotating coordinate system in Fig. 2-17(a) and in the laboratory system in Fig. 2-17(b). Our discussions so far in Chapter 2 suggest three ways of inverting the magnetization: adiabatic inversion, a 180° pulse (twice as long as a 90° pulse), and a sudden rotation of the field by 180°.

We note that for the geometry we have been considering (a nearly constant field along the z axis and a smaller rotating component in the xy plane), we have obtained a transverse component of the magnetization which rotates at the frequency of the rotating field. This behavior is generally encountered and is not limited to adiabatic rapid passage. As a result of the coherence of $\mathbf{H}_1$ and the rotating magnetization, the experimental equipment frequently measures either the component of $\mathbf{M}$ in phase with $\mathbf{H}_1$ or the component lagging $\mathbf{H}_1$ by 90°. In the frame rotating at ω we will again take x' as the axis parallel to $\mathbf{H}_1$. Then the in-phase component will lead to a susceptibility

$$\chi' = \frac{M_{x'}}{H_1}, \tag{2-45}$$

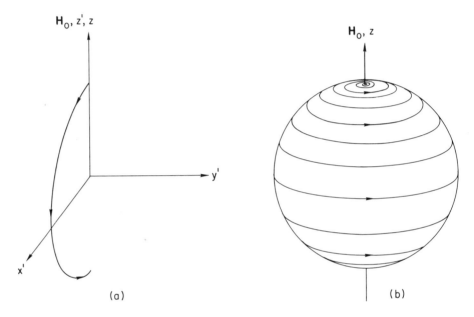

FIG. 2-17   The path of the tip of the magnetization vector during an adiabatic rapid passage. Case (a) is for the coordinate system rotating with $\mathbf{H}_1$, and case (b) shows the path in the laboratory system.

which is termed dispersion. The lagging component leads to another susceptibility,

$$\chi'' = -\frac{M_{y'}}{H_1}, \tag{2-46}$$

which is called absorption. A factor of 2 usually appears in the denominator because a linearly polarized field of amplitude $2H_1$ is assumed in most definitions. If the time dependence is written in terms of $e^{i\omega t}$, these definitions allow us to write the transverse magnetization as $\chi\mathbf{H}_1$ with $\chi = \chi' - i\chi''$, the complex susceptibility.

Since in adiabatic rapid passage starting with $H_0 > \omega/\gamma$ the magnetization follows $\mathbf{H}_e$, it will only have x' and z' components and hence to a first approximation χ'' will be zero and χ' will have a value which reaches a maximum, M_0/H_1, at resonance. From the cosine of the angle between $\mathbf{H}_e$ and $\mathbf{H}_1$ we have

$$\chi' = \frac{M_0}{[H_1^2 + (H_0 - \omega/\gamma)^2]^{1/2}}. \tag{2-47}$$

The sign will be negative if we are originally at a field below resonance. Actually, although χ'' is always much smaller than the maximum value of χ', it is not zero. The reason for this can be seen if we return to Figs. 2-13, 2-14, and 2-15 where we showed the path of $\mathbf{M}$ for an adiabatic process. We note that if $\mathbf{M}$ starts along $\mathbf{H}$ it will precess about $\mathbf{H}_e$ so that it makes an average angle of $\Omega/\gamma H$ with $\mathbf{H}$. This angle constitutes an average nonzero value of $M_{y'}$ for the case of adiabatic rapid passage and has a sense such that $M_{y'}$ is negative. Thus χ'' looks qualitatively similar to χ' but has a peak which is weaker by the factor $|(d/dt)(H_0 - \omega/\gamma)|/\gamma H_1^2$ which is much less than one. The expression for χ'' is

$$\chi'' = \frac{H_1 \left| \dfrac{d}{dt}(H_0 - \omega/\gamma) \right|}{\gamma[H_1^2 + (H_0 - \omega/\gamma)^2]^{3/2}}. \tag{2-48}$$

The form of the signals proportional to χ' and χ'' for adiabatic rapid passage are shown in Fig. 2-18. We see the "bell-shaped" resonances, the phase difference in χ' upon starting above and below resonance, and at the right we see the effect of returning through resonance so quickly that no relaxation has occurred.

As shown in Eq. (2-22) the energy of the spin system is $-\mathbf{M} \cdot \mathbf{H}$. The power absorbed by the dipoles, P, is the time derivative of this quantity

$$P = \frac{d}{dt}(-\mathbf{M} \cdot \mathbf{H}) = -\mathbf{M} \cdot \frac{d\mathbf{H}}{dt} - \mathbf{H} \cdot \frac{d\mathbf{M}}{dt}. \tag{2-49}$$

The first term represents the absorption of energy from the time-varying magnetic field, including any rotating or oscillating component. The second term is the power absorbed from the lattice, that is, by relaxation. For a rapid process the second term is zero, as can be seen mathematically by replacing $d\mathbf{M}/dt$ by $\gamma \mathbf{H} \times \mathbf{M}$. For adiabatic rapid passage $d\mathbf{H}/dt$ has a rotating component leading $\mathbf{H}_1$ by 90°. This means that power will be absorbed because of the nonzero value of χ''. This absorption of power from the rotating field integrated over the whole sweep will account for the total energy required to invert the magnetization, $2\mathbf{M} \cdot \mathbf{H}_0$, where $\mathbf{H}_0$ has the value corresponding to magnetic resonance. The energy absorbed is independent of the rate of sweep, as long as it is adiabatic and rapid, and no contribution occurs from $d\mathbf{H}_0/dt$.

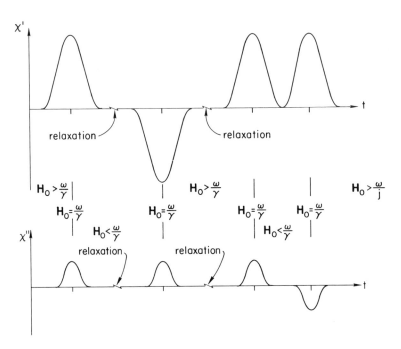

FIG. 2-18   The dispersion and absorption signals resulting from adiabatic rapid passage. Starting at thermal equilibrium with the magnetic field above the value for magnetic resonance, we obtain the signals on the left by sweeping the field down through resonance (or the frequency up). If after the sweep we delay the return until relaxation has occurred, we obtain the second pair of signals, in which weak absorption still occurs but for which the dispersion is inverted. The last two sweeps are the same as the first two except that the return sweep is made before any relaxation can occur. Note that in this case there is no net absorption.

Because electronic paramagnets usually have rather short relaxation times, the conditions for observation of free induction decay or adiabatic rapid passage are not as common as those for a technique known as slow passage. In slow passage the sweep is so slow that relaxation maintains a constant magnetization in the coordinate system rotating with the time-varying field. Using the usual geometry of fields with a constant component along z and a small rotating one in the xy plane, we have the effective field in a system rotating with $\mathbf{H}_1$ at the frequency ω given by [see Eq. (2-19)]

$$\mathbf{H}_e = H_1 \mathbf{i}' + \left(H_0 - \frac{\omega}{\gamma} \right) \mathbf{k}' . \tag{2-50}$$

The Bloch equations in this reference system are

$$\frac{d' M_{x'}}{dt} = \gamma (\mathbf{H}_e \times \mathbf{M})_{x'} - \frac{M_{x'}}{T_2} ,$$

$$\frac{dM_{y'}}{dt} = \gamma (\mathbf{H}_e \times \mathbf{M})_{y'} - \frac{M_{y'}}{T_2} , \tag{2-51}$$

$$\frac{dM_{z'}}{dt} = \gamma (\mathbf{H}_e \times \mathbf{M})_{z'} + \frac{1}{T_1} (M_0 - M_{z'}) .$$

It will now be our purpose to solve these equations under slow-passage conditions. Introducing the value of $\mathbf{H}_e$, we obtain

$$\frac{d' M_{x'}}{dt} = -(\gamma H_0 - \omega) M_{y'} - \frac{M_{x'}}{T_2} ,$$

$$\frac{d' M_{y'}}{dt} = (\gamma H_0 - \omega) M_{x'} - \gamma H_1 M_{z'} - \frac{M_{y'}}{T_2} , \tag{2-52}$$

$$\frac{d' M_{z'}}{dt} = \gamma H_1 M_{y'} + \frac{M_0 - M_{z'}'}{T_1} .$$

The slow-passage solutions are independent of time in the rotating system with its nearly constant field. Thus we have

$$\frac{d' M_{x'}}{dt} = \frac{d' M_{y'}}{dt} = \frac{d' M_{z'}}{dt} = 0 . \tag{2-53}$$

This gives

$$\frac{1}{T_2} M_{x'} + (\gamma H_0 - \omega) M_{y'} = 0 ,$$

$$(\gamma H_0 - \omega) M_{x'} - \frac{1}{T_2} M_{y'} - \gamma H_1 M_{z'} = 0 , \tag{2-54}$$

$$\gamma H_1 M_{y'} - \frac{1}{T_1} M_{z'} = -\frac{M_0}{T_1} .$$

Straightforward solution of these algebraic equations gives

$$M_{x'} = \frac{\gamma H_1 (\gamma H_0 - \omega) T_2^2}{1 + (\gamma H_0 - \omega)^2 T_2^2 + \gamma^2 H_1^2 T_1 T_2} M_0,$$

$$M_{y'} = \frac{-\gamma H_1 T_2}{1 + (\gamma H_0 - \omega)^2 T_2^2 + \gamma^2 H_1^2 T_1 T_2} M_0, \qquad (2\text{-}55)$$

$$M_{z'} = \frac{1 + (\gamma H_0 - \omega)^2 T_2^2}{1 + (\gamma H_0 - \omega)^2 T_2^2 + \gamma^2 H_1^2 T_1 T_2} M_0.$$

Writing these in terms of the complex susceptibility, we obtain

$$\chi' = \frac{M_{x'}}{H_1} = \frac{\gamma(\gamma H_0 - \omega) T_2^2 M_0}{1 + (\gamma H_0 - \omega)^2 T_2^2 + \gamma^2 H_1^2 T_1 T_2},$$

$$\qquad (2\text{-}56)$$

$$\chi'' = -\frac{M_{y'}}{H_1} = \frac{\gamma T_2 M_0}{1 + (\gamma H_0 - \omega)^2 T_2^2 + \gamma^2 H_1^2 T_1 T_2} = \frac{\chi'}{(\gamma H_0 - \omega) T_2},$$

which for small values of H_1, that is, $\gamma^2 H_1^2 T_1 T_2 \ll 1$, become

$$\chi'' = \frac{\gamma T_2}{1 + (\gamma H_0 - \omega)^2 T_2^2} M_0,$$

$$\chi' = (\gamma H_0 - \omega) T_2 \chi'', \qquad (2\text{-}57)$$

$$M_z = M_0.$$

Note that because we have continued to use only a properly rotating $\mathbf{H}_1$ our χ will be twice as big as the value commonly used.

Plots of χ'' and χ' versus $(\chi H_0 - \omega) T_2$ for $\gamma^2 H_1^2 T_1 T_2 \ll 1$ are shown in Fig. 2-19. This particular dependence on field or frequency is referred to as a Lorentzian line shape. Also shown is another useful line shape function, the Gaussian. For large values of H_1 the Bloch equations and their slow-passage solutions are not necessarily a good description. Low-viscosity liquids obey the Bloch equations even for large H_1, and some insight into the behavior of other systems can be obtained by studying the saturation behavior of the Bloch equations for slow passage. Saturation occurs when the precessional frequency, γH_1, becomes greater than the corresponding relaxation frequencies, $1/T$, or, more precisely,

$$\gamma^2 H_1^2 T_1 T_2 \gtrsim 1. \qquad (2\text{-}58)$$

Even under conditions of saturation we find that the absorption has a Lorentzian shape,

$$\chi'' = \frac{\gamma \tilde{T}_2 M_0}{\sqrt{1 + \gamma^2 H_1^2 T_1 T_2}} \frac{1}{1 + (\gamma H_0 - \omega)^2 \tilde{T}_2^2}, \qquad (2\text{-}59)$$

where

$$\tilde{T}_2 = \frac{T_2}{\sqrt{1 + \gamma^2 H_1^2 T_1 T_2}}. \qquad (2\text{-}60)$$

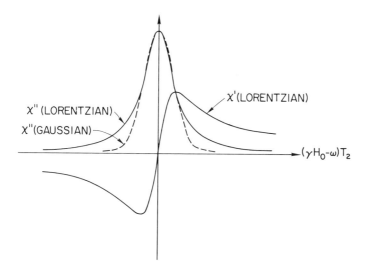

FIG. 2-19   The absorption and dispersion obtained by solving Bloch's equations for slow passage. The resultant shape is termed Lorentzian. For contrast the Gaussian line shape for absorption is drawn with the same maximum value and the same width at half of the maximum amplitude. These line shapes are the ones most frequently employed because they are simple and constitute a reasonable approximation to the shapes actually observed.

The maximum value of χ'' occurs for $\omega = \gamma H_0$ and is $\gamma \tilde{T}_2 M_0 / \sqrt{1 + \gamma^2 H_1^2 T_1 T_2}$. The absorption signal will be proportional to the corresponding magnetization, $\chi'' H_1$, for a linear detector. The maximum in this magnetization is proportional to H_1 for $\gamma^2 H_1^2 T_1 T_2 \ll 1$, has its greatest value of $\frac{1}{2} M_0 \sqrt{T_2/T_1}$ at $\gamma^2 H_1^2 T_1 T_2 = 1$, and decreases as H_1^{-1} for $\gamma^2 H_1^2 T_1 T_2 \gg 1$. Although the line shape remains Lorentzian, the width gets larger as a result of saturation. The simplest definition of the width for our present purposes is the field (or frequency) spacing between the half-amplitude points of χ'', which we will call ΔH_0. This implies $(\gamma H_0 - \omega)^2 \tilde{T}_2^2 = 1$, or

$$\Delta H_0 = \frac{2}{\gamma \tilde{T}_2} = \frac{2}{\gamma T_2} \sqrt{1 + \gamma^2 H_1^2 T_1 T_2}. \qquad (2\text{-}61)$$

The relationship $\chi' = (\gamma H_0 - \omega)T_2\chi''$ allows us to write

$$\chi' = \gamma \tilde{T}_2 M_0 \frac{(\gamma H_0 - \omega)\tilde{T}_2}{1 + (\gamma H_0 - \omega)^2 \tilde{T}_2^2} \qquad (2\text{-}62)$$

and thus to see that the dispersion also has a Lorentzian shape at all values of H_1. The maximum and the minimum values of χ' occur at $H_0 = \omega/\gamma \pm 1/\gamma \tilde{T}_2$, at which points $|\chi'|$ has the value $\frac{1}{2}\gamma \tilde{T}_2 M_0$. Thus in contrast with the case of χ'' the maximum in-phase magnetization, $\chi' H_1$, increases linearly with H_1 if $\gamma^2 H_1^2 T_1 T_2 \ll 1$ and approaches a constant value of $\frac{1}{2}M_0\sqrt{T_2/T_1}$ for $\gamma^2 H_1^2 T_1 T_2 \gg 1$. We also note from Eq. (2-55) that, although $M_z = M_0$ for $\gamma^2 H_1^2 T_1 T_2 \ll 1$, it becomes proportional to H_1^{-2} on magnetic resonance for $\gamma^2 H_1^2 T_1 T_2 \gg 1$.

The behaviors we have just described for the absorption and dispersion are not always quantitatively correct but indicate in a simple and qualitative way the nature of saturation. The significance may be somewhat clearer if we examine the power absorbed by the spin system per unit volume [see Eq. (2-49)]:

$$P = -\mathbf{M} \cdot \frac{d\mathbf{H}}{dt} - \mathbf{H} \cdot \frac{d\mathbf{M}}{dt}. \qquad (2\text{-}63)$$

In slow passage, energy cannot accumulate in the spin system so

$$\mathbf{H} \cdot \frac{d\mathbf{M}}{dt} = -\mathbf{M} \cdot \frac{d\mathbf{H}}{dt} \qquad (2\text{-}64)$$

or $P = 0$. By straightforward algebra we can show that the power absorbed from the rotating field, P_H (and hence the power given off to the lattice by relaxation), is

$$P_H = \omega \chi'' H_1^2. \qquad (2\text{-}65)$$

From this we see that the power absorbed at resonance will approach a constant value as H_1 is increased, that is, under saturating conditions. We will encounter this characteristic again in Section 2-4.

Although we have indicated that slow passage is the most common mode of observation of electron paramagnetic resonance, we have not described the most common way of utilizing this behavior, the method of field modulation. Instead of detecting χ' and χ'' directly, or something depending multiplicatively on them, an additional oscillating component of the magnetic field is applied parallel to $\mathbf{H}_0$. All other components of the field are as we have used them already on several occasions. The amplitude of this modulation field is usually kept less than the line width. Thus, in addition to signals near zero frequency depending on χ' and χ'', we will have signals near the modulation frequency whose amplitudes depend on the derivatives of χ' and χ''. The use of phase-sensitive detection thus leads to signals proportional to $d\chi'/dH$ and $d\chi''/dH$. These quantities are shown in Fig. 2-20 for slow passage and a Lorentzian line shape. The introduction of another frequency and another field complicates the types of possible processes (adiabatic rapid, sudden, slow), as has been demonstrated in an extensive study by Weger [7].

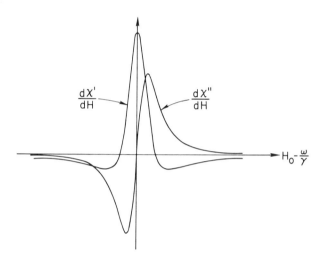

FIG. 2-20   The derivative of the absorption and dispersion for a Lorentzian line shape such as is shown in Fig. 2-19. These are the types of signals obtained by using small-amplitude field modulation and phase-sensitive detection.

2–3 Quantum-Mechanical Time-Dependent Perturbation Theory

In Sections 2–1 and 2–2 we gave descriptions of magnetic resonance which were classical in appearance. However, we derived the basic equation of motion from a quantum-mechanical theorem involving expectation values. But the expectation value of $\boldsymbol{\mu}$, although providing much insight into magnetic resonance, does not constitute a thorough quantum-mechanical description of magnetic resonance. We will attempt to give a more detailed quantum-mechanical presentation in this section. For simplicity we will again ignore all effects of relaxation.

Our purpose will be to solve the time-dependent Schrödinger equation,

$$\mathcal{H}\psi = -\frac{\hbar}{i}\frac{\partial \psi}{\partial t}, \tag{2-66}$$

where

$$\mathcal{JC} = \gamma\hbar\mathbf{H}\cdot\mathbf{J}, \tag{2-67}$$

$$\mathbf{H} = 2H_1\mathbf{i}\cos\omega t + H_0\mathbf{k}.$$

We have chosen to use a linearly polarized oscillating magnetic field of amplitude $2H_1$ rather than the circularly polarized field employed in Sections 2–1 and 2–2. This is a rather simple form for the time-dependent Schrödinger equation, one which admits exact solutions [10]. However, since the exact solutions cannot easily be generalized to apply to the more complex paramagnetic entities that we will consider later, and because perturbation theory can be so generalized and has clear physical inter-pretations, we will employ time-dependent perturbation theory. The Hamiltonian is written as the sum of two terms, a large static term and the time-dependent perturbation:

$$\mathcal{JC} = \mathcal{JC}_0 + \mathcal{JC}_1,$$

$$\mathcal{JC}_0 = \gamma\hbar H_0 J_z, \tag{2-68}$$

$$\mathcal{JC}_1 = \gamma\hbar(2H_1\cos\omega t)J_x.$$

The zero-order eigenfunctions are $\Phi_M \exp[-(i/\hbar)E_M t]$, where

$$\mathcal{JC}_0\Phi_M = E_M\Phi_M, \tag{2-69}$$

$$E_M = \gamma\hbar H_0 M \qquad (M = -J, -J+1, \cdots, J-1, J).$$

Following the usual procedure [11], we expand ψ in terms of the Φ's with time-varying coefficients,

$$\psi = \sum_{M''} a_{M''}(t)\Phi_{M''}\exp\left(-\frac{i}{\hbar}E_{M''}t\right), \tag{2-70}$$

and substitute into Eq. (2-66). Using Eq. (2-69), multiplying by $\Phi_{M'}$, and integrating gives

$$i\hbar\dot{a}_{M'}\exp\left(-\frac{i}{\hbar}E_{M'}t\right) = \sum_{M''} a_{M''}\langle M'|\mathcal{JC}_1|M''\rangle\exp\left(-\frac{i}{\hbar}E_{M''}t\right). \tag{2-71}$$

Let us calculate the amplitude corresponding to the state M' if the system was initially in a stationary state M. Assuming that $\mathcal{JC}_1$ is a perturbation is equivalent to saying that the $a_{M''}$ are never far from their initial values, $a_{M''}(0) = \delta_{M''M}$. Therefore we can write

$$\dot{a}_{M'} = (i\hbar)^{-1}\langle M'|\mathcal{JC}_1|M\rangle\exp(i\omega_{M'M}t), \tag{2-72}$$

where

$$\omega_{M'M} = \frac{1}{\hbar}(E_{M'} - E_M). \tag{2-73}$$

For our problem

$$\mathcal{H}_1 = \gamma\hbar H_1[\exp(i\omega t) + \exp(-i\omega t)]J_x; \tag{2-74}$$

hence we obtain by integrating Eq. (2-72)

$$a_{M'}(t) = -\gamma H_1\langle M'|J_x|M\rangle \left\{\frac{\exp[i(\omega_{M'M}+\omega)t]}{\omega_{M'M}+\omega} + \frac{\exp[i(\omega_{M'M}-\omega)t]}{\omega_{M'M}-\omega}\right\}_0^t. \tag{2-75}$$

Near magnetic resonance the denominator of one of the two terms in the braces of Eq. (2-75) will be small and that term will dominate the expression for $a_{M'}$. Thus we may write (assuming $\omega_{M'M} > 0$)

$$|a_{M'}(t)|^2 = \gamma^2 H_1^2 |\langle M'|J_x|M\rangle|^2 \xi(\omega_{M'M}-\omega, t), \tag{2-76}$$

where ξ is given by

$$\xi(\omega_{M'M}-\omega, t) = 4\frac{\sin^2[(\omega_{M'M}-\omega)t/2]}{(\omega_{M'M}-\omega)^2} \tag{2-77}$$

and is shown in Fig. 2-21.

Equation (2-76) gives the probability that at a time t the system will be in stationary state M' if it originally was in state M. For this rather idealized calculation we have confined our attention to lines with an infinitesimal width. For this we would find at magnetic resonance the probability proportional to t^2. However, all transitions are broadened in some manner. Let us take this to be a distribution of $v_{M'M} = \omega_{M'M}/2\pi$, where the relative density of v values in the range from $v_{M'M}$ to $v_{M'M}+dv_{M'M}$ is given by $g(v_{M'M})dv_{M'M}$, where

$$\int g(v_{M'M})dv_{M'M} = 1. \tag{2-78}$$

We then may write the probability for the transition from stationary state M to M' as $w_{MM'}t$, where

$$w_{MM'} = \frac{1}{t}\gamma^2 H_1^2 \int_0^\infty |\langle M'|J_x|M\rangle|^2 \xi(2\pi v_{M'M}-2\pi v, t)g(v_{M'M})dv_{M'M}. \tag{2-79}$$

The integral can be evaluated simply if t is long enough so that ξ is a sharper function of $v_{M'M}$ than is g, for then $\xi(2\pi v_{M'M}-2\pi v, t)$ may be replaced by $t\delta(v_{M'M}-v)$ and

$$w_{MM'} = \gamma^2 H_1^2 |\langle M'|J_x|M\rangle|^2 g(v). \tag{2-80}$$

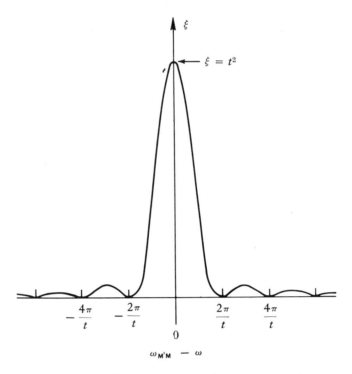

FIG. 2-21 The function $\xi(\omega_{M'M}-\omega, t)$ against $\omega_{M'M}-\omega$ for a particular value of t.

The matrix element can be evaluated using the following equations (see Appendix A):

$$J_x = \tfrac{1}{2}(J_+ + J_-),\tag{2-81}$$

$$\langle M'|J_\pm|M\rangle = \sqrt{J(J+1)-M(M\pm1)}\,\delta_{M'M\pm1},\tag{2-82}$$

so that

$$w_{MM\pm1} = \tfrac{1}{4}\gamma^2 H_1^2[J(J+1)-M(M\pm1)]g(\nu)\tag{2-83}$$

and all others are zero. The transition rate is the same in either sense, as is evident since $w_{MM+1} = w_{M+1M}$. Although the transitions vary in intensity as a function of M, this would not be observable as a variation of the magnetic resonance signal because all of these transitions correspond to $\Delta M = \pm1$ and therefore occur at the same field or frequency,

$$\Delta E = \gamma\hbar H_0|\Delta M| = \gamma\hbar H_0 = h\nu.\tag{2-84}$$

In more complex situations it might be necessary to define a different $g(v)$ for each transition. This refinement is generally unnecessary, however, for the usual experimental techniques and theoretical approximations.

The validity of Eq. (2-83) requires that $t \gg T_2$, which is the requirement that the function ξ be sharper than $g(v)$, where T_2 is given in terms of the width of $g(v)$, $\Delta v \simeq 1/T_2$. In order for the assumption that all the a_M are zero but one to be valid we must also require $t \ll 1/w_{max}$. The utility of Eq. (2-83) if $t > 1/w_{max}$ is discussed by Abragam [12].

2–4 Rate Equations and Saturation

In Section 2–3 we calculated the probability per unit time, w_{ij}, that a paramagnet will make a transition between any two of its stationary states, i and j [see Eq. (2-83)]. For a large number of such paramagnets the total number of transitions occurring in unit time is given by $N_i w_{ij}$, where N_i is the number in state i at the time in question. This is one of the contributions to the change in the populations of the stationary states. In particular it arises from the coupling of the magnetic dipoles to the time-varying field. The magnetic dipoles are also coupled to the lattice degrees of freedom, and population changes due to the resulting relaxation can also occur. If we define W_{ij} as the probability per unit time of a transition from i to j occurring because of the coupling of a paramagnet to the lattice, we find that the total number of transitions directly from i to j is given by $N_i(w_{ij} + W_{ij})$. The rate equations are the differential equations obtained by writing down all contributions to the rate of change of the populations of the states of the system:

$$\frac{dN_i}{dt} = -N_i \sum_j (w_{ij} + W_{ij}) + \sum_j N_j (w_{ji} + W_{ji}). \qquad (2\text{-}85)$$

In addition there is the equation for conservation of the number of magnetic dipoles, $\Sigma_i N_i = N$.

Because of their simplicity and the ease of their interpretation, solutions of the rate equations are useful in describing magnetic resonance. We will illustrate this by discussing the two-level system obtained if $J = \frac{1}{2}$. Figure 2-22 shows the energy levels and the rates.

The rate equations are

$$\frac{dN_1}{dt} = -N_1(w_{12} + W_{12}) + N_2(w_{21} + W_{21}),$$

$$\frac{dN_2}{dt} = N_1(w_{12} + W_{12}) - N_2(w_{21} + W_{21}), \qquad (2\text{-}86)$$

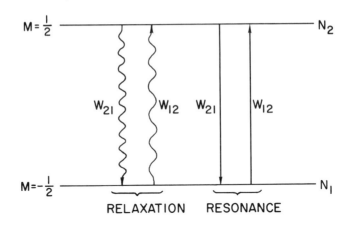

FIG. 2-22   Energy levels, populations, and transition rates for $J = \frac{1}{2}$.

together with

$$N_1 + N_2 = N. \qquad (2\text{-}87)$$

Only one of the rate equations is independent, and it [plus Eq. (2-87)] defines N_1 and N_2. Let us examine the steady-state behavior of such a system, that is, $dN_1/dt = dN_2/dt = 0$. Thus we have

$$\frac{N_2}{N_1} = \frac{w_{12} + W_{12}}{w_{21} + W_{21}}. \qquad (2\text{-}88)$$

The thermal equilibrium values of the populations occur when no radiation field is present, that is, for $w_{12} = w_{21} = 0$. But the ratio N_2/N_1 in thermal equilibrium is

$$\frac{N_2}{N_1} = \exp\left(-\frac{E_2 - E_1}{kT}\right), \qquad (2\text{-}89)$$

as expected from Maxwell-Boltzmann statistics. Thus W_{12} and W_{21} are not independent but are related by

$$\frac{W_{12}}{W_{21}} = \exp\left(-\frac{E_2 - E_1}{kT}\right). \qquad (2\text{-}90)$$

It is perhaps not so surprising to find W_{12} and W_{21} related as to find them unequal. What leads to the different relaxation rate upward and downward? The answer is that the lattice has an energy spectrum and the populations of the lattice states are also governed by the Maxwell-Boltzmann statistics.

In order for a transition to occur from 2 to 1, the lattice must make one or more transitions such as to increase the population of its higher energy states. Then the fact that there is a greater population of lattice states capable of making an upward transition than a downward one will result in Eq. (2-90). In other words, an upward transition for the magnetic dipoles can occur only from a stimulated process but spontaneous processes can occur for downward transitions (spontaneously phonons can only be created). Quantitatively we can write

$$\frac{W_{12}}{W_{21}} = \frac{\overline{n(v)}}{\overline{n(v)}+1} = \frac{B\rho}{A+B\rho}, \tag{2-91}$$

where $\overline{n(v)}$ is the mean phonon number [13], A and B are the Einstein coefficients [14], and ρ is the phonon energy per unit volume and unit frequency interval.

If in contrast we set $W_{12} = W_{21} = 0$, we obtain

$$\frac{N_2}{N_1} = \frac{w_{12}}{w_{21}}, \tag{2-92}$$

and since $w_{12} = w_{21}$ we find the populations equal. The equality of the transition rate in the two senses comes from Eq. (2-83). This may seem questionable in light of our comments in the previous paragraph with regard to coupling to the lattice. In fact w_{12} and w_{21} are not precisely equal. However, in typical microwave fields the effective temperature describing the photon numbers is so large that for all practical purposes the ratio is unity. Equality of populations is not the behavior we obtained in Section 2–1 for the same problem. We found there that M_z, which is proportional to $N_1 - N_2$ in the present calculations, varied sinusoidally with angular frequency γH_1 for magnetic resonance. The failure of the solutions of the rate equations to have time variations at the frequency γH_e is a result of the neglect of coherence in the effects of the time-dependent field and follows from the use of populations alone to specify the system.

For the case of relaxation plus transitions arising from time-varying fields, we may write [see Eq. (2-88)]

$$-N_1(w_{12} + W_{12}) + N_2(w_{21} + W_{21}) = 0. \tag{2-93}$$

If we define the population difference, n, by $n \equiv N_1 - N_2$, we have

$$-W_{12}(\tfrac{1}{2})(N+n) + W_{21}(\tfrac{1}{2})(N-n) - wn = 0,$$

$$n = \frac{1}{1+w/(\tfrac{1}{2})(W_{12}+W_{21})} \frac{W_{21}-W_{12}}{W_{21}+W_{12}} N = \frac{1}{1+w/(\tfrac{1}{2})(W_{12}+W_{21})} n_0, \tag{2-94}$$

where n_0 is the thermal equilibrium value of n, and $w = w_{12} = w_{21}$. Thus we see that for large w the population difference approaches zero and saturation occurs. This is the same behavior as obtained in Eq. (2-55) for M_z.

We can make a connection between the solution of the rate equations and that of the Bloch equations by calculating the power absorbed by the spin system in the two cases. The net power absorbed from the field is

$$P_H = nhvw. \qquad (2\text{-}95)$$

Using Eq. (2-94) for n and Eq. (2-83) with $J = \frac{1}{2}$ for w (a linearly polarized oscillating field of amplitude $2H_1$ is assumed), we obtain

$$w = \tfrac{1}{4}\gamma^2 H_1^2 g(v), \qquad (2\text{-}96)$$

which yields the power absorbed:

$$P_H = \tfrac{1}{4}\gamma^2 H_1^2 hv n_0 g(v) \, \frac{1}{1 + \tfrac{1}{4}\gamma^2 H_1^2 g(v)/(\tfrac{1}{2})(W_{12} + W_{21})}. \qquad (2\text{-}97)$$

Using a rotating field of amplitude H_1 we have previously shown [Eq. (2-65)] that

$$P_H = \omega \chi'' H_1^2. \qquad (2\text{-}98)$$

Rewriting Eq. (2-56) for χ'' in another way, we obtain

$$\chi'' = \frac{\gamma T_2 M_0}{1 + (\gamma H_0 - \omega)^2 T_2^2} \, \frac{1}{1 + \gamma^2 H_1^2 T_1 T_2/[1 + (\gamma H_0 - \omega)^2 T_2^2]}. \qquad (2\text{-}99)$$

Equations (2-98) and (2-99), together with the expression for M_0 in terms of n_0, $M_0 = \frac{1}{2}\gamma\hbar n_0$, allow us to write

$$P_H = \frac{\tfrac{1}{2}\gamma^2 H_1^2 \hbar \omega n_0 T_2}{1 + (\gamma H_0 - \omega)^2 T_2^2} \, \frac{1}{1 + \gamma^2 H_1^2 T_1 T_2/[1 + (\gamma H_0 - \omega)^2 T_2^2]}. \qquad (2\text{-}100)$$

Comparing Eqs. (2-97) and (2-100), we see that they are identical if $g(v)$ has the Lorentzian shape,

$$g(v) = \frac{2T_2}{1 + (\gamma H_0 - 2\pi v)^2 T_2^2}, \qquad (2\text{-}101)$$

and the relationship between T_1, W_{12}, and W_{21} is

$$W_{12} + W_{21} = \frac{1}{T_1}. \qquad (2\text{-}102)$$

However, Eq. (2-65), which appears above as Eq. (2-98), is much more general than the Bloch equations. It depends only on the geometry of $\mathbf{H}_0$

and $\mathbf{H}_1$ and the definition of the complex susceptibility. The specific form shown here assumes a rotating field of amplitude H_1. If we again define T_1 by $T_1(W_{12} + W_{21}) = 1$ and use $n_0 = 2M_0/\gamma\hbar$, we find from Eqs. (2-97) and (2-98)

$$\chi'' = \tfrac{1}{2}\gamma M_0 g(v) \frac{1}{1 + \tfrac{1}{2}\gamma^2 H_1^2 T_1 g(v)}. \tag{2-103}$$

Equation (2-103) equates terms obtained by considering linearly polarized and rotating fields. This is meaningful since only the properly rotating component of the linearly polarized field made contributions to w. Thus Eq. (2-103) is valid if it is remembered that the χ's were defined in terms of a rotating field (more frequently a value half this size is used). It is more general than the Bloch equations in that line shapes other than Lorentzian may be used. The Lorentzian line shape shown in Fig. 2-19 has an appreciable intensity in the "wings" of the line, the region of the curves which are more than one half-width from the peak of the absorption. In contrast to this behavior a Gaussian shape is often employed to describe a system with very little intensity in the "wings". The Gaussian shape is often encountered experimentally when there is a random distribution of resonance frequencies for noninteracting dipoles. The Gaussian shape function is

$$g(v) = \frac{2\sqrt{\pi}}{\delta} \exp\left[\frac{-(\gamma H_0 - 2\pi v)^2}{\delta^2} \right] \tag{2-104}$$

which is also shown in Fig. 2-19. Experimentally most line shapes that are observed are Lorentzian or Gaussian, or seem to be intermediate between the two.

When the term $\tfrac{1}{2}\gamma^2 H_1^2 T_1 g(v)$ is much less than unity, Eq. (2-103) shows that χ'' is independent of H_1. This is the condition leading to the neglect of saturation and, by Eq. (2-94) as modified for Eq. (2-97), to the equality of n and n_0. Under such circumstances the time-varying components of $\mathbf{M}$ are linearly related to $\mathbf{H}_1$. This condition then allows χ' and χ'' to be related by the Kramers-Kronig relations [15]:

$$\chi'(v) = \chi'(\infty) + \frac{2}{\pi} \int_0^\infty \frac{v' \chi''(v')}{v'^2 - v^2} \, dv',$$

$$\chi''(v) = -\frac{2v}{\pi} \int_0^\infty \frac{\chi'(v') - \chi'(\infty)}{v'^2 - v^2} \, dv', \tag{2-105}$$

where the Cauchy principal values are to be used. For our purposes we shall usually be able to take $\chi'(\infty) = 0$. Relations (2-105) hold very generally for complex quantities describing the response of physical systems to harmonic stimuli. They would enable us to calculate $\chi'(v)$ for the χ'' given in Eq. (2-103) except for the effects of saturation.

2–5 Experimental Techniques

It is the purpose of this section to indicate how the complex susceptibilities or rotating magnetizations are observed. The sophisticated microwave spectrometers developed for this purpose have been analyzed in detail in a number of publications; specific references are listed at the end of this section. We will concentrate on explaining the basic principles, using very primitive spectrometers.

Perhaps the simplest experiment conceptually is illustrated in Fig. 2-23, which represents a transmission spectrometer. A klystron generates microwaves that are transmitted down a rectangular waveguide in a TE_{10} mode. The microwave energy falls upon a crystal rectifier, which we suppose to be operating in the square-law region. Thus the crystal current is directly proportional to the microwave power falling on it. A paramagnetic crystal glued to the end of a stick is placed inside the waveguide through a hole in the narrow face, and the external magnetic field is varied through the resonance condition $H_0 = \omega/\gamma$.

An interesting facet of this simple spectrometer (which definitely is not a sensitive one) is that the microwave magnetic field experienced by the

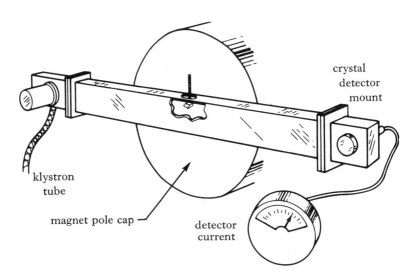

FIG. 2-23 Sketch of an extremely simple transmission spectrometer for detection of electron paramagnetic resonance, with a cutaway view showing a paramagnetic crystal inserted into the waveguide.

crystal can be made nearly a rotating field by proper positioning of the sample and elimination of reflections. To see that the microwave field is a rotating one, we note in Fig. 2-24 the magnetic field pattern for a TE_{10} mode, viewed perpendicular to the broad face of the waveguide. This magnetic field pattern propagates down the waveguide at the guide phase velocity. It is evident that, as the field pattern flows down the waveguide, the magnetic field at the position of the crystal in Fig. 2-24 will rotate in a counterclockwise direction. Such a simple spectrometer is useful to demonstrate, for a given direction of the external H_0 field, the sign of the electronic magnetic moment, as considerably greater absorption occurs in the crystal position for which the H_1 field rotates in the same sense as the Larmor precession about H_0. (There is a small absorption for the opposite sense because reflections build up small-intensity standing waves charactized by an oscillating H_1 with both rotating components present, and because if the crystal is not positioned perfectly H_1 will be elliptically rather than circularly polarized even with no reflections.)

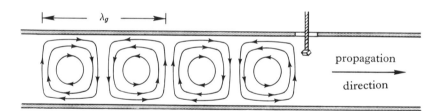

FIG. 2-24　Magnetic field pattern propagating through the waveguide. The paramagnetic crystal shown experiences a rotating magnetic field as the wave passes by. The quantity λ_g is the wavelength in the waveguide.

A plot of crystal current as a function of external field will now result in a curve such as Fig. 2-25, because the detector current is proportional to the power falling on the detector crystal, and at resonance an amount of power, $\omega\chi''H_1^2$, per unit sample volume, is absorbed from the train of microwaves. Because of this absorption from the power that otherwise would fall on the detector, Fig. 2-25 is in effect an inversion of Fig. 2-19 for χ''.

The effects of noise inherent in the crystal detector and in the klystron can be reduced by the technique of field modulation discussed briefly at the end of Section 2-2. If a small magnetic field sinusoidally varying at an audio or radio frequency is superimposed on H_0, we see from Fig. 2-25 that a component of detector current at that frequency will in general exist in the neighborhood of the resonance. In fact, if the modulation amplitude is smaller than the magnetic resonance width, a simple Taylor expansion shows that this component will be proportional to the derivative of χ'' with respect to H_0 or ω_0. By beating this signal with a reference signal at the modulation frequency, a d-c signal will be obtained proportional to $d\chi''(\omega_0)/d\omega_0$. Although the derivative response is sometimes inconvenient to interpret and although occasionally one is required to integrate it to obtain χ'', the technique has one important advantage—it accepts only the noise within a narrow bandwidth near the modulation frequency. By adjusting to very long times of observation, one can make this bandwidth as small as is desired, but in practical cases it is seldom less than 0.1 sec^{-1}. Workers in electron paramagnetic resonance, as in nuclear magnetic resonance, quickly learn to deal directly with the derivative, which is actually more sensitive to slight tendencies toward structure in the curve of χ'' versus frequency than is the χ'' curve itself.

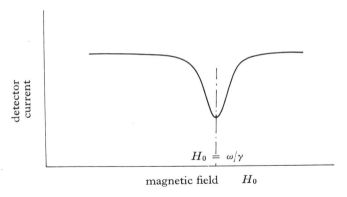

FIG. 2-25 Detector current as a function of H_0, showing the absorption of power at magnetic resonance as the simple spectrometer of Fig. 2-23 would measure it.

Greater sensitivity for small to modest numbers of paramagnets is obtained by using a resonant cavity. The advantage of any such resonant structure is that the standing-wave pattern set up within it leads to very large H_1 field values. In general the signal ultimately observed is increased by a factor Q, which is the quality factor of the cavity:

$$Q = \frac{2\pi \text{ (stored energy)}}{\text{cavity energy losses per cycle}}. \tag{2-106}$$

In typical EPR spectrometers the cavity Q may be anywhere from about 1000 to approximately 20,000. It is clear, however, that a larger sample will also increase the energy absorption. If it should happen that the sample is so large as to determine the cavity Q through the paramagnetic losses rather than through the normal losses in the walls, the cavity response is quite a complicated function of χ. This situation is usually avoided if at all possible. In normal cases the cavity Q will be slightly altered by the paramagnetic losses as the magnetic resonance is traversed. This can be observed either as a change in power transmitted through the cavity or as a change in power reflected from the cavity. Quite often it is desirable to set up a microwave bridge in which the cavity and sample form one arm and the paramagnetic resonance introduces an unbalance, which permits observation of a resonant susceptibility.

To understand how the cavity can indicate the dependence of the susceptibility on H_0, it is perhaps simplest to set up an equivalent lumped-parameter circuit for the cavity. Let the impedance of the cavity be

$$Z = R + i\left(\omega L - \frac{1}{\omega C}\right), \tag{2-107}$$

where R, L, and C are the equivalent resistance, inductance, and capacitance of the cavity. Since not all the volume occupied by the cavity magnetic energy is filled with the sample, we use a filling factor, η, to write

$$L = L_0[(1-\eta) + \eta(1+4\pi\chi)] = L_0(1 + 4\pi\eta\chi), \tag{2-108}$$

where $1 + 4\pi\chi$ is the permeability of the sample, and $0 < \eta < 1$.

Let $\omega_r = 1/(L_0 C)^{1/2}$ be the cavity resonant frequency when the sample is off magnetic resonance. Then

$$Z = R + \frac{iL_0(\omega^2 - \omega_r^2)}{\omega + iL_0\omega 4\pi\eta\chi}, \tag{2-109}$$

and, putting in the complex form for χ, we have the cavity impedance:

$$Z = R + 4\pi\eta\omega L_0\chi'' + i\left(4\pi L_0\omega\eta\chi' + \frac{L_0}{\omega}(\omega^2 - \omega_r^2)\right). \tag{2-110}$$

The Q of such a simple RLC circuit is $\omega L/R$. At circuit resonance $\omega = \omega_r$, we find

$$Z_r = R(1 + 4\pi\eta Q_0\chi'') + i4\pi L_0\omega\eta\chi', \tag{2-111}$$

where $Q_0 = \omega L_0/R$. Since the resistive term fixes the energy dissipation, Eq. (2-111) shows directly the way in which the resonant structure augments by a factor Q the effect of χ''.

But Eq. (2-111) also makes clear another problem, because the reactive term shifts the cavity resonance from ω_r; if χ' varies to sufficiently large values near magnetic resonance, the cavity will be appreciably detuned. There are at least two common ways of avoiding this effect. One is to use the cavity as an element in a microwave bridge so tuned as to be sensitive to resistive unbalance but not to reactive unbalance. Another method is to stabilize the klystron frequency on the cavity. Then the klystron frequency shifts as χ' varies so that the reactive term in Z is always zero. Again, two common experimental procedures are in use for stabilizing on the cavity. The Pound stabilizer [16] is quite effective. Another system, used in some commercial spectrometers, simply introduces a small modulation of the klystron reflector voltage at about 10 kHz. As the klystron drifts off the cavity resonance, there is a reflected signal at the modulation frequency. Precisely on cavity resonance, the reflected signal is zero at that frequency. If the reflected signal is phase-sensitively detected, an error signal is obtained which can be used to retune the klystron to the cavity resonance. This is automatic frequency control (or afc).

It should perhaps be emphasized explicitly that any of the experimental arrangements of the cavity, microwave bridge, and other components can achieve the reduction in detector and/or klystron noise by magnetic field modulation and coherent detection, as discussed earlier in this section. It is clear that, to reproduce faithfully the derivative of χ'', the field modulation should be a small fraction of the magnetic resonance width, ΔH_0, and, if a stabilization system employing klystron frequency modulation is used, the modulation amplitude and frequency must be less than the magnetic resonance width expressed as a frequency, $\Delta v_0 = \gamma \Delta H_0 / 2\pi$. When such conditions are not met, the spectrometer response may still be interpretable in terms of χ, but not without careful analysis.

Our discussion of experimental techniques can be so short primarily because there is available an extensive literature on the subject to which reference can be made. The following are good sources of information about experimental techniques:

1. C. P. Poole, Jr., *Electron Spin Resonance, A Comprehensive Treatise on Experimental Techniques*, Interscience, New York, 1967. As its name implies, this book contains a large amount of information.

2. R. S. Alger, *Electron Paramagnetic Resonance: Techniques and Applications*, Interscience, New York, 1968. On a par with Poole's book.

3. T. L. Squires, *An Introduction to Electron Spin Resonance*, Academic, New York, 1964. A simple introductory discussion of experimental techniques.

4. R. S. Anderson, *Electron Spin Resonance*, Methods of Experimental Physics (D. Williams, ed.), Academic, New York, 1962, Vol. 3, p. 441.

5. T. H. Wilmshurst, *Electron Spin Resonance Spectrometers*, Plenum, New York, 1968.

2–6 Supplemental Bibliography

Two references stand out for the clarity of their treatment of material such as is contained in Sections 2–1 to 2–4:

1. C. P. Slichter, *Principles of Magnetic Resonance, with Examples from Solid State Physics*, Harper and Row, New York, 1963.

2. A. Abragam, *The Principles of Nuclear Magnetism*, Oxford, New York, 1961.

References Cited in Chapter 2

[1] R. H. Dicke and J. P. Wittke, *Introduction to Quantum Mechanics*, Addison-Wesley, Reading, Mass., 1960, p. 125; E. Merzbacher, *Quantum Mechanics*, 2nd ed., Wiley, New York, 1970, p. 337.

[2] H. Goldstein, *Classical Mechanics*, Addison-Wesley, Reading, Mass.,1951, p. 133; C. P. Slichter, *Principles of Magnetic Resonance*, Harper and Row, New York, 1963, p. 11.

[3] H. Goldstein, *Classical Mechanics*, Addison-Wesley, Reading, Mass., 1951, p. 168.

[4] R. H. Dicke and J. P. Wittke, *Introduction to Quantum Mechanics*, Addison-Wesley, Reading, Mass., 1960, p. 203.

[5] F. Bloch, *Phys. Rev.* **70**, 460 (1946); A. Abragam, *The Principles of Nuclear Magnetism*, Oxford, New York, 1961, p. 44; C. P. Slichter, *Principles of Magnetic Resonance*, Harper and Row, New York, 1963, p. 28.

[6] E. Merzbacher, *Quantum Mechanics*, 2nd ed., Wiley, New York, 1970, p. 68.

[7] M. Weger, *Bell System Tech. J.* **39**, 1013 (1960).

[8] See also C. P. Slichter, *Principles of Magnetic Resonance*, Harper and Row, New York, 1963, p. 21; A. Abragam, *The Principles of Nuclear Magnetism*, Oxford, New York, 1961, p. 34.

[9] J. G. Powles, *Proc. Phys. Soc.* **71**, 497 (1958).

[10] A. Abragam, *The Principles of Nuclear Magnetism*, Oxford, New York, 1961, p. 22.

[11] R. H. Dicke and J. P. Wittke, *Introduction to Quantum Mechanics*, Addison-Wesley, Reading, Mass., 1960, p. 237; E. Merzbacher, *Quantum Mechanics*, 2nd ed., Wiley, New York, 1970, p. 450.

[12] A. Abragam, *The Principles of Nuclear Magnetism*, Oxford, New York, 1961, p. 28.

[13] J. S. Blakemore, *Solid State Physics*, Saunders, Philadelphia, 1969, p. 103; R. A. Levy, *Principles of Solid State Physics*, Academic, New York, 1968, p. 135.

[14] D. Bohm, *Quantum Theory*, Prentice-Hall, Englewood Cliffs, N.J., 1951, p. 425.

[15] A. Abragam, *The Principles of Nuclear Magnetism*, Oxford, New York, 1961, p. 93.

[16] C. P. Poole, Jr., *Electron Spin Resonance*, Interscience, New York, 1967, p. 195.

CHAPTER 3

Ligand or Crystal Fields

In Chapters 1 and 2 we saw that the existence of angular momentum implied the simultaneous presence of a magnetic dipole moment. Together they make possible the phenomenon of magnetic resonance. In these early chapters, however, we used only a very simple isotropic paramagnet. In the next three chapters we will discuss noninteracting paramagnetic entities in more detail and will learn their relationship to the electron paramagnetic resonance spectra that they produce. In this way we will see that, although the results of Chapter 2 are sound, they are much simpler in detail than those usually encountered. Our plan is to develop a description (that of crystal-field theory) of the energy levels and wave functions for some typical paramagnetic entities in this chapter. Then in Chapter 4 we will develop the spin Hamiltonian description of the lower energy states of the paramagnet. In Chapter 5 we will relate EPR spectra to the spin Hamiltonian and hence to the paramagnetic entity itself.

3–1 Paramagnets and Transition-Group Ions

As indicated in Section 1–3, free atoms or ions and free molecules may be paramagnetic. For atoms and ions the paramagnetic entities are only slightly more complex than those assumed in Chapter 2, differing primarily by the occasional addition of nuclear interactions producing hyperfine structure. Molecules are more complicated because they lack spherical symmetry, as do paramagnetic entities in crystalline solids. In the next three chapters we will consider primarily the case of fixed crystals, although much of what we learn will be useful for free paramagnets, for liquids, or for other cases in which motion is important. Thus we now consider point imperfections in solids, category 4 of Section 1–3.

These point imperfections represent regions in a crystal where some changes occur in the normal positions and types of atomic constituents. These different or displaced atoms and their neighbors form a molecule-like complex which is located in a crystalline matrix. For our purposes we are interested only in those with magnetic dipole moments. It is hard to generalize about paramagnetic imperfections. Hence, let us specialize to cases in which the magnetic moment occurs because of an incomplete atomic shell. If a prospective incomplete shell consists of *s* or *p* electrons, the electrons are likely to be lost or the shell to be filled in the solid. However, the inner *d* or *f* shells are more impervious to their environment and therefore are much more likely to be incomplete when in crystalline surroundings. For this reason, and others to be mentioned, we shall examine transition-group impurity ions in crystals. Other paramagnetic entities are usually somewhat similar and a little simpler.

The transition-group elements are those elements in the periodic table for which *d* or *f* electron shells are incomplete. They constitute the most common causes of magnetism and represent roughly one half of all of the elements. We are here interested in these elements when acting as dilute impurities in crystals. Since there is some change in the energy of various kinds of orbitals in a crystal, the impurities for which the *d* or *f* shells are incomplete may be slightly different from the atoms. Actually this difference is very small. Table 3-1 lists the five transition groups and some of their properties. At present the most commonly studied transition groups are the iron group, consisting of scandium, titanium, vanadium, chromium, manganese, iron, cobalt, nickel, and copper, and the rare earths.

Table 3-1

The Transition Groups

Transition Group	Iron	Palladium	Platinum	Rare Earth	Actinide
Incomplete shell	3*d*	4*d*	5*d*	4*f*	5*f* (6*d*)
Elements at ends	Sc–Cu	Y–Ag	Lu–Au	La–Yb	Th–No
Atomic numbers at ends	21–29	39–47	71–79	57–70	90–102

To understand transition-group impurities it is necessary to know what happens when these relatively complicated ions are placed in a nonspherical environment. This crystalline environment can be regarded most simply as an additional electrostatic potential acting on the electrons of the ion, a potential lacking spherical symmetry. More accurately we should try to obtain wave functions for the ion and its neighbors in the crystal. Either approach must make considerable use of the point symmetry of the imperfection. For this reason the most efficient and elegant way to handle such problems is to employ group theory. For two reasons, however, we will not use this approach. First, we want the book to be accessible to readers whose knowledge of group theory is not adequate for the group theoretical approach. Second, since our interest is primarily in laying the foundations and not in constructing the elaborate edifice, we do not usually need group theory and in fact should probably avoid it so as not to miss the pertinent physical features.

3-2 Free Atoms and Ions

The first step we must take is to obtain an understanding of the free transition-group ion. Then we will attempt to blend the crystalline effects into our description. The free-ion description which we will use will not be exact, although it can be refined in obvious ways. It will have the advantage of providing a simple approach for limiting cases. Only nonrelativistic quantum mechanics together with the largest effects of electronic spin will be employed.

The most important potential energy terms in the Hamiltonian for a free atom or ion arise from Coulomb interactions. The largest non-electrostatic term is the spin-orbit interaction arising from the Zeeman interaction of the electron spin with the magnetic field produced by the motion of the nuclear charge relative to the electron. This is the largest magnetic term and the only one which we will consider at present. The resultant Hamiltonian is

$$\mathcal{H} = -\sum_i \frac{\hbar^2}{2m} \nabla_i^2 - \sum_i \frac{Ze^2}{r_i} + \sum_{i>j} \frac{e^2}{r_{ij}} \sum_i \xi(r_i) \mathbf{l}_i \cdot \mathbf{s}_i. \tag{3-1}$$

The dominant contribution to this Hamiltonian is obtained from the first three terms: the kinetic energy (the first term) and an effective spherical potential consisting of the nuclear attraction (the second term) plus an average screening by the electron-electron interactions (a spherically symmetric average of the third term). This leads to the solution of a Hamiltonian consisting of a sum of identical or nearly identical spherically symmetric Hamiltonians for each electron. Thus the angular momentum, l_i, of each electron is a good quantum number, as is the principal quantum number, n_i, and the magnetic quantum number, m_i. The individual electron eigenfunctions are called orbitals. By the Pauli principle, only two electrons with opposite spins can occupy each orbital. In this way we arrive at the configuration which specifies the total energy and the states of all of the electrons. The energy is the sum of the individual electron energies, and the ion wave functions are Slater determinants. There generally are a great many states of the ion with the same energy in this approximation, all of which correspond to the same configuration.

The configuration with the lowest energy is usually separated from the next higher energy configuration by about 10,000 cm^{-1} or more. The magnitude of the separation and the answer as to which configuration is lowest depend on whether the ion is free or is in a crystal. The states in which we will have the greatest interest arise from the splitting of this lowest configuration as a result of the remaining terms in the Hamiltonian. We will always make the approximation that this splitting is small relative to the spacing between the lowest two configurations.

We now have two simple choices. One is to assume that the difference between the electron-electron interaction and its spherical average will produce bigger splittings than the spin-orbit interaction, and the other is to assume the opposite. The spin-orbit interaction is small for light nuclei because of the smaller nuclear charge. Thus for light elements the electron-electron interaction is considered next. This is called Russell-Saunders or L-S coupling. For heavy nuclei the reverse is often a good approximation; it is called j-j coupling. Russell-Saunders coupling is a reasonably good approximation for most of the paramagnetic entities of interest to us.

The electron-electron interaction will cause nonvanishing matrix elements between states for which the orbitals of two electrons differ. This means that the orbital angular momenta for the individual electrons are no longer good quantum numbers. However, no spin-dependent operators have yet been employed, so the orbital angular momentum, $\mathbf{L} = \Sigma_i \mathbf{l}_i$, is not coupled to the spin and hence has eigenvalues, L, which are good quantum numbers. For the same reason that individual orbitals can no longer be defined, individual spin functions no longer exist, but the total spin, S, is a good quantum number (along with M_L and M_S).

The result of these considerations is that all of the terms (a term is a group of states specified by L and S) from the lowest configuration will in general have different energies because the electrons interact to different extents, depending on L and S. The lowest energy terms will be those for which the electrons stay farthest from each other. This will occur for a spatial wave function which has the greatest tendency to change sign on the pairwise interchange of electrons (such a wave function must have a vanishingly small probability of having the electrons arbitrarily close to each other). Since the Pauli principle requires the full wave function, spatial times spin, to be odd under particle interchange, we would expect the lower energy terms to be those with the higher spin (the higher the spin, the more even character the spin wave function has under pairwise electron interchange). This is a slight generalization of the first of Hund's rules.

The second of Hund's rules specifies that the maximum L consistent with the maximum of S will characterize the lowest term. Figures 3-1 and 3-2 show the behavior of the lower energy levels for an atom or ion with two d electrons in addition to closed shells (such as Ti^{2+} or V^{3+}). On the left side of Fig. 3-1 we show the 45-fold degenerate lowest configuration (we take the $3d$ electrons to be lower in energy than the $4s$ electrons since this is the situation found for iron-group ions in solids), breaking up into the five terms allowed by coupling of angular momenta and the Pauli principle. The wave functions for the terms can be obtained by using angular momentum raising or lowering operators (see Appendix A) and orthogonalization to go from the wave functions with the extreme values

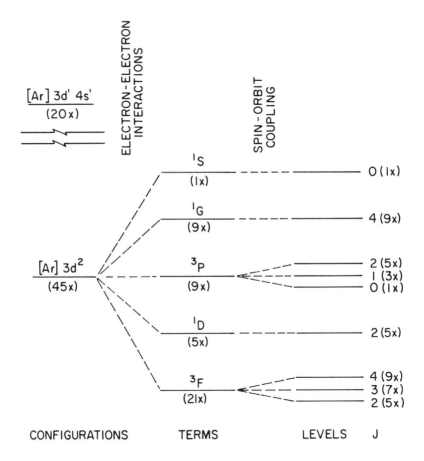

FIG. 3-1 A schematic energy level diagram for the lowest states of an ion with two $3d$ electrons beyond the closed-shell argon core to various degrees of accuracy. On the left we show the two lowest levels for the orbital approximation. The lowest configuration is taken to be $[Ar]3d^2$ since in crystals the $3d$ level is lower than the $4s$. The symbol $[Ar]$ stands for $1s^2 2s^2 2p^6 3s^2 3p^6$, the argon ground configuration. The 45-fold degenerate ground configuration breaks up into five terms as a result of the electron-electron Coulomb interactions. Employing L-S coupling, the spin-orbit interaction splits the terms into energy levels characterized by J and shown on the right.

of M_L and M_S to the remainder. Use of the Clebsch-Gordon or vector addition coefficients will produce the same result.

The spacing of the terms in Fig. 3-1 was chosen for convenience only. The actual behavior, assuming the electron-electron interactions to be a perturbation to the central-field problem, is shown in Fig. 3-2. Here the Racah parameters, B and C, are sufficient to specify the full range of possibilities [1]. The ratio B/C is usually about $1/4$ for iron-group ions.

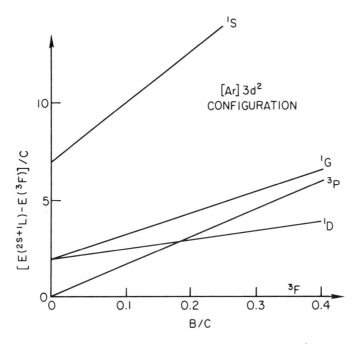

FIG. 3-2   The energies of the terms resulting from the [Ar]$3d^2$ configuration, plotted as a function of the ratio of the Racah parameters, B and C. Only these two parameters are required to describe the effect of electrostatic interactions among the electrons. A typical value for B/C is $\frac{1}{4}$ for iron-transition-group ions.

The final step is to include the spin-orbit interaction as a perturbation to all that has preceded. Since L and S are good quantum numbers for a term, and since only matrix elements between wave functions for a single term are needed in the lowest-order perturbation approach, the operator $\sum_i \xi(r_i)\mathbf{l}_i \cdot \mathbf{s}_i$ can be replaced by $\lambda \mathbf{L} \cdot \mathbf{S}$. The levels created by the splitting of a term by $\lambda \mathbf{L} \cdot \mathbf{S}$ are characterized by their total angular momentum, J. This is shown on the right of Fig. 3-1 for the [Ar] $3d^2$

configuration. (By the symbol [Ar] $3d^2$ we mean the closed-shell configuration of argon plus two $3d$ electrons.)

For the case of *j-j* coupling the spin-orbit interaction is considered
before the electron-electron interaction. Since $\Sigma_i \xi(r_i) \mathbf{l}_i \cdot \mathbf{s}_i$ is the sum of
one-electron operators, we still have good quantum numbers for individual
electrons. However, l_i and s_i are no longer good quantum numbers,
although j_i still is. The addition of electron-electron interactions then

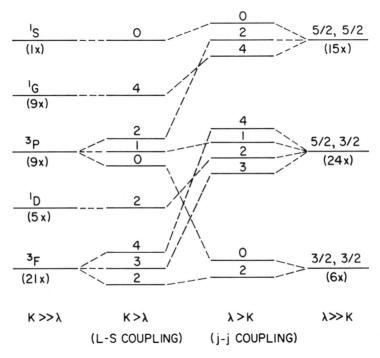

FIG. 3-3   A schematic energy level diagram for an ion with a [Ar]$3d^2$ configuration. On the left is shown the extreme *L-S* coupling limit, and on the right
is the extreme *j-j* coupling limit. The two intermediate cases have the levels
labeled by their *J* values. The levels on the right are labeled by the two *j* values
of the two electrons. The symbol λ is the spin-orbit coupling constant, and *K*
is characteristic of the strength of the electron-electron interactions (*K* is of the
order of the splitting between terms).

couples the $\{\mathbf{j}_i\}$, resulting in *J* (and M_J) being the only valid quantum
numbers. The relationship to the Russell-Saunders limit is shown in the
schematic energy level diagram of Fig. 3-3, in which we have introduced *K*

and λ as quantities characterizing the strength of the electron-electron interaction and the spin-orbit interaction, respectively.

These two limiting cases, L-S and j-j coupling, can be understood with relative ease. The energies can be calculated using the lowest order of perturbation theory, and the wave functions by considerations of the coupling of angular momenta. A very similar approach will be adopted in the next section, where the increased complexity will make the examination of simple limiting cases the only practical approach for us.

3-3 The Crystal-Field Description of Transition-Group Ions in Crystals

The simplest reasonable description that we can offer for an ion in a crystal is to say that the crystal produces an electric field at the site of the ion. Since this field originates from the charged particles making up the crystal, it must have the same point symmetry as the ion site (making allowance for distortions by the presence of the ion). This crystal field will introduce an additional term into our atomic Hamiltonian If the parameter characterizing the strength of the crystal-field interaction is Δ, the results will depend on the relationship of Δ, λ, and K. Six limiting cases are now possible, depending on the relative order of these three parameters (see Section 3-5).

There is sometimes more than one parameter describing the crystal-field splitting, just as there are actually two parameters describing the electron-electron interaction for an $[Ar]\, 3d^n$ ion. If the symmetry is cubic, only one parameter appears for the crystal field. Others occur for lower symmetries, and these are frequently smaller than the parameter which corresponds to the single cubic one. For reasons of simplicity and to choose the dominant effect, we will work primarily with cubic symmetry.

In this and the next section we will explore the behavior of a single electron (or a single electron plus a closed-shell ion core) in a cubic crystal. In this section we will use the crystal-field approach. In Section 3-4 we will discuss briefly a more accurate description in which the electrons occupy molecular orbitals extending over the ion and its nearer neighbors. The term ligand-field theory has been applied to a theory with characteristics from crystal-field theory and molecular orbital theory.

Consider an electron in a central potential to which we will add a perturbing crystal field. For the present we neglect the spin-orbit interaction. If the electron is in an s orbital, there is no degeneracy which can be removed by the crystal field. However, the threefold degeneracy of a p orbital can be lifted by the crystal field. The free-ion term for a single p electron outside of closed shells is ^2P (under the influence of spin-orbit interaction this splits into the $^2P_{1/2}$ and $^2P_{3/2}$ levels). The angular part of the electron orbitals are the spherical harmonics, $|l, m\rangle$, which for the p orbitals are as follows:

$$|1, 1\rangle = -\tfrac{1}{2}\sqrt{3/2\pi}\, e^{i\phi} \sin\theta = -\tfrac{1}{2}\sqrt{3/2\pi}\, (\sin\theta\cos\phi + i\sin\theta\sin\phi)$$

$$= -\tfrac{1}{2}\sqrt{3/2\pi}\, \frac{x+iy}{r},$$

$$|1, 0\rangle = \sqrt{3/4\pi}\cos\theta = \sqrt{3/4\pi}\,\frac{z}{r}, \qquad\qquad (3\text{-}2)$$

$$|1, -1\rangle = \tfrac{1}{2}\sqrt{3/2\pi}\, e^{-i\phi}\sin\theta = \tfrac{1}{2}\sqrt{3/2\pi}\, (\sin\theta\cos\phi - i\sin\theta\sin\phi)$$

$$= \tfrac{1}{2}\sqrt{3/2\pi}\,\frac{x-iy}{r},$$

where the phases are chosen as in Condon and Shortley [2]. Inclusion of the $e^{-i\omega t}$ time dependence shows that $|1, 1\rangle$ and $|1, -1\rangle$ are rotating waves in the positive and negative sense about the z axis. To understand the interaction with an electrostatic field when spin-orbit coupling is negligible it is better to replace the rotating waves by standing waves, thereby obtaining real wave functions instead of imaginary ones. A convenient choice is

$$|1, x\rangle = -\frac{1}{\sqrt{2}}|1, 1\rangle + \frac{1}{\sqrt{2}}|1, -1\rangle = \sqrt{3/4\pi}\,\frac{x}{r},$$

$$|1, y\rangle = \frac{i}{\sqrt{2}}|1, 1\rangle + \frac{i}{\sqrt{2}}|1, -1\rangle = \sqrt{3/4\pi}\,\frac{y}{r}, \qquad (3\text{-}3)$$

$$|1, z\rangle = |1, 0\rangle = \sqrt{3/4\pi}\,\frac{z}{r}.$$

These will frequently be characterized by x, y, and z, respectively, since the latter are the factors having the angular dependence. It is useful to show these functions diagramatically. We will do this by plotting along r the absolute value of the amplitude of the angular wave function against θ and ϕ. Thus for $|1, z\rangle$ we have the diagram of Fig. 3-4, where the phase of the angular wave function is indicated for the two lobes. Since this function has axial symmetry about the z axis, is it not necessary to show the dependence in any other plane. If the associated radial wave function is combined with $|1, z\rangle$ to give the total orbital wave function, the electron probability density is seen to be greatest along $\pm z$ and contours of constant electron probability density also look somewhat like Fig. 3-4. As a result we can make relative arguments about the influence of the crystal field on p orbitals.

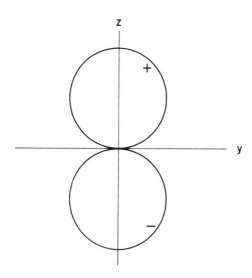

FIG. 3-4 The $|1, z\rangle$ or p_z function plotted in the yz plane. This and all similar functions depend on the spherical polar angles, θ and ϕ. Hence we plot the value of the function along the radius vector versus θ and ϕ. The p functions are axially symmetric, and the sign of the function is indicated for each lobe. The contours of constant electron probability also resemble this plot.

Consider the crystal field produced by two point negative charges, one placed on the positive z axis and the other the same distance from the ion on the negative z axis. An electron occupying a $|1, z\rangle$ function will have its greatest density closer to the negative charges than will an electron in either $|1, x\rangle$ or $|1, y\rangle$. Thus the energy of the $|1, z\rangle$ state will be highest, and the energies for $|1, x\rangle$ and $|1, y\rangle$ are identical. Showing only the splitting, but no shift, we have the results of Fig. 3-5 If in fact negative charges existed along all three axes, x, y, and z, and their negatives, but with unequal spacings, we would find in general that the x, y, and z states all had different energies.

We have already mentioned two competing effects for a one-electron system, the crystal-field and the spin-orbit interaction. Schematically the relationship is shown in Fig. 3-6. The splitting due to the crystal field we will call Δ, and that resulting from the spin-orbit interaction is $\frac{3}{2}\lambda$. Thus the relationship of λ and Δ determines what limiting case, if any, is

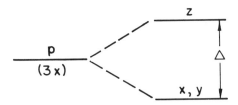

FIG. 3-5 Splitting of the threefold degenerate p orbitals by two negative charges on the positive and the negative z axis. Since an electron in a $|1, z\rangle$ orbital will approach the negative charges more, its energy will be raised. The $|1, x\rangle$ and $|1, y\rangle$ functions are equivalent and are farther from the charges on the average.

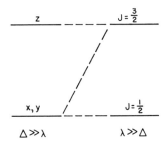

FIG. 3-6 The energy levels for a single p electron resulting from the axial crystal field assumed for Fig. 3-5 and the spin-orbit interaction. Although only two levels exist in the two limits shown, for intermediate cases there are three levels. The quantities λ and Δ are the spin-orbit coupling parameter and the crystal-field splitting, respectively.

reasonable. For a system with more than one electron in unfilled shells (but not just one hole) we must include at least one more parameter, K, defining the splitting due to the Coulomb interaction of the electrons. Also, for our approach (considering the effect of the crystal field on the one-electron orbitals) to be valid we must require that $\lambda \ll \Delta$.

The electrons of most interest for the understanding of transition-group paramagnetism with crystal-field effects dominating spin-orbit effects are the d electrons. Let us carry through arguments similar to those we just gave for a single p electron for the case of a single d electron. The free-ion term is ^2D, and the five degenerate orbitals can be written in terms of spherical harmonics as follows:

$$|2, 2\rangle = \tfrac{1}{4}\sqrt{15/2\pi} \ e^{i2\phi} \sin^2 \theta = \tfrac{1}{4}\sqrt{15/2\pi} \ \frac{(x+iy)^2}{r^2}$$

$$= \tfrac{1}{4}\sqrt{15/2\pi} \ [(x^2 - y^2) + i2xy] \frac{1}{r^2},$$

$$|2, 1\rangle = -\tfrac{1}{2}\sqrt{15/2\pi} \ e^{i\phi} \sin \theta \cos \theta = -\tfrac{1}{2}\sqrt{15/2\pi} \ \frac{z(x+iy)}{r^2}$$

$$= -\tfrac{1}{2}\sqrt{15/2\pi} \ (zx + izy) \frac{1}{r^2},$$

$$|2, 0\rangle = \tfrac{1}{2}\sqrt{5/4\pi} \ (3 \cos^2 \theta - 1) = \tfrac{1}{4}\sqrt{5/\pi} \ \frac{3z^2 - r^2}{r^2}, \qquad (3\text{-}4)$$

$$|2, -1\rangle = \tfrac{1}{2}\sqrt{15/2\pi} \ e^{-i\phi} \sin \theta \cos \theta = \tfrac{1}{2}\sqrt{15/2\pi} \ \frac{z(x-iy)}{r^2}$$

$$= \tfrac{1}{2}\sqrt{15/2\pi} \ (zx - iyz) \frac{1}{r^2},$$

$$|2, -2\rangle = \tfrac{1}{4}\sqrt{15/2\pi} \ e^{-i2\phi} \sin^2 \theta = \tfrac{1}{4}\sqrt{15/2\pi} \ \frac{(x-iy)^2}{r^2}$$

$$= \tfrac{1}{4}\sqrt{15/2\pi} \ [(x^2 - y^2) - i2xy] \frac{1}{r^2}.$$

Replacing the rotating waves appropriate in spherical symmetry with the standing waves which are usually more convenient in crystals, we obtain:

$$|2, xy\rangle = -\frac{i}{\sqrt{2}} |2, 2\rangle + \frac{i}{\sqrt{2}} |2, -2\rangle = \tfrac{1}{2}\sqrt{15/\pi} \ \frac{xy}{r^2},$$

$$|2, yz\rangle = \frac{i}{\sqrt{2}} |2, 1\rangle + \frac{i}{\sqrt{2}} |2, -1\rangle = \tfrac{1}{2}\sqrt{15/\pi} \ \frac{yz}{r^2},$$

$$|2, zx\rangle = -\frac{1}{\sqrt{2}} |2, 1\rangle + \frac{1}{\sqrt{2}} |2, -1\rangle = \tfrac{1}{2}\sqrt{15/\pi} \ \frac{zx}{r^2}, \qquad (3\text{-}5)$$

$$|2, x^2 - y^2\rangle = \frac{1}{\sqrt{2}} |2, 2\rangle + \frac{1}{\sqrt{2}} |2, -2\rangle = \tfrac{1}{4}\sqrt{15/\pi} \ \frac{x^2 - y^2}{r^2},$$

$$|2, 3z^2 - r^2\rangle = |2, 0\rangle = \tfrac{1}{4}\sqrt{5/\pi} \ \frac{3z^2 - r^2}{r^2}.$$

The five functions are seen to be proportional to xy, yz, zx, $x^2 - y^2$, and $3z^2 - r^2$, and these polynomials are frequently employed to characterize the functions since they have the same angular dependence. We should bear in mind that, if the same factor is removed from each, the last two should actually be $\frac{1}{2}(x^2 - y^2)$ and $(1/2\sqrt{3})(3z^2 - r^2)$.

As we did for p orbitals in Fig, 3-4, we may also express the angular properties of d orbitals by diagrams. The properties for $|2, xy\rangle$, $|2, x^2 - y^2\rangle$, and $|2, 3z^2 - r^2\rangle$ are shown in Fig. 3-7. The other two can be obtained from $|2, xy\rangle$ by cyclic permutation of the x, y, and z axes. The cross section for $|2, xy\rangle$ at 45° to the x and y axes is the same as shown for the zy plane for $|2, x^2 - y^2\rangle$. Note that all except $|2, 3z^2 - r^2\rangle$ have the same maximum value. The function $|2, 3z^2 - r^2\rangle$ has axial symmetry. Even the individual lobes of the other functions lack axial symmetry.

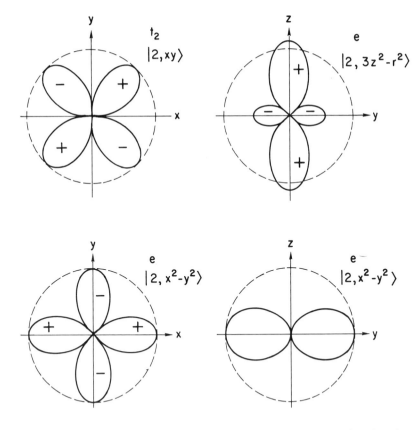

FIG. 3-7   Plots of the angular properties of d orbitals. The yz and zx functions are analogous to the xy function. Only the $3z^2 - r^2$ function is axial; the others have lobes with cross sections like the $x^2 - y^2$ function.

Our choice of these particular standing waves is most appropriate for cubic symmetry, and we will confine our attention to this high symmetry temporarily. In cubic symmetry a cyclic permutation of the cubic axes (taken to be x, y, and z) will leave the system invariant. We see that the functions $|2, xy\rangle$, $|2, yz\rangle$, and $|2, zx\rangle$ are therefore equivalent because they transform into each other as a result of such cyclic permutations. We will label these three orbitals as t_2 orbitals. (Actually they are t orbitals in T symmetry, t_g orbitals in T_h symmetry, t_2 orbitals in O and T_d symmetry, and t_{2g} orbitals in O_h symmetry. The symbol γ_5 or $d\varepsilon$ is sometimes used.)

It is equally obvious that the three functions $x^2 - y^2$, $y^2 - z^2$, and $z^2 - x^2$ are equivalent. As is evident from the fact that their sum is zero, the three functions are not linearly independent (a quick calculation shows that they are not orthogonal, an equivalent result). However, one can make two orthogonal functions which, if they have the same normalization, can be taken as

$$x^2 - y^2,$$

$$\frac{1}{\sqrt{3}}[(z^2 - x^2) - (y^2 - z^2)] = \frac{1}{\sqrt{3}}(3z^2 - r^2). \tag{3-6}$$

Thus we find that $|2, x^2 - y^2\rangle$ and $|2, 3z^2 - r^2\rangle$ are always degenerate in cubic symmetry, and they will be labeled e orbitals (again e in T, O, and T_d symmetry and e_g in T_h and O_h; in this case γ_3 or $d\gamma$ is used by some authors).

It is now an easy matter to decide what would happen to the d-orbital energy level in cubic crystal fields. Two levels, t_2 and e, result, and we must determine their order. We assume first that the transition-group ion is surrounded by six negative point charges, each placed equidistant from the ion along the positive and negative cubic axes. This is octahedral symmetry, O_h, with the ion being six coordinated (the same symmetry as the Na or Cl sites in a NaCl crystal). In this case the relative energies of the t_2 and e orbitals can be seen by examining Fig. 3-7. The orbitals involving $|2, x^2 - y^2\rangle$ and $|2, 3z^2 - r^2\rangle$ have large electron densities in the direction of the negative ions. In contrast, $|2, xy\rangle$, $|2, yz\rangle$, and $|2, zx\rangle$ have their maxima along directions midway between the directions to two of the negative charges. In this way we conclude that the e orbitals are higher in energy than the t_2 orbitals. Thus the splitting of the energy levels is as shown in Fig. 3-8(a), where the magnitude of the splitting is called Δ (or $10Dq$ by some authors).

In contrast, if we consider eight-coordinated cubic symmetry with point negative charges at the corners of the cube and the paramagnetic ion at the body center of the cube (as for the Ca site in CaF_2), we conclude that the e orbitals efficiently avoided the negative charges but the t_2 orbitals were less diligent. Thus the energy level diagram is as shown in Fig. 3-8(b).

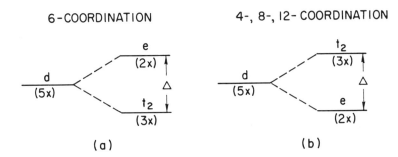

FIG. 3-8 The splitting of the d orbitals in cubic symmetry. In (a) the cubic field has the sense expected for six negative charges along the cubic axes. In (b) the sense is reversed, as expected, for four negative charges on the corners of a tetrahedron centered on the ion. The same sense results from eight negative charges on the corners of a cube or twelve negative charges in the center of the edges of a cube when the cube is centered on the ion.

The same ordering occurs also for four-coordinated cubic symmetry (as for the Zn site in the zinc blende structure of ZnS), since two interpenetrating tetrahedra with charges on the vertices create eight-coordination, and for twelve-coordinated cubic symmetry, since the charges then lie along $\langle 110 \rangle$ directions, as do the lobes of the t_2 orbitals.

Although we will concentrate on incomplete-d-shell ions in cubic symmetry, for which there is only one crystal-field parameter, Δ, let us briefly discuss the effects of lower symmetry. Consider as an example the case of six-coordination but with an additional crystal field of tetragonal symmetry. We can view such a field as a compression or extension of the two negative charges on the z axis. If it is a compression, then $|2, 3z^2 - r^2\rangle$ will be raised in energy relative to $|2, x^2 - y^2\rangle$. Also $|2, yz\rangle$ and $|2, zx\rangle$ will be higher than $|2, xy\rangle$. The energy level diagram is roughly as shown in Fig. 3-9, where the two limits of pure cubic and pure axial symmetry are shown. Actually the tetragonal field requires two parameters to describe its effect within an incomplete d-shell configuration (in addition to the cubic parameter). For the majority of transition-group impurities in tetragonal symmetry in crystals, the tetragonal fields are weak. In fact the tetragonal field frequently does not exceed the spin-orbit interaction even when the cubic field does. Somewhat similar results apply to other symmetries lower than cubic.

Before we return to cubic symmetry and treat the problem of a single d electron in a more plausible manner, some remarks about the perturbing potentials used previously will be helpful. We have considered primarily the sources of the potential and not the potential itself. If the potential

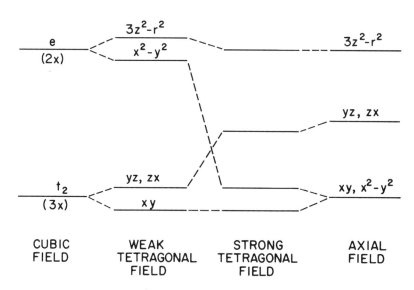

FIG. 3-9　The *d*-orbital energy level diagram for various combinations of a cubic and a tetragonal crystal field.

is calculated [3] in the region of the *d* electron, which is inside the region of the negative charges, then *V* can be expanded as a series of spherical harmonics. By virtue of the characteristics of coupled angular momenta and the Wigner-Eckart theorem, it turns out that very few terms in the expansion are needed and symmetry eliminates many of these. Thus for cubic symmetry and *d* electrons we have just one term,

$$V \propto Y_4^0(\theta, \phi) + \sqrt{5/14} \, [Y_4^4(\theta, \phi) + Y_4^{-4}(\theta, \phi)], \qquad (3\text{-}7)$$

and for tetragonal symmetry we introduce $Y_2^0(\theta, \phi)$ and $Y_4^0(\theta, \phi)$ in addition (recall that two parameters were needed to specify a tetragonal field). Actual computations using crystal-field theory make frequent use of this approach [4].

3–4 The Molecular Orbital Treatment of Transition-Group Ions

The atoms and ions of the crystal, particularly those near the transition-group ion, provide additional force centers which influence the electronic states of the free transition-group ion. The result is that the electrons occupy molecular orbitals, not atomic ones [5]. The molecular orbitals are spread over a molecular complex consisting of the impurity, its nearest neighbors (ligands), and possibly other close neighbors. If the atoms do not overlap each other very greatly, we may argue that near any atom the wave function of an electron will appear atomic. Thus to a reasonable approximation we may write the molecular orbital as a linear combination of atomic orbitals (LCAO) centered on the various atoms making up the complex. This description may seem to be quite different from crystal-field theory. Nevertheless the two approaches are equivalent in many respects [6].

Let us examine first the problem of a p electron on an ion midway between two other ions. This was the case we first examined in crystal-field theory, where we took the end ions to be negatively charged, thus implying that they were highly electronegative and nonmetallic. We now assume that only one s orbital on the two atoms and the p orbitals on the central ion are important. The geometry of the atoms and the angular dependences of the wave functions are shown in Fig. 3-10. We are assuming that our molecular orbitals are of the form

$$\psi = a\psi_{s_1} + b\psi_{s_2} + \sum_i c_i\psi_{p_i} \qquad (i = x, y, z). \qquad (3\text{-}8)$$

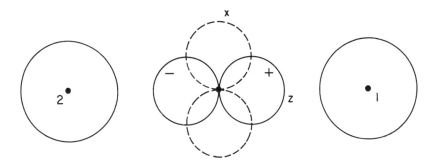

FIG. 3-10   The geometry used to discuss the molecular orbital treatment of the splitting of p orbitals arising from two negative ions along the positive and the negative z axis. Note that the p_z function can mix with the two s orbitals, but the nodal plane of p_x or p_y prevents any such mixing.

We wish to solve the eigenvalue problem in which the matrices of the Hamiltonian are calculated using ψ_{s_1}, ψ_{s_2}, and $\{\psi_{p_i}\}$ as a basis. The Hamiltonian we choose to obtain molecular orbitals is the analog of the central potential in the atomic case. This Hamiltonian excludes the electron-electron interaction, except as an effective potential, and the spin-orbit interaction. The resultant one-electron Hamiltonian has axial symmetry. This means that it can have matrix elements only if the product of the two basis functions is also axial. In this way all matrix elements among s_1, s_2, and p_z may exist, but the nodal plane of p_x and p_y causes them to have no matrix elements with each other or any of the other functions. Similarly the linear combination $\psi_{s_1} - \psi_{s_2}$ has the same alternation of sign when crossing a plane perpendicular to the axis through the central ion as does ψ_{p_z}. Thus the product $(\psi_{s_1} - \psi_{s_2})\psi_{p_z}$ is always positive and will give matrix elements in general, whereas there will be no matrix elements between $\psi_{s_1} + \psi_{s_2}$ and ψ_{p_z}. With just one off-diagonal matrix element between our basis functions, we need only solve a 2×2 eigenvalue problem. Neglecting both the overlap of ψ_{s_1} and ψ_{s_2} and the matrix element of $\mathcal{H}$ between them, we have

$$\begin{vmatrix} \mathcal{H}_{11} - E & \sqrt{2}\,\mathcal{H}_{1z} - \sqrt{2}\,SE \\ \sqrt{2}\,\mathcal{H}_{1z} - \sqrt{2}\,SE & \mathcal{H}_{zz} - E \end{vmatrix} = 0, \tag{3-9}$$

where

$$\psi = \frac{a}{\sqrt{2}}(\psi_{s_1} - \psi_{s_2}) + c\psi_{p_z}, \tag{3-10}$$

and

$$\begin{aligned} \mathcal{H}_{11} &\equiv \langle \psi_{s_1} | \mathcal{H} | \psi_{s_1} \rangle = \langle \psi_{s_2} | \mathcal{H} | \psi_{s_2} \rangle, \\ \mathcal{H}_{1z} &\equiv \langle \psi_{s_1} | \mathcal{H} | \psi_{p_z} \rangle = -\langle \psi_{s_2} | \mathcal{H} | \psi_{p_z} \rangle, \\ \mathcal{H}_{zz} &\equiv \langle \psi_{p_z} | \mathcal{H} | \psi_{p_z} \rangle, \\ S &\equiv \langle \psi_{s_1} | \psi_{p_z} \rangle = -\langle \psi_{s_2} | \psi_{p_z} \rangle. \end{aligned} \tag{3-11}$$

If we also neglect S (a less obvious assumption but one which leaves the main features of the argument intact), we obtain the solution

$$E = \tfrac{1}{2}(\mathcal{H}_{zz} + \mathcal{H}_{11}) \pm \tfrac{1}{2}[(\mathcal{H}_{zz} - \mathcal{H}_{11})^2 + 8\mathcal{H}_{1z}^2]^{1/2} \tag{3-12}$$

and the corresponding ratio for the composition of the wave function:

$$\frac{c}{a} = -\frac{\mathcal{H}_{11} - E}{\sqrt{2}\,\mathcal{H}_{1z}}. \tag{3-13}$$

To be consistent with real situations and our assumptions in the crystal field analysis, we take $\mathcal{H}_{zz} > \mathcal{H}_{11}$. Actually $\mathcal{H}_{zz}$ is approximately the central ion p-orbital energy when free, and $\mathcal{H}_{11}$ is nearly the s-electron energy for the outer ions. Equation (3-12) indicates that the molecular orbital energy levels are somewhat more than half the atomic energy difference above and below the average atomic energy. Thus we have the results shown in Fig. 3-11. For $|\mathcal{H}_{1z}|$ small compared to the atomic energy difference, $|c/a| \gg 1$ and c/a is negative. Thus the wave function is primarily ψ_{p_z} with nodes between its lobes and the two s functions. This is the antibonding orbital; the lower, primarily s function is the bonding orbital. The p_x and p_y orbitals have nearly the same energy as in the free ion. Hence the antibonding character of p_z causes it to have a higher energy (and to have an admixture of neighboring s orbitals) than the p_x and p_y orbitals, the result previously obtained using crystal-field concepts and shown in Fig. 3-5.

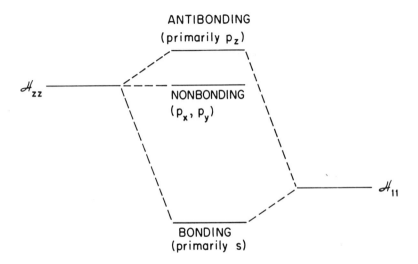

FIG. 3-11   The splitting of the p orbitals from the molecular orbital point of view. Note that the p_z orbital is raised above the p_x and p_y orbitals because it is an antibonding orbital.

The molecular orbital method can be applied to an ion with an incomplete d shell surrounded by six atoms along the cubic axes as in Fig. 3-12. If only bonding with tightly held s electrons on the six neighbors is considered, the two e orbitals will form bonding and antibonding orbitals with the s orbitals (see Fig. 3-13). By contrast the nodal planes of the t_2 orbitals prevent bonding, and only nonbonding orbitals result (Fig. 3-13). The electrons "from the neighbor" fill the bonding orbitals, and the nonbonding t_2 and higher antibonding e orbitals are available to accomodate the d electrons. Thus the two levels are as shown in Fig. 3-8(a).

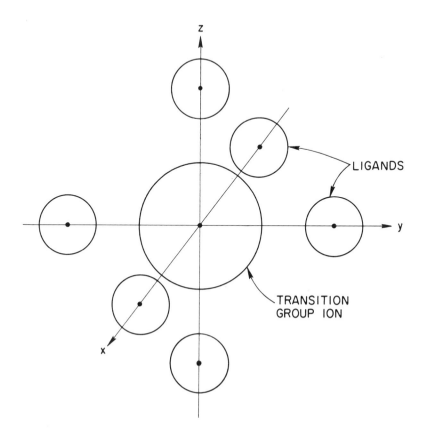

FIG 3-12   The geometry used for the molecular orbital treatment of an ion in
a cubic and six-coordinated environment.

3–5 Ions with Several *d* Electrons

Sections 3–3 and 3–4 give some insight into how to treat an ion with
a single *d* electron beyond the closed shells. Introducing more than one
electron adds the complications of the electron-electron Coulomb interactions. Of the six possible permutations of λ (the spin-orbit coupling
parameter), Δ (the cubic crystal-field splitting parameter), and K (a parameter typical of the splittings due to electron-electron interactions) only
three limiting cases are usually discussed. The other three possible cases
correspond to *j-j* coupling in the free transition-group ion, a situation which
arises only for the heaviest ions ($n = 5$ and above). For ions with Russell-
Saunders coupling ($K \gg \lambda$) we may insert Δ in three simple ways into the

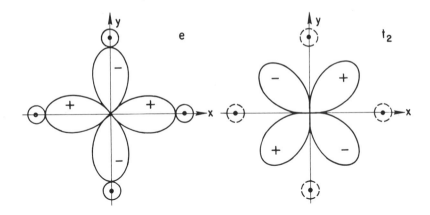

FIG. 3-13 Plots of e and t_2 orbitals for the geometry of Fig. 3-12, showing that the e orbital can mix with the ligand s orbitals whereas the t_2 orbitals cannot. Thus an antibonding, primarily e orbital is above the nonbonding t_2 orbital, and the energies are as in Fig. 3-8(a).

inequality. If $\Delta \gg K \gg \lambda$, we have what is called the strong crystal-field case. If $K \gg \Delta \gg \lambda$, we have the weak crystal-field case. A case intermediate between these two is often treated, ignoring the spin-orbit interaction at least initially. A rather different approach is employed for $K \gg \lambda \gg \Delta$, the case applied most frequently to the rare-earth ions. The strong and weak crystal-field cases describe nicely the iron transition group and to a lesser extent also ions from the palladium and platinum group.

We will now attempt to develop an approximate description of the weak and strong field cases, one which is simple but yet has many of the features of more elaborate theoretical treatments [7]. Our approach will give very useful information about the ground states which play the dominant role in electron paramagnetic resonance. We developed some preliminary ideas for this discussion in Section 3–2. The spin function corresponding to the maximum possible spin for a configuration is a function which is even under all two-particle interchanges. Thus the associated spatial function is odd under such interchanges and the electrons avoid each other. In this way we argue that the higher the spin of a term the lower is its energy. The statement works well for the ground term but not so well for higher ones. In a cubic crystal the d orbitals are split into t_2 and e orbitals. As indicated in Fig. 3-8 a six-coordinated ion will be lower in energy by Δ for each electron that can be taken from an e orbital and put into a t_2 orbital. We are thus faced with two sometimes competing effects. In either extreme limit we can easily write down many of the characteristics of the ground state. Table 3-2 gives the results for

Table 3-2

Properties of the Ground Cubic Crystal-Field State for Several d Electrons
(Six-Coordination)

Number of d Electrons	Weak Field			Strong Field		
	Configuration	Spin	Orbital Degeneracy	Configuration	Spin	Orbital Degeneracy
1	t_2^1	$\frac{1}{2}$	$3\times$	←		
2	t_2^2	1	$3\times$	←		
3	t_2^3	$\frac{3}{2}$	$1\times$	←		
4	$t_2^3 e^1$	2	$2\times$	t_2^4	1	$3\times$
5	$t_2^3 e^2$	$\frac{5}{2}$	$1\times$	t_2^5	$\frac{1}{2}$	$3\times$
6	$t_2^4 e^2$	2	$3\times$	t_2^6	0	$1\times$
7	$t_2^5 e^2$	$\frac{3}{2}$	$3\times$	$t_2^6 e^1$	$\frac{1}{2}$	$2\times$
8	$t_2^6 e^2$	1	$1\times$	←		
9	$t_2^6 e^3$	$\frac{1}{2}$	$2\times$	←		

ions with 1 to 9 d electrons in a six-coordinated cubic environment. The weak field case ($\Delta \ll K$) is obtained by putting electrons into orbitals for which the Pauli principle will allow maximum spin (but otherwise, placing them in the lowest orbitals). In contrast, for the strong field case ($\Delta \gg K$) the electrons are placed in the lowest orbitals (maximizing the spin consis-

Table 3-3

Properties of the Ground Cubic Crystal-Field State for Several d Electrons
(Four-, Eight-, Twelve-Coordination)

Number of d Electrons	Weak Field			Strong Field		
	Configuration	Spin	Orbital Degeneracy	Configuration	Spin	Orbital Degeneracy
1	e^1	$\frac{1}{2}$	$2\times$	←		
2	e^2	1	$1\times$	←		
3	$e^2 t_2^1$	$\frac{3}{2}$	$3\times$	e^3	$\frac{1}{2}$	$2\times$
4	$e^2 t_2^2$	2	$3\times$	e^4	0	$1\times$
5	$e^2 t_2^3$	$\frac{5}{2}$	$1\times$	$e^4 t_2^1$	$\frac{1}{2}$	$3\times$
6	$e^3 t_2^3$	2	$2\times$	$e^4 t_2^2$	1	$3\times$
7	$e^4 t_2^3$	$\frac{3}{2}$	$1\times$	←		
8	$e^4 t_2^4$	1	$3\times$	←		
9	$e^4 t_2^5$	$\frac{1}{2}$	$3\times$	←		

tent with this orbital placement). The orbital degeneracy represents the number of equivalent ways of obtaining the configuration with the indicated spin.

The closely related results for four-, eight-, and twelve-coordination, where the order of t_2 and e is inverted, are shown in Table 3-3. Because of the similarity of electron and hole behavior, the two tables are seen to be the same if one of them is reversed (i.e., $d^n \rightarrow d^{10-n}$). Many of the most useful qualitative features of the transition-group ions for electron paramagnetic resonance are contained in these two tables. The tables express the ground states in terms of crystal-field configurations which are strictly correct only in the extreme strong field limit. In weak fields other crystal-

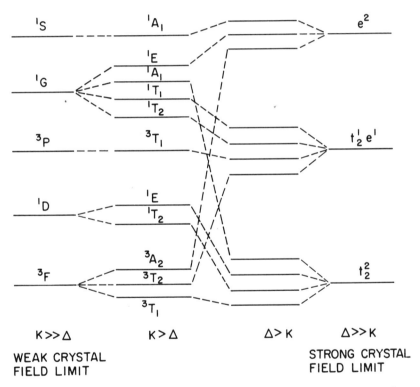

FIG. 3-14 A schematic energy level diagram for the configuration $[Ar]3d^2$ for various relative magnitudes of the term splitting K and the cubic crystal-field splitting Δ for six-coordination. Spin-orbit coupling is neglected. Note that the state formed from the ground strong-field configuration with spins aligned is the lowest state throughout. This explains why in Table 3-2 the d^2 configuration is the same in both strong and weak field. If the symmetry were actually O_h (full cubic symmetry), a subscript g would conventionally appear on all state designations except those for terms, that is, $^1A_{1g}$, $^3T_{2g}$, e_g, etc.

field configurations may arise from the d^n free-ion configuration, which can be mixed in. This "configuration interaction" is present only for t_2^2, $t_2^5 e^2$, $e^2 t_2^1$, and $e^4 t_2^4$ among the configurations employed in weak field (all ground configurations which occur only for strong fields can mix with other of these crystal-field configurations).

For some people any advantages of simplicity associated with the arguments leading to Tables 3-2 and 3-3 may be outweighed by the incompleteness of the results and the questionable approximations involved. A more detailed but still merely qualitative description can be given by schematic energy level diagrams (correlation diagrams) such as the example for d^2 given in Fig. 3-14. A diagram having a similar appearance was employed in Fig. 3-3 when comparing K and λ for free d^2 ions.

Quantitative versions of Fig. 3-14, called Tanabe-Sugano diagrams, have been calculated for certain values of C/B, the ratio of the two Racah parameters specifying the interelectronic Coulomb interaction [8]. As an example the behavior for a d^2 configuration and $C/B = 4.42$ is shown in Fig. 3-15.

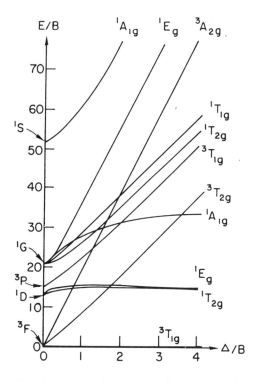

FIG. 3-15 The Tanabe-Sugano diagram analogous to Fig. 3-14. This plot assumes a ratio of $C/B = 4.42$ for the Racah parameters.

One of the first steps in generating diagrams such as Figs. 3-14 and 3-15 is to decide how the terms split in a cubic field. This is analogous to finding out how the energy levels of a single d electron split, since one d electron produces a ^2D term. The result is that S and P terms do not split, D terms split into a doublet and a triplet, and an F term splits into two triplets and a singlet (spin degeneracy is nowhere included). The levels are ordered so that the ground state is always as predicted from Tables 3-2 and 3-3 for weak fields.

All of our considerations for incomplete multielectron configurations have been for cubic symmetry. If we consider lower symmetry, we have two or more independent crystal-field parameters and the results become more complicated and more difficult to display. Frequently, however, we may consider departures from a cubic crystal field as perturbations to the solutions already described or implied.

3–6 The Ground State and Its Relationship to Electron Paramagnetic Resonance

Our considerations in Sections 3–1 through 3–5 were based on a Hamiltonian consisting of electronic kinetic energy, electrostatic interactions between charged particles, and the spin-orbit interaction. We now wish to include the Zeeman interaction of Eq. (1-4) and to determine the energy levels produced from the ground state. This is the principal problem in electron paramagnetic resonance, and the explanations are numerous and differ considerably, depending on the system under study. However, to illustrate the relationships we will consider a $3d^1$ configuration (in addition to closed shells) and tetragonal symmetry (see Fig. 3-9) with the spin-orbit interaction parameter λ smaller than either of the crystal-field splitting parameters, Δ or δ (see Fig. 3-16). Applying the tetragonal crystal field to the ground term yields the energy levels shown in Fig. 3-16. Let us consider the effect of the spin-orbit interaction in modifying these eigenfunctions in first order and then determine the effect of the Zeeman interaction on the resultant functions.

Table 3-4 shows the results of operating on the five d orbitals with the orbital angular momentum operators, where the latter are expressed in terms of x, y, and z components for convenience (see Appendix A), $L_x = -i[y(\partial/\partial z) - z(\partial/\partial y)]$, $L_y = -i[z(\partial/\partial x) - x(\partial/\partial z)]$, and $L_z = -i[x(\partial/\partial y) - y(\partial/\partial x)]$. The spin-orbit interaction within a single term can be expressed as

$$\lambda \mathbf{L} \cdot \mathbf{S} = \lambda L_z S_z + \tfrac{1}{2}\lambda L_x(S_+ + S_-) + \frac{1}{2i}\lambda L_y(S_+ - S_-), \qquad (3-14)$$

where $\lambda = \pm \xi_{3d}/2S$, since it is the ground term (plus if less than half full, minus otherwise). The quantity ξ_{3d} is the expectation value of $\xi(r_i)$ of

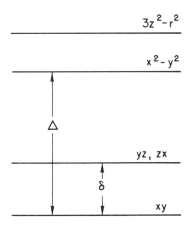

FIG. 3-16 Energy level diagram for a single *d* electron in tetragonal symmetry. The energies of the two states mixed into the ground state by spin-orbit interaction in first order are shown.

Eq. (3-1), averaged over the $3d$ radial functions. When we include the spin, we will designate the basis functions as $|2, xy, \pm\rangle$, where the $\pm$ sign represents the sign of M_S for the z axis along the tetragonal axis. The ground state is a spin doublet which is approximately of the form $|2, xy, \pm\rangle$. Using first-order perturbation theory, we obtain first-order eigenfunctions $|\pm\rangle$, given by

$$|\pm\rangle = |2, xy, \pm\rangle + \sum_{i,\alpha} \frac{\langle 2, i, \alpha|\lambda\mathbf{L}\cdot\mathbf{S}|2, xy, \pm\rangle}{E_{xy}-E_i} |2, i, \alpha\rangle. \quad (3-15)$$

By using Eq. (3-14) and Table 3-4, we obtain the result for Eq. (3-15) as

$$|\pm\rangle = |2, xy, \pm\rangle \pm \frac{i\lambda}{\Delta} |2, x^2-y^2, \pm\rangle - \frac{i\lambda}{2\delta} |2, zx, \mp\rangle \mp \frac{\lambda}{2\delta} |2, yz, \mp\rangle.$$

$$(3-16)$$

So far in this chapter we have overlooked one of the most important aspects of the crystal field, the quenching of orbital angular momentum. We can see from an inspection of Table 3-4 that no matrix elements of **L** exist between the approximate ground-state functions $|2, xy, \pm\rangle$. This consequence of the presence of the crystal field is referred to as the quenching of the orbital angular momentum and is of common occurrence among ions of the iron transition group. The presence of the spin-orbit interaction as a perturbation causes small first-order matrix elements

Table 3-4

Operation of Orbital Angular Momentum on d Orbitals

$|\;\rangle$	$L_x|\;\rangle$	$L_y|\;\rangle$	$L_z|\;\rangle$
xy	izx	$-iyz$	$-2i[\tfrac{1}{2}(x^2-y^2)]$
yz	$i[\tfrac{1}{2}(x^2-y^2)]+i\sqrt{3}[(1/2\sqrt{3})(3z^2-r^2)]$	ixy	$-izx$
zx	$-ixy$	$i[\tfrac{1}{2}(x^2-y^2)]-i\sqrt{3}[(1/2\sqrt{3})(3z^2-r^2)]$	iyz
$\tfrac{1}{2}(x^2-y^2)$	$-iyz$	$-izx$	$2ixy$
$(1/2\sqrt{3})(3z^2-r^2)$	$-i\sqrt{3}yz$	$i\sqrt{3}zx$	0

of $\mathbf{L}$ of the order of λ/Δ, and thus reintroduces some Zeeman splitting from the orbital magnetic moment. Using Eq. (3-16), we can show that

$$\langle\pm|L_z|\pm\rangle = \mp\frac{4\lambda}{\Delta}, \qquad \langle\pm|S_z|\pm\rangle = \pm\tfrac{1}{2},$$

$$\langle\pm|L_x|\pm\rangle = -\frac{\lambda}{\delta}, \qquad \langle\pm|S_x|\pm\rangle = \tfrac{1}{2}, \qquad\qquad (3\text{-}17)$$

$$\langle\pm|L_y|\pm\rangle = \mp i\frac{\lambda}{\delta}, \qquad \langle\pm|S_y|\pm\rangle = \pm i\tfrac{1}{2},$$

where all other matrix elements of $\mathbf{L}$ or $\mathbf{S}$ are zero. From Eq. (3-17) we can calculate the matrix elements of [see Eq. (1-4)] $\mathcal{H} = \beta(\mathbf{L}+g_e\mathbf{S})\cdot\mathbf{H}$. These are

$$\langle\pm|\mathcal{H}|\pm\rangle = \left(\pm\tfrac{1}{2}g_e\mp 4\frac{\lambda}{\Delta}\right)\beta H_z,$$

$$\langle\pm|\mathcal{H}|\mp\rangle = \left(\tfrac{1}{2}g_e - \frac{\lambda}{\delta}\right)\beta H_x \pm i\left(\tfrac{1}{2}g_e - \frac{\lambda}{\delta}\right)\beta H_y. \qquad (3\text{-}18)$$

This leads to a 2×2 determinantal eigenvalue equation whose solutions are

$$E = \pm\tfrac{1}{2}\sqrt{[g_e - 8(\lambda/\Delta)]^2\cos^2\theta + [g_e - 2(\lambda/\delta)]^2\sin^2\theta}\,\beta H \equiv \pm\tfrac{1}{2}g\beta H, \quad (3\text{-}19)$$

where θ is the angle between $\mathbf{H}$ and the tetragonal z axis. The g factor is different from the free-electron value, g_e, and is anisotropic as a result of the small contribution of orbital angular momentum. The g value for $\mathbf{H}$ parallel to z is $g_\parallel$, which is $g_e - 8(\lambda/\Delta)$ in this case. Similarly for a field perpendicular to z the g value is $g_e - 2(\lambda/\delta)$ and is designated $g_\perp$. For this simple case the g values are below the free-electron value since $\lambda>0$. This is commonly the case if the shell is less than half-filled, since then $\lambda>0$, but the g values are greater than the free-spin value if the shell is more than half full (λ is then negative).

3–7 Rare Earths

As mentioned in Section 3–5, the rare earths require an approach different from the methods discussed so far. In this case, we have $K\gg\lambda\gg\Delta$ as our most appropriate limiting case. This means that the crystal field is a perturbation to the free-ion properties, which in turn are taken as the results of Russell-Saunders coupling. Although we will not discuss this topic extensively, we will illustrate the main features by a simple example.

Consider an ion with a $4f^1$ configuration such as might occur for Ce^{3+}, and assume that the ion is in a cubic crystal at a six-coordinated site. The spin-orbit interaction couples the orbital angular momentum of 3 and the spin of $\frac{1}{2}$, giving two states with $J = \frac{5}{2}$ and $J = \frac{7}{2}$. The $J = \frac{5}{2}$ state is lower. The sixfold degeneracy of this lower state is partially lifted by the cubic crystal field, and two states result, an excited one with a fourfold degeneracy and a lowest twofold degenerate state. The lowest state can be shown to have the form [9]

$$\psi_\pm = \frac{1}{\sqrt{6}} |\tfrac{5}{2}, \pm\tfrac{5}{2}\rangle - \sqrt{\tfrac{5}{6}} |\tfrac{5}{2}, \mp\tfrac{3}{2}\rangle. \tag{3-20}$$

Using Eqs. (1-8) and (1-9), we find that the Hamiltonian describing the interaction of any $J = \frac{5}{2}$ state with the magnetic field is

$$\mathcal{H} = \tfrac{6}{7}\beta \mathbf{H} \cdot \mathbf{J}. \tag{3-21}$$

Calculating the matrix elements of the Hamiltonian of Eq. (3-21) between the states specified by Eq. (3-20), we obtain

$$\langle \psi_\pm | \mathcal{H} | \psi_\pm \rangle = \mp\tfrac{5}{7}\beta H. \tag{3-22}$$

All other matrix elements are zero (the magnetic field has been taken along a cubic axis, which is then defined as the z axis, since the results are isotropic). By comparison of Eqs. (3-22) and (1-12) we see that the energy is the same as would be obtained from a two-level system with an (spin) angular momentum of $\frac{1}{2}$ and a g value of 10/7. This convention is used almost exclusively in electron paramagnetic resonance since it is more closely associated with the experimental observations. Thus for our present problem we say that the ground state has a g value of $10/7 = 1.43$, and we would essentially ignore its true wave function and talk as if it were a system with angular momentum of $\frac{1}{2}$ arising from spin alone.

3–8 Kramers' Theorem

As a result of the fact that the Hamiltonians which we use are invariant under time reversal when no magnetic field is applied, we find certain required degeneracies. A theorem, called Kramers' theorem, states that all systems with an odd number of electrons can have only even degeneracies in zero field. Thus the lowest degeneracy is twofold.

The time-reversal operator K causes all processes which evolve in time to flow backward. Thus K operating on linear or angular momentum reverses the sign. In addition, K has the effect of taking the complex conjugate and thus reverses running and rotating waves (see Section 3–3). For the spin angular momentum $\mathbf{S}$ and the spin functions for one electron we have

$$S_z |\tfrac{1}{2}, \pm\tfrac{1}{2}\rangle = \pm\tfrac{1}{2} |\tfrac{1}{2}, \pm\tfrac{1}{2}\rangle. \tag{3-23}$$

The time-reversed spin functions are obtained by applying the time reversal operator to Eq. (3-23). Thus we have

$$KS_z|\tfrac{1}{2}, \pm\tfrac{1}{2}\rangle = \pm\tfrac{1}{2}K|\tfrac{1}{2}, \pm\tfrac{1}{2}\rangle. \tag{3-24}$$

But since $KS = -SK$ we obtain

$$S_zK|\tfrac{1}{2}, \pm\tfrac{1}{2}\rangle = \mp\tfrac{1}{2}K|\tfrac{1}{2}, \pm\tfrac{1}{2}\rangle. \tag{3-25}$$

Thus $K|\tfrac{1}{2}, \pm\tfrac{1}{2}\rangle$ must be a phase factor times $|\tfrac{1}{2}, \mp\tfrac{1}{2}\rangle$:

$$K|\tfrac{1}{2}, \pm\tfrac{1}{2}\rangle = \lambda_\pm|\tfrac{1}{2}, \mp\tfrac{1}{2}\rangle, \tag{3-26}$$

where $|\lambda_\pm| = 1$. Similarly we have

$$S_\pm|\tfrac{1}{2}, \mp\tfrac{1}{2}\rangle = |\tfrac{1}{2}, \pm\tfrac{1}{2}\rangle \tag{3-27}$$

and the corresponding equation after time reversal:

$$KS_\pm|\tfrac{1}{2}, \mp\tfrac{1}{2}\rangle = K|\tfrac{1}{2}, \pm\tfrac{1}{2}\rangle. \tag{3-28}$$

But $KS_\pm = -S_\mp K$ results from our definition of K, so that we have

$$-S_\mp K|\tfrac{1}{2}, \mp\tfrac{1}{2}\rangle = K|\tfrac{1}{2}, \pm\tfrac{1}{2}\rangle. \tag{3-29}$$

Using Eqs. (3-26) and (3-27), we obtain $\lambda_\pm = -\lambda_\mp$ from Eq. (3-29). Application of K again to Eq. (3-26) yields

$$K^2|\tfrac{1}{2}, \pm\tfrac{1}{2}\rangle = \lambda_\pm K|\tfrac{1}{2}, \mp\tfrac{1}{2}\rangle = \lambda_\pm\lambda_\mp|\tfrac{1}{2}, \pm\tfrac{1}{2}\rangle = -|\tfrac{1}{2}, \pm\tfrac{1}{2}\rangle. \tag{3-30}$$

We can apply this to an n-electron system consisting of either a product of n one-electron wave functions (spin and orbital), a Slater determinant, or a sum of Slater determinants. In any case we obtain

$$K^2\Psi = (-1)^n\Psi. \tag{3-31}$$

Finally, let us consider the Schrödinger equation for a system whose Hamiltonian is invariant to time reversal, $K\mathcal{H} = \mathcal{H}K$. Let us assume that a singly degenerate ground state can occur. Then we have

$$\mathcal{H}\Psi_j = E_j\Psi_j, \qquad K\mathcal{H}\Psi_j = \mathcal{H}K\Psi_j = E_jK\Psi_j. \tag{3-32}$$

Thus we must have

$$K\Psi_j = a\Psi_j \tag{3-33}$$

and $|a| = 1$ since the state is nondegenerate and $K\Psi_j$ has the same eigenvalue as Ψ_j. We may operate on Eq. (3-33) with K and obtain

$$K^2\Psi_j = K(a\Psi_j) = a^*K\Psi_j = a^*a\Psi_j = \Psi_j. \tag{3-34}$$

The only way in which Eqs. (3-31) and (3-34) can be consistent is for n to be an even integer. Thus no nondegenerate states can occur for an odd-electron system as stated by Kramers' theorem.

The two functions that must be degenerate for an odd-electron system are those connected by K. Generally these Kramers conjugate functions are related by reversing the signs of all M values and taking the complex conjugate of the coefficients. For example, the two functions of Eq. (3-20) are Kramers conjugates.

3–9 The Jahn-Teller Theorem

The properties of the ground states of ions with several d electrons implied by Tables 3-2 and 3-3 can be very useful in anticipating the general nature of any resultant EPR spectra. However, in the form given they are somewhat misleading because some of the ground states are listed as possessing a two- or threefold orbital degeneracy. It is known that in general these degeneracies cannot persist, and we wish to explain why this is true and what happens so that the actual nature of the EPR spectra can be at least roughly anticipated.

The Jahn-Teller theorem states that a nonlinear molecule or molecular complex having electronic degeneracy will spontaneously distort to a nuclear configuration of lower symmetry such that only twofold Kramers degeneracy, if any, remains. In practice the interaction between spin angular momentum and the nuclear coordinates is so weak that we need

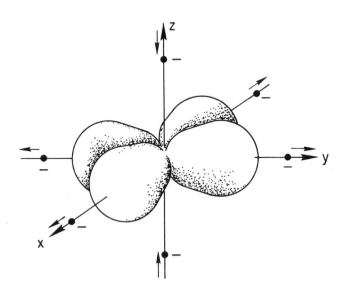

FIG. 3-17   The distortion which lowers the energy of the $x^2 - y^2$ state. The energy of the $3z^2 - r^2$ state would be raised by this distortion. It is just these electrostatic forces which cause the Jahn-Teller effect.

consider only orbital degeneracy. The reason for this behavior is that one of several degenerate states does not interact equally with all of its neighbors. To illustrate this consider a single electron in an e orbital of a six-coordinated ion (see Figs. 3-7 and 3-8). The electron could occupy either of the degenerate states, $|2, x^2-y^2\rangle$ or $|2, 3z^2-r^2\rangle$ (or any linear combination of these two). Consider first the electron in $|2, x^2-y^2\rangle$ shown in Fig. 3-17. The energy of the electron will be reduced as a result of the distortion shown in Fig. 3-17. This is a consequence of a reduced Coulomb interaction with the four point negative charges in the xy plane. This particular distortion will raise the energy of the $|2, 3z^2-r^2\rangle$ state, and the negative of this distortion will lower $|2, 3z^2-r^2\rangle$ and raise $|2, x^2-y^2\rangle$. This distortion, as shown in Fig. 3-17, is known as $-Q_3$, and the energy levels for the system are given in Fig. 3-18. Other interactions within the complex will change the initial linear dependence on Q_3, producing minima in the energy corresponding to a significant distortion from the high-symmetry nuclear configuration. This distortion is tetragonal and results in an energy level diagram similar to that of Fig. 3-9. A physical situation similar to our example is Ag^{2+} ($4d^9$). At temperatures near $4°K$ several equivalent tetragonally distorted ions are observed [10]. For a more

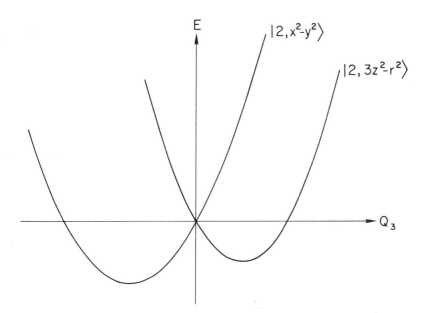

FIG. 3-18   The energies of the x^2-y^2 and $3z^2-r^2$ states as a function of the distortion shown in Fig. 3-17 (the distortion there is taken as negative). Elastic restoring forces eventually cause the energy to increase, giving minima for a nonzero distortion.

thorough discussion of the Jahn-Teller effect in general see the reviews by Sturge, Ham, and Müller [11].

3–10 Supplemental Bibliography

The general subject of ligand or crystal fields has been discussed in a large number of books and articles. Treatments possessing great rigor and based largely on group theory are available as well as qualitative and semiquantitative discussions of the principles. Chemists have been particularly active in the latter effort.

1. J. S. Griffith, *The Theory of Transition-Metal Ions*, Cambridge, 1961. Probably the most authoritative and complete work on crystal-field theory. It may be somewhat difficult for beginners.

2. C. J. Ballhausen, *Introduction to Ligand Field Theory*, McGraw-Hill, New York, 1962. An extensive and very readable treatment.

3. L. E. Orgel, *Introduction to Transition Chemistry*, Wiley, New York, 1960. A very clear discussion of the main features of crystal-field theory, using only a minimum of mathematics and a number of simple and useful approximations.

4. B. N. Figgis, *Introduction to Ligand Fields*, Wiley, New York, 1966. An easily read and clear description of the main features of crystal-field theory.

5. H. Watanabe, *Operator Methods in Ligand Field Theory*, Prentice-Hall, Englewood Cliffs, N.J., 1966. A very complete discussion for a small book. Rigorous and containing many useful tables and figures.

6. T. M. Dunn, D. S. McClure, and R. G. Pearson, *Some Aspects of Crystal Field Theory*, Harper and Row, New York, 1965. A good introduction.

7. C. J. Ballhausen and H. B. Gray, *Molecular Orbital Theory*, Benjamin, New York, 1965. A good introduction to the molecular orbital method.

8. D. S. McClure, "Electronic Spectra of Molecules and Ions in Crystals. Part II: Spectra of Ions in Crystals," in *Solid State Physics* (F. Seitz and D. Turnbull, eds.), Academic, New York, 1959, Vol. 9, p. 399. Discusses both crystals fields and molecular orbitals.

References Cited in Chapter 3

[1] R. Stevenson, *Multiplet Structure of Atoms and Molecules*, Saunders, Philadelphia, 1965, p. 40.

[2] E. U. Condon and G. H. Shortley, *The Theory of Atomic Spectra*, Cambridge, 1953, p. 52.

[3] M. T. Hutchings, "Point-Charge Calculations of Energy Levels of Magnetic Ions in Crystalline Electric Fields," in *Solid State Physics* (F. Seitz and D. Turnbull, eds.), Academic, New York, 1964, Vol. 16, p. 227.

[4] C. J. Ballhausen, *Introduction to Ligand Field Theory*, McGraw-Hill, New York, 1962; J. S. Griffith, *The Theory of Transition-Metal Ions*, Cambridge, 1961.

[5] C. J. Ballhausen and H. B. Gray, *Molecular Orbital Theory*, Benjamin, New York, 1965.
[6] J. S. Griffith, *J. Chem. Phys.* **41**, 576 (1964).
[7] L. E. Orgel, *Introduction to Transition Chemistry*, Wiley, New York, 1960, p. 42.
[8] B. N. Figgis, *Introduction to Ligand Fields*, Wiley, New York, 1966, p. 161.
[9] K. R. Lea, M. J. M. Leask, and W. P. Wolf, *J. Phys. Chem. Solids* **23**, 1381 (1962). The authors present numerical results for the energies and eigenfunctions in cubic symmetry for $J \leq 8$.
[10] J. Sierro, *J. Phys. Chem. Solids* **28**, 417 (1967).
[11] M. D. Sturge, "The Jahn-Teller Effect in Solids," in *Solid State Physics* (F. Seitz, D. Turnbull, and H. Ehrenreich, eds.), Academic, New York, 1967, Vol. 20, p. 92; F. S. Ham, "Jahn-Teller Effects in Electron Paramagnetic Resonance Spectra," in *Electron Paramagnetic Resonance* (S. Geschwind, ed.), Plenum, New York, 1972, p. 1; K. A. Müller, "Jahn-Teller Effects in Magnetic Resonance," in *Magnetic Resonance and Relaxation* (R. Blinc, ed.), North Holland, Amsterdam, 1967, p. 192.

CHAPTER 4

The Effective Spin Hamiltonian

In Chapter 3 we introduced the concepts which in principle should allow us to describe the properties of the lowest set of states of most paramagnetic entities. We are primarily interested in the states within a few reciprocal centimeters of the ground state since they are accessible to electron paramagnetic resonance at microwave frequencies and with reasonable magnetic field values (actually any group of states within a few reciprocal centimeters of each other and capable of being adequately populated might be considered). We will refer to this set of states as the ground manifold. In Chapter 3 we introduced contributions to the Hamiltonian which are too numerous, too complicated, and too far away in terms of computations from the actual ground manifold energies and wave functions to be directly useful in discussing and understanding actual EPR data. Hence we introduce here, as is often done,* an effective Hamiltonian, one which is intended to give valid results only for the ground manifold of states. In this chapter we will develop this spin Hamiltonian, as it is called, and apply it in Chapter 5 to the description of EPR spectra.

4–1 The Ground Manifold and the Effective Spin

Because of the large energy differences only the lowest energy level resulting from a first-order crystal-field splitting or a first-order spin-orbit splitting can lead to the ground manifold of states. Let us examine the origin of the states arising from such a lowest level and in this way determine the transformation properties of the lowest manifold of states. In Section 3–5 (Tables 3-2 and 3-3) we determined the orbital degeneracy of the ground state of an ion with an incomplete d shell in a cubic crystal field. Similar arguments could be applied to lower symmetries such as the tetragonal case shown in Fig. 3-9. Some of these ground states will be

---

* Recall that the exchange interaction in the form $-2J\mathbf{S}_1\cdot\mathbf{S}_2$ is an effective Hamiltonian, the spin-otbit interaction in the form $\lambda\,\mathbf{L}\cdot\mathbf{S}$ is an effective Hamiltonian for spherical symmetry and a given atomic term, and electron-electron interactions in atoms are often approximated by a central potential which is part of an effective Hamiltonian. Treatment of nuclear motion in molecules using the adiabatic approximation employs an effective potential consisting of the electronic energy.

orbital singlets, and for these the only degeneracy arises from the spin of the ion. Even though the wave functions will not generally be just the several spin functions times a common orbital function (see Section 3–6), they will have the transformation properties of spin angular momentum eigenfunctions or properties so similar that for practical purposes they are the same. Thus the ground manifold is said to have an effective spin, usually called just spin, which in this case equals the actual spin of the crystal-field ground state.

Considering the crystal-field ground states as before, we find that the remaining ions are orbitally degenerate. Two things may occur here. The Jahn-Teller theorem described in Section 3–9 suggests that a spontaneous distortion will occur, and we may now be in a situation similar to the one described in the previous paragraph (for an exception see Section 10–4). Another limiting possibility is that the spin-orbit interaction will dominate any tendency to distort. Again the states arising from the spin-orbit interaction transform like angular momenta or in a very similar manner.

For ions with incomplete f-electron shells, the crystal field produces ground states which transform either like angular momentum eigenfunctions of $J = \frac{3}{2}$ or less or in a very similar manner with one exception. For even-electron systems it is possible to have a twofold degenerate (or nearly degenerate) state which can only very crudely be described by $S = \frac{1}{2}$. The so-called non-Kramers doublets with axial symmetry have been discussed by several authors [1].

For the case of most other paramagnetic entities, it is difficult to see how orbital angular momentum can contribute to the degeneracy. Thus only the spin degeneracy remains, and the ground manifold has the transformation properties of the spin eigenfunctions [for an exception in which additional degeneracy occurs see G. D. Watkins and F. S. Ham, *Phys. Rev.* Bl, 4071 (1970)].

Thus we will ascribe an effective spin S to the ground manifold. We usually set $2S + 1$ equal to the ground manifold degeneracy except for the non-Kramers doublets. Henceforth we will consider explicitly only ground manifolds which indeed have transformation properties identical, for the point symmetry involved, to those of spin eigenfunctions (Section 10–4 is excepted).

4–2 The Spin Hamiltonian

Although the ground manifold transforms like spin angular momentum eigenfunctions, it will not have the simple isotropic behavior of a free spin. As we have seen by example in Section 3–6 and as we will see in greater detail in later sections, the energy levels for the ground manifold may depend on the angle between the crystalline axes and the magnetic field, as well as having other properties not possessed by a free spin. Because the ground manifold energies can be rather complicated, we require an identical complicated behavior of the energy of the effective spin states. To ensure our ability to treat the most general case we introduce an effective Hamiltonian, called the spin Hamiltonian, which operates only upon the effective spin functions and which will reproduce the full range of possible behavior of the ground manifold.

Since it operates on the eigenfunctions for a given (effective) spin, the spin Hamiltonian must consist of spin operators for the electronic spins and for any nuclear spins which make a significant contribution to the paramagnetism. In addition the components of the magnetic field, an electric field, and a stress may be included (for the latter two, see Chapter 8 in this book). Each independent term in the spin Hamiltonian will be multiplied by a constant which is not restricted by the considerations of this section but which in principle can be calculated theoretically (see Sections 4–3 and 4–4) or measured experimentally (see Chapter 5). Each of these independent terms must be invariant under the point symmetry operations of the paramagnetic entity. This invariance is a necessary characteristic of the Hamiltonian (effective or otherwise) when both the fields and the spin operators are transformed (not just the operators alone).

The independent terms in the spin Hamiltonian consist of each of the fields or angular momentum operators raised to a certain power (except for terms present exclusively to eliminate average energy shifts, which are meaningless in this application). Thus, if we restrict ourselves to magnetic fields, electronic spin, and the nuclear spin of a nucleus at the symmetry point, a term in the spin Hamiltonian can be written symbolically as $H^a S^b I^c$. As an example $H_x S_x + H_y S_y + H_z S_z$ is such a term with $a = 1, b = 1$, and $c = 0$, and is, of course, proportional to the Zeeman-interaction Hamiltonian for free spins. We wish now to consider a variety of restrictions on a, b, and c, some required and some merely good approximations.

We discussed the time-reversal operator in Section 3–8 and noted that it caused all circulations to reverse. Since magnetic fields and angular momenta result from circulations, they must change sign under the operation of time reversal. Since the spin Hamiltonian must be invariant under time reversal, we see that $a + b + c$ must be an even integer.

Because the (effective) spin and the nuclear spin have values S and I, we can use the usual vector addition triangular inequality [2] to place upper limits on b and c as follows: $b \leq 2S$ and $c \leq 2I$. Since the energy splitting as a result of externally applied fields (including stress) is small compared to the energy spacing between the ground manifold and any excited manifolds, it is usually necessary to consider only terms in the Hamiltonian which are linear in the fields. For example, the interaction with an external magnetic field arises from the Hamiltonian $\beta(\mathbf{L} + 2\mathbf{S}) \cdot \mathbf{H}$. Even for fields as large as 100 kG the Zeeman splitting is only about 10 cm^{-1}, a value comparable to that allowed for the spread in the ground manifold and normally very small compared to the separation from any higher state. Thus by perturbation theory arguments a quadratic term in H in the effective spin Hamiltonian would be very small. For the present case this usually means $a \leq 1$.

The magnetic dipole interaction of the nuclear spin with the angular momentum of the paramagnetic entity can be described by saying that the nucleus produces a magnetic field at the ion which depends on M_I. Thus, as above, we restrict the nuclear magnetic field to linear terms or $c \leq 1$ for magnetic dipole interactions. Actually other multipole interactions can occur, but usually the electric quadrupole interaction is the only other one producing measurable effects. Therefore generally $c \leq 2$. Summing up, we have

$$a + b + c = 2n \qquad (n > 0, \text{ integer}),$$

$$b \leq 2S, \qquad c \leq 2I, 2, \qquad a \leq 1. \tag{4-1}$$

Finally we would expect that the larger the quantities a, b, and c become, the smaller the term in the spin Hamiltonian becomes. Thus when all have their maximum value the resulting terms may be negligible. We show symbolically in Table 4-1 the types of terms which can occur for various values of S and I and still satisfy the limitations imposed by Eq. (4-1).

Table 4-1
Types of Allowed Terms in the Spin Hamiltonian as Limited by Eq. (4-1)

S \ I	0	$\frac{1}{2}$	≥ 1
$\frac{1}{2}$	HS	SI, HI, HS	I^2, SI, HI, HS, HSI^2
1	S^2, HS	SI, S^2, HI, HS, HS^2I	$I^2, SI, S^2, S^2I^2, HI, HS, HSI^2, HS^2I$
$\frac{3}{2}$	S^2, HS, HS^3	$SI, S^2, S^3I, HI, HS, HS^2I, HS^3$	$I^2, SI, S^2, S^2I^2, S^3I, HI, HS, HSI^2, HS^2I, HS^3, HS^3I^2$

In addition to the types of terms in Table 4-1, it has been found useful to employ S^4, S^6, and occasionally HS^5, S^5I, HS^7, S^7I when the value of S allows. Some of the types of terms shown symbolically in Table 4-1 are in fact not observed.

Since the three vectors $\mathbf{H}$, $\mathbf{S}$, and $\mathbf{I}$ are all axial vectors, we may investigate the transformation properties with little regard for which vectors are involved (and that only because of the commutation relations for the spins). That is, we will treat *HS*, *SI*, and *HI* in the same way. In doing this we can regard **S** and **I** as irreducible tensor operators [3] of the first rank. These are combined to form irreducible tensor operators of rank *b* and *c*, respectively, and the resultant operators are classified according to their transformation properties for the particular point symmetry. Products of components of **H** are similarly classified. As many invariants as possible are obtained by combining the three types of quantities (invariant under point symmetry operations). Each of these invariants can be an independent term in the spin Hamiltonian.

Using group theory, one can quickly and easily (if character tables are available [4]) determine the number of independent terms of each type allowed by a given symmetry. This information alone often makes it possible to determine the form of the operator by inspection; in other words, frequently the difficulty is not to think of terms consistent with the symmetry, but rather to be certain that one has all the terms of a given type. For this reason we give in Table 4-2 the number of independent terms that can occur for each type of operator as a function of the 32 crystallographic point symmetry groups, various axial symmetries, and full spherical symmetry. The only point groups which can occur in crystals are the crystallographic point groups. For molecules, however, many other groups are possible in addition to the ones included in Table 4-2. In Fig. 4-1

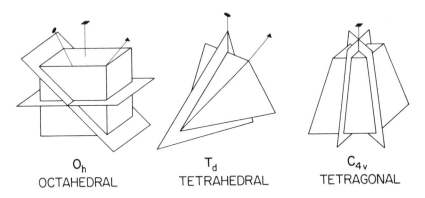

| O_h | T_d | C_{4v} |
| OCTAHEDRAL | TETRAHEDRAL | TETRAGONAL |

FIG. 4-1　Three different kinds of point symmetry. For each point group an object is shown that is invariant under all of the symmetry operations of that point group. Typical symmetry operations are also shown. Thus the cube is invariant against rotation about three fourfold axes, four threefold axes, and six twofold axes. It is also unchanged as a result of reflection in any of the three planes perpendicular to the fourfold axes, or any of the six planes perpendicular to the twofold axes. Similarly the regular tetrahedron is invariant under the operations of the point group T_d, a cubic symmetry. The right square pyramid is invariant under the operations of C_{4v}, one of the tetragonal point groups.

Table 4-2

The Number of Independent Terms of a Given Type Allowed by Symmetry in a Spin Hamiltonian

Point Group	Symbolic Operator Type	A^2	A^4	A^6	AB	AB^3	AB^5	AB^7	A^2B^2	A^2BC
Spherical		0	0	0	1	0	0	0	1	1
Cubic	$\{O_h, O, T_d$	0	1	1	1	1	2	2	2	2
	$\ T_h, T$	0	1	2	1	2	3	4	3	4
Hexagonal	$\{D_{6h}, D_6, C_{6v}, D_{3h}$	1	1	2	2	2	3	5	3	5
	$\ C_{6h}, C_6, C_{3h}$	1	1	3	3	3	5	9	5	9
Tetragonal	$\{D_{4h}, D_4, C_{4v}, D_{2d}$	1	2	2	2	3	5	6	4	6
	$\ C_{4h}, S_4, C_4$	1	3	3	3	5	9	11	7	11
Trigonal	$\{D_{3d}, D_3, C_{3v}$	1	2	3	2	4	6	8	5	8
	$\ S_6, C_3$	1	3	5	3	7	11	15	9	15
Orthorhombic	D_{2h}, D_2, C_{2v}	2	3	4	3	6	9	12	7	12
Monoclinic	C_{2h}, C_2, C_s	3	5	7	5	11	17	23	13	23
Triclinic	C_i, C_1	5	9	13	9	21	33	45	25	45
Axial	$\{D_{\infty h}, C_{\infty v}$	1	1	1	2	2	2	2	3	5
	$\ C_{\infty h}$	1	1	1	3	3	3	3	5	9

we show three objects: a cube, a regular tetrahedron, and a right square pyramid. Each object is invariant under the point group shown. Also given are typical rotation axes and reflection planes which characterize the symmetry. For more detail on the crystallographic point groups consult reference 5.

We note from Table 4-2 that 14 general kinds of spin Hamiltonians are allowed for the symmetries shown. If electric fields are also allowed, this would in fact produce a unique spin Hamiltonian for each point symmetry (at least among this set), resulting in the satisfying consequence that all point symmetries could be distinguished by their spin Hamiltonians. (In fact, of course, with limited spin values and many terms too small to be observed, one normally cannot make a complete distinction.) Table 4-2 will not give the correct number for situations in which powers of the components of H higher than 1 appear, although, as pointed out in the discussion leading to Eq. (4-1), such cases should be uncommon. (It is still easy to calculate the result, as it simply involves adding the number of terms for $A^2 X$, AX, and X if $a = 2$, where X contains the spin-operator part. Similar but more complicated procedures would apply for $a > 2$.)

It is particularly easy to write down the actual terms in the Hamiltonian for small powers of the operators and high symmetries. To illustrate the consequences of the approach we have outlined, we will determine most of the terms in spin Hamiltonians employed in practice.*

Let us consider the quadratic and bilinear forms first, that is, $a + b + c = 2$. These include all but three of the terms needed for values of S up to 1. The other three terms are observed to be small. This spin Hamiltonian can be written as

$$\mathcal{H} = \mathbf{S} \cdot \mathbf{D} \cdot \mathbf{S} + \beta \mathbf{H} \cdot \mathbf{g} \cdot \mathbf{S} + \mathbf{S} \cdot \mathbf{A} \cdot \mathbf{I} - \beta_n \mathbf{H} \cdot \mathbf{g}_n \cdot \mathbf{I} + \mathbf{I} \cdot \mathbf{Q} \cdot \mathbf{I}, \qquad (4\text{-}2)$$

where $\mathbf{D}$, $\beta\mathbf{g}$, $\mathbf{A}$, $-\beta_n \mathbf{g}_n$, and $\mathbf{Q}$ are the tensors which couple the indicated vectors, and the independent elements of the coupling tensors are the coefficients of the independent terms in the spin Hamiltonian. (Actually these quantities are not second-rank tensors since they form invariants by contraction with axial vectors rather than polar vectors. However, throughout the book we will use the tensor properties only for rotations of the coordinate system. In this case they behave like tensors and we will

---

* Alternatively one can use group theory to determine the independent terms, particularly if tables of coupling coefficients are available [4]. One then uses linear combinations of the products of the components of H to form bases of irreducible representations of the point group. Similarly the irreducible tensor operators of rank b for $\mathbf{S}$ and the ones of rank c for $\mathbf{I}$ are used as bases of irreducible representations. If the direct product of an irreducible representation of H^a with one from S^b and then one from I^c contains the completely symmetric representation at least once, the bases are coupled appropriately, tabulated coupling coefficients being used to give the desired invariant term(s).

continue to use the term tensor in this context.) The maximum possible number of coefficients occurs for triclinic symmetry, cases devoid of symmetry or having only inversion symmetry. In this case there are nine independent terms for the bilinear form. In other words, all nine elements of the $\mathbf{g}$, $\mathbf{A}$, and $\mathbf{g}_n$ tensors can be present and independent of each other. For the quadratic forms there are only five independent elements in the coupling tensor. The reason for the difference is that four possible terms in the spin Hamiltonian which appear to be quadratic are not. The commutation relations eliminate three of these: the skew-symmetric components of the coupling tensor. A fourth term is missing because $S_x^2 + S_y^2 + S_z^2 = S(S+1)$, a constant within a manifold of states of constant S, with a similar expression for I. By a rotation of the coordinates the coupling tensor $\mathbf{D}$ or $\mathbf{Q}$ can be brought into diagonal form with two independent diagonal elements and three Euler angles to specify the orientation of the principal axes, a total of five parameters. A similar transformation can be performed for the other coupling tensors except that only the symmetric part is diagonal and there are three independent diagonal elements or principal values. Thus in triclinic symmetry each coupling tensor for bilinear or quadratic terms in the spin Hamiltonian has its own principal axis system, with each principal axis system different and no simple relationships among them.

For monoclinic symmetry (C_{2h}, C_2, C_s) one principal axis is determined by symmetry. It is either normal to the reflection plane or parallel to the twofold axis of rotation. This removes two of the off-diagonal elements for the quadratic and bilinear coupling tensors and two skew-symmetric components of the bilinear form. In addition to the skew-symmetric components for triclinic and monoclinic symmetry, there is also a single skew-symmetric component for each symmetry in four other rows of Table 4-2. These symmetries are $C_{\infty h}$, S_6, C_3, C_{4h}, S_4, C_4, C_{6h}, C_6, and C_{3h}. These skew-symmetric components for the bilinear forms in the spin Hamiltonian are believed to play a minor role, if any, in observed properties [6]. This point will be discussed further in Chapter 5. Similar behavior occurs for more complicated forms containing two or more of the vectors $\mathbf{H}$, $\mathbf{S}$, and $\mathbf{I}$ (T_h and T symmetries also produce such terms in general).

For orthorhombic symmetry (D_{2h}, D_2, C_{2v}) we see from Table 4-2 that three terms for each bilinear form and two for each quadratic form are required. In orthorhombic symmetry three orthogonal directions are determined uniquely (by the twofold axes and the reflection planes), and these are principal axes for all coupling tensors. Thus only the three independent diagonal elements are parameters for the bilinear forms, and no skew-symmetric components exist. The quadratic terms have only two diagonal elements because the sum of the squares of the components is a scalar. The form of the spin Hamiltonian for orthorhombic symmetry and for cases involving operators of the types HS, SI, and S^2 is

$$\mathcal{H} = \beta(g_x H_x S_x + g_y H_y S_y + g_z H_z S_z) + A_x S_x I_x + A_y S_y I_y + A_z S_z I_z$$
$$+ D[S_z^2 - \tfrac{1}{3}S(S+1)] + E(S_x^2 - S_y^2), \qquad (4\text{-}3)$$

a special case of Eq. (4-2). The two S^2 terms have been written in the conventional form, which is quite generally allowed since $S_x^2 + S_y^2 + S_z^2 = S(S+1)$ and terms producing uniform shifts in the energy are not included. The quantity $-\tfrac{1}{3}S(S+1)$ causes the "center of gravity" of the energy levels to be fixed. Since z has no special significance, it is possible to write the S^2 terms in Eq. (4-3) in the same form as shown but with the axes playing different roles. This can be seen from

$$D[S_z^2 - \tfrac{1}{3}S(S+1)] + E(S_x^2 - S_y^2)$$
$$= -\tfrac{1}{2}(D - 3E)[S_x^2 - \tfrac{1}{3}S(S+1)] - \tfrac{1}{2}(D+E)(S_y^2 - S_z^2)$$
$$= -\tfrac{1}{2}(D + 3E)[S_y^2 - \tfrac{1}{3}S(S+1)] + \tfrac{1}{2}(D-E)(S_z^2 - S_x^2). \qquad (4\text{-}4)$$

If both D and E are present in a spin Hamiltonian, it is often convenient to analyze the transformations of Eq. (4-4) and to choose a form for which one constant is as small as possible. Convenient approximations may then result (see Section 5–2).

If the symmetry is tetragonal (D_{4h}, D_4, C_{4v}, D_{2d}, C_{4h}, S_4, and C_4), one quadratic form and two bilinear forms are allowed, in addition to the skew-symmetric bilinear form allowed in C_{4h}, S_4, and C_4 symmetry. If the tetragonal axis is taken as the z axis, the correspondent of Eq. (4-3), ignoring any skew-symmetric terms, is now

$$\mathcal{H} = g_{\parallel}\beta H_z S_z + g_{\perp}\beta(H_x S_x + H_y S_y) + A S_z I_z + B(S_x I_x + S_y I_y)$$
$$+ D[S_z^2 - \tfrac{1}{3}S(S+1)]. \qquad (4\text{-}5)$$

A similar form is appropriate for the trigonal and hexagonal symmetries except that the z axis is then the threefold or sixfold axis, respectively. Axial symmetry ($D_{\infty h}$, $C_{\infty v}$, $C_{\infty h}$) also has this form.

For cubic symmetry (O_h, O, T_d, T_h, T) and spherical symmetry there are no quadratic forms and only one bilinear form. Thus the Hamiltonian corresponding to Eqs. (4-3) and (4-5) is

$$\mathcal{H} = g\beta \mathbf{H} \cdot \mathbf{S} + A \mathbf{S} \cdot \mathbf{I}. \qquad (4\text{-}6)$$

Two second-rank operators included in Eq. (4-2) are not present in Eqs. (4-3), (4-5), and (4-6). These are of the forms HI and I^2. The HI terms include at least the interaction of the nuclear magnetic dipole moment with the magnetic field and are often taken to be only this contribution,

$$\mathcal{H} = -g_n \beta_n \mathbf{H} \cdot \mathbf{I}, \qquad (4\text{-}7)$$

where the negative sign is present since it is not canceled by the negative charge of the electron, as in the case of electrons, and g_n is the nuclear g factor for free nuclei. However, the more general form found in Eq. (4-2) is allowed and is occasionally employed. The I^2 terms can be handled in the same way as were the S^2 terms.

The next most important terms in analyzing EPR spectra are the higher powers of components of **S**. They are now sufficiently complicated in general that we will discuss only the cases of highest symmetry. For spherical symmetry there are no S^4 or S^6 terms. For cubic symmetry there is one fourth-order term; this can be written down by inspection except for the constant part, which keeps the average energy constant:

$$\mathcal{H} = \tfrac{1}{6}a\{S_x^4 + S_y^4 + S_z^4 - \tfrac{1}{5}S(S+1)[3S(S+1)-1]\}. \tag{4-8}$$

The coefficient $\tfrac{1}{6}a$ is chosen to conform to the convention usually employed for iron transition-group ions. For rare-earth ions the conventions are not as definite or used as widely, and the reader is cautioned to check each author's conventions carefully when comparisons are made. Likewise in axial or hexagonal symmetry only one S^4 term appears. If the rotational axis is taken as z, then again we have by inspection an operator of the form S_z^4, which, including the convention for the coefficient usually employed for the iron group and adding quantities that keep the average energy constant, is written as

$$\mathcal{H} = \frac{1}{180} F[35S_z^4 - 30S(S+1)S_z^2 + 25S_z^2 - 6S(S+1) + 3S^2(S+1)^2]. \tag{4-9}$$

For D_{4h}, D_4, D_{4v}, and D_{2d} symmetries the quartic spin operators are the sum of Eqs. (4-8) and (4-9), where z is the tetragonal axis and x and y are determined by twofold axes or mirror planes. The result for D_{3d}, D_3, and C_{3v} symmetry is also a combination of Eqs. (4-8) and (4-9), but now z in Eq. (4-9) is taken as the threefold axis and the axes of the three Cartesian coordinates in Eq. (4-8) all make an angle of $\cos^{-1} 1/\sqrt{3}$ with z. Their orientations are determined by the twofold axes or mirror planes. Transforming Eq. (4-8) to a coordinate system with z along the trigonal axis and x and y perpendicular to it, we obtain the final spin Hamiltonian in the form

$$\mathcal{H} = \frac{1}{180}(F-a)[35S_z^4 - 30S(S+1)S_z^2 + 25S_z^2 - 6S(S+1) + 3S^2(S+1)^2]$$

$$+ \frac{a\sqrt{2}}{36}[S_z(S_+^3 + S_-^3) + (S_+^3 + S_-^3)S_z], \tag{4-10}$$

where $S_\pm = S_x \pm iS_y$.

As already mentioned, no sixth-order term appears in spherical symmetry (in fact, no terms having only electronic spin operators appear), but again one term occurs for O_h, O, and T_d symmetry (it is usually required only for the f^7 configuration such as is obtained for Eu^{2+} and Gd^{3+}). This term can be taken proportional to $S_x^6 + S_y^6 + S_z^6$ if it is realized that a shift of the average energy will result, as will splittings like those produced by the quartic term of Eq. (4-8). The term is not very useful in this form, and hence it is conventionally expressed in terms of irreducible tensor operators [7]:

$$\mathcal{H} = B_6(O_6^0 - 21O_6^4), \qquad (4\text{-}11)$$

where the operators O_6^0 and O_6^4 are listed in Table VIII, p. 254, of Hutchings [7], and in Table 16, p. 864, of Abragam and Bleaney [7]. The single axial term may be taken proportional to S_z^6, where z is the symmetry axis and the average energy is not fixed. Other fourth- and sixth-order spin operators have been tabulated as well [7].

The spin Hamiltonian terms which we have discussed so far, except the skew-symmetric bilinear forms, were introduced into the theory very early. More recently interest has been shown in the presence of other terms such as AB^3. No AB^3 terms can exist in spherical symmetry, but one such term occurs for O_h, O, and T_d symmetries. These terms can be written [8] [only HS^3 and S^3I are allowed by the limitations of Eq. (4-1)] as follows:

$$\mathcal{H} = u\beta\{H_xS_x^3 + H_yS_y^3 + H_zS_z^3 - \tfrac{1}{5}[3S(S+1)-1]\mathbf{H}\cdot\mathbf{S}\}$$
$$+ U\{I_xS_x^3 + I_yS_y^3 + I_zS_z^3 - \tfrac{1}{5}[3S(S+1)-1]\mathbf{I}\cdot\mathbf{S}\}. \qquad (4\text{-}12)$$

For the uncommon cubic symmetries T_h and T another HS^3 term is permitted; this has the form

$$\mathcal{H} \propto H_x[S_x(S_y^2 - S_z^2) + (S_y^2 - S_z^2)S_x] + H_y[S_y(S_z^2 - S_x^2) + (S_z^2 - S_x^2)S_y]$$
$$+ H_z[S_z(S_x^2 - S_y^2) + (S_x^2 - S_y^2)S_z]. \qquad (4\text{-}13)$$

For lower symmetries the results frequently become rather complicated. Expressions similar to Eq. (4-12) can be written for HS^5 and IS^5 terms.

In spherical symmetry we have encountered only AB terms so far. One A^2B^2 term is also allowed, which for S^2I^2 has the form of the quadrupole interaction studied in free atoms and ions [9]:

$$\mathcal{H} \propto 3(\mathbf{S}\cdot\mathbf{I})^2 + \tfrac{3}{2}\mathbf{S}\cdot\mathbf{I} - S^2I^2. \qquad (4\text{-}14)$$

For crystals terms of the type I^2 are usually referred to as the quadrupole interaction. Both I^2 and S^2I^2 terms may be proportional to the quadrupole moment of the nucleus. Again in lower symmetry many more complicated forms can occur for A^2B^2.

4–3 Calculation of the Spin Hamiltonian Using Perturbation Theory

In Chapter 8 we will apply the methods used in Section 4–2 to the description of paramagnetic entities under stress or in electric fields. However, the remaining chapters will typically use the spin Hamiltonian to provide an understanding of electron paramagnetic resonance. Before embarking on that goal we will discuss the coefficients of the operators in the spin Hamiltonian.

It is possible, at least in principle, to calculate the spin Hamiltonian, but the nature of such a calculation would vary from one system to the next. The method suggested in Section 4–2 is more general and quickly provides the experimentalist with a compact and convenient way of expressing his results, as well as yielding much insight into the methods of data analysis. However, in that approach we have no information about the magnitudes of the parameters in the spin Hamiltonian and it provides no insight into the physical mechanisms responsible for these parameters. We will now present a derivation of the spin Hamiltonian for a certain class of paramagnetic systems. Although both the form of the operators and the values of the parameters are obtained, this approach is difficult to generalize.

Abragam and Pryce [10, 11] introduced the spin Hamiltonian by a modified perturbation procedure for degenerate systems. The reader is referred to Pryce's article [10] for an elegant description of this technique. Our purpose here is to formulate the problem in a less elegant and less compact fashion but one which may be easier to understand because of its explicit detail.

In most elementary treatments of degenerate perturbation theory [12] the first step is to diagonalize the matrix of the perturbing Hamiltonian within the manifold of degenerate states. Sometimes the degeneracy is not removed in first order, and second-order removal is required. Following Pryce, we will remove the degeneracy by including first- and second-order effects on an equal footing (higher orders could also be included). This is important in the present case because it leads directly to the concept of the spin Hamiltonian and because the second-order effects are often comparable to the first-order ones.

Specifically we shall consider a system for which the unperturbed Hamiltonian, $\mathcal{H}_0$, consists of all of the kinetic energy and Coulomb interaction terms, including the crystal field. For incomplete d shells we discussed this problem briefly in Section 3–5. We wish to restrict ourselves further to a ground manifold of states with no orbital degeneracy. The degeneracy of the ground manifold is thus $2S+1$, and the spin is a good quantum number of $\mathcal{H}_0$, since no spin-dependent terms are included. The perturbing Hamiltonian will include all of the smaller terms in the total Hamiltonian, such as the spin-orbit interaction, and can be written in the form

$$\mathcal{H}_1 = \sum_\alpha F_\alpha T_\alpha, \tag{4-15}$$

where F_α is an operator which operates on spatial variables only, and T_α is an operator operating on spin variables only. That we have solved the spin-independent unperturbed problem can be expressed by

$$\mathcal{H}_0 \phi_n = E_n \phi_n, \tag{4-16}$$

where ϕ_n is a function of spatial variables only, and $n = 0$ designates the ground-state singlet whose associated spin degeneracy we wish to remove with the perturbation. The total wave function for one of the states of the unperturbed ground manifold is $\phi_0 \chi_j$, where the χ_j are the spin functions (we are discussing the actual spin here). If we further assume that the wave functions are made up entirely of wave functions of a single atomic term (so that the χ_j's are the only spin functions required), we can write the wave function for the perturbed system as

$$\psi = \sum_j a_j \phi_0 \chi_j + \sum_{n \neq 0} \sum_j b_{nj} \phi_n \chi_j. \tag{4-17}$$

Substituting Eq. (4-17) for ψ into the Schrödinger equation, we obtain

$$(\mathcal{H}_0 + \mathcal{H}_1 - E)(\sum_j a_j \phi_0 \chi_j + \sum_{n \neq 0} \sum_j b_{nj} \phi_n \chi_j) = 0, \tag{4-18}$$

or in a more useful form

$$\sum_j a_j (E_0 - E + \mathcal{H}_1) \phi_0 \chi_j + \sum_{n \neq 0} \sum_j b_{nj} (E_n - E + \mathcal{H}_1) \phi_n \chi_j = 0, \tag{4-19}$$

where $\mathcal{H}_1$ may be replaced by the expression in Eq. (4-15). Let us define two matrix elements as follows:

$$\langle n | F_\alpha | m \rangle \equiv \int \phi_n^* F_\alpha \phi_m \, d\tau,$$
$$\langle i | T_\alpha | j \rangle \equiv \int \chi_i^* T_\alpha \chi_j \, d\sigma, \tag{4-20}$$

where $\int d\tau$ is the integral over all spatial coordinates, and $\int d\sigma$ is the integral (sum) over all spin coordinates. Then, by multiplying Eq. (4-19) by $(\phi_0 \chi_i)^*$ and integrating over all variables, we have

$$\sum_j a_j [(E_0 - E)\delta_{ij} + \sum_\alpha \langle 0 | F_\alpha | 0 \rangle \langle i | T_\alpha | j \rangle]$$

$$+ \sum_{n \neq 0} \sum_j b_{nj} \sum_\alpha \langle 0 | F_\alpha | n \rangle \langle i | T_\alpha | j \rangle = 0. \tag{4-21}$$

Similarly, if we multiply by $(\phi_m \chi_i)^*$ and integrate over all variables, we have

$$\sum_j a_j \sum_\alpha \langle m|F_\alpha|0\rangle\langle i|T_\alpha|j\rangle + \sum_j b_{mj}(E_m - E)\delta_{ij}$$

$$+ \sum_{n\neq 0}\sum_j b_{nj}\sum_\alpha \langle m|F_\alpha|n\rangle\langle i|T_\alpha|j\rangle = 0 \qquad (m\neq 0). \qquad (4\text{-}22)$$

If we solve Eq. (4-22) to first order, we have

$$b_{mi} = -\sum_j a_j \sum_\alpha \frac{\langle m|F_\alpha|0\rangle}{E_m - E_0}\langle i|T_\alpha|j\rangle, \qquad (4\text{-}23)$$

where we replace E by E_0 in the denominator since any refinement would be of second order and above. Substituting Eq. (4-23) into Eq. (4-21), we obtain

$$\sum_j a_j [(E_0 - E)\delta_{ij} + \sum_\alpha \langle 0|F_\alpha|0\rangle\langle i|T_\alpha|j\rangle$$

$$-\sum_{\alpha,\alpha'}\sum_{n\neq 0}\frac{\langle 0|F_\alpha|n\rangle\langle n|F_{\alpha'}|0\rangle}{E_n - E_0}\sum_k \langle i|T_\alpha|k\rangle\langle k|T_{\alpha'}|j\rangle] = 0. \qquad (4\text{-}24)$$

We may make use of

$$\sum_k \langle i|T_\alpha|k\rangle\langle k|T_{\alpha'}|j\rangle = \langle i|T_\alpha T_{\alpha'}|j\rangle$$

and the convention of measuring the energy from E_0 to conclude that Eq. (4-24) will have nontrivial solutions for the a_i only if the operator $\mathcal{H}_s$ satisfies the eigenvalue equation

$$\mathcal{H}_s\chi = E\chi, \qquad (4\text{-}25)$$

where χ is a linear combination of the χ_i, and

$$\mathcal{H}_s = \sum_\alpha \langle 0|F_\alpha|0\rangle T_\alpha - \sum_{\alpha,\alpha'}\sum_{n\neq 0}\frac{\langle 0|F_\alpha|n\rangle\langle n|F_{\alpha'}|0\rangle}{E_n - E_0}T_\alpha T_{\alpha'}. \qquad (4\text{-}26)$$

The operator in Eq. (4-26) is called the spin Hamiltonian. It is possible to include still higher orders of perturbation theory in removing the degeneracy, and in this way we can obtain additional terms in the spin Hamiltonian, such as those involving the fourth power of the spin operators, as well as higher-order corrections to the parameters for existing operators.

Let us examine the form of the spin Hamiltonian of Eq. (4-26) if we consider the perturbing Hamiltonian:

$$\mathcal{H}_1 = \lambda\mathbf{L}\cdot\mathbf{S} + \beta(\mathbf{L} + g_e\mathbf{S})\cdot\mathbf{H}. \qquad (4\text{-}27)$$

Equation (4-27) contains the spin-orbit interaction in the form appropriate within a given term and the electronic Zeeman interaction. As we saw in

Chapter 3, the orbital functions are standing waves in crystals, and thus for singlet states

$$\langle 0|\mathbf{L}|0\rangle = 0, \tag{4-28}$$

just as for the one-electron example of Section 3–6. This is referred to as the quenching of the orbital angular momentum. Thus we have

$$\sum_\alpha \langle 0|F_\alpha|0\rangle T_\alpha = g_e\beta\mathbf{H}\cdot\mathbf{S}. \tag{4-29}$$

The terms of Eq. (4-27) involving $\mathbf{L}$ make the second-order contribution,

$$-\sum_{\alpha,\alpha'}\left[\sum_{n\neq 0}\frac{\langle 0|F_\alpha|n\rangle\langle n|F_{\alpha'}|0\rangle}{E_n-E_0}\right]T_\alpha T_{\alpha'} = -\sum_{\alpha,\alpha'}\left[\sum_{n\neq 0}\frac{\langle 0|L_\alpha|n\rangle\langle n|L_{\alpha'}|0\rangle}{E_n-E_0}\right]$$

$$(\lambda S_\alpha+\beta H_\alpha)(\lambda S_{\alpha'}+\beta H_{\alpha'}). \tag{4-30}$$

Defining the quantity $\Lambda_{\alpha\alpha'}=\Lambda_{\alpha'\alpha}$ by

$$\Lambda_{\alpha\alpha'}\equiv\sum_{n\neq 0}\frac{\langle 0|L_\alpha|n\rangle\langle n|L_{\alpha'}|0\rangle}{E_n-E_0}, \tag{4-31}$$

we may write

$$\mathcal{H}_S = -\lambda^2\sum_{\alpha,\alpha'}\Lambda_{\alpha\alpha'}S_\alpha S_{\alpha'}+\beta\sum_{\alpha,\alpha'}H_\alpha(g_e\delta_{\alpha\alpha'}-2\lambda\Lambda_{\alpha\alpha'})S_{\alpha'}-\beta^2\sum_{\alpha,\alpha'}\Lambda_{\alpha\alpha'}H_\alpha H_{\alpha'}. \tag{4-32}$$

We can see the relationship to the first two terms of the spin Hamiltonian of Eq. (4-2) except that now we have a way, at least in principle, to calculate the components of the coupling tensors. The last term of Eq. (4-32) is, of course, also allowed by the arguments leading to Eq. (4-2) but is normally not included, since it represents an equal shift of all energy levels and is therefore unobservable in electron paramagnetic resonance. It does, however, lead to the Van Vleck temperature-independent paramagnetism [13].

We could now take the expression for the *g* tensor given in Eq. (4-32) and apply it to the case of Section 3–6. The answer would be the same as we obtained there in Eq. (3-19). This illustrates the fact that the spin Hamiltonian operating on the effective spin functions and the true Hamiltonian operating on the true eigenfunctions give the same energy (recall that we modified the wave functions in Section 3–6 to first order in the spin-orbit interaction).

4–4 The Parameters in the Spin Hamiltonian

In Section 4–3 we indicated how to calculate a few of the parameters in the spin Hamiltonian in one of the simple limiting approximations which can be applied to incomplete *d*-shell ions in crystals. We should add that it is just as easy (in principle if not algebraically) to include several spin operators, for example, one or more nuclear spins. In this section we will consider in more detail the parameters in the spin Hamiltonian and the mechanisms for their existence.

The g tensor obtained in Eq. (4-32) for the ground manifold of an orbital singlet, assuming that the spin-orbit interaction is a perturbation and that L-S coupling is valid, has the form

$$g_{\alpha\alpha'} = g_e\delta_{\alpha\alpha'} - 2\lambda \sum_{n\neq 0} \frac{\langle 0|L_\alpha|n\rangle\langle n|L_{\alpha'}|0\rangle}{E_n - E_0}. \qquad (4\text{-}33)$$

Since λ is normally small compared to the appropriate values of $E_n - E_0$, we would expect the principal values of the g tensor to have the form

$$g_{x,y,z} = g_e - c\frac{\lambda}{\Delta E}, \qquad (4\text{-}34)$$

where ΔE is a typical energy separation and c is a constant which is usually in the range of 1 to 10. (If λ is large enough, perturbation theory carried only to second order may not be adequate [14].) Thus for such a system the g factor is near the free-spin value of 2.0023. Since $|\langle 0|L_\alpha|n\rangle|^2/(E_n - E_0) > 0$, we find that the g shift, $g - g_e$, is less than zero for a paramagnetic ion whose unfilled shell is less than half full (since λ is then positive). The g shift is correspondingly positive if the shell is more than half full. These comments should not be generalized uncritically to more complicated paramagnets.

Although such orbital singlets are common enough to justify emphasizing their properties, we considered in Section 3–7 a case which displays drastically different g values. In that case the spin-orbit interaction is not a perturbation but the crystalline field is.

Contributions to the g factors may be made by other terms in the Hamiltonian or by effects not completely described by crystal-field theory. An example is the configuration interaction occurring in covalent crystals [15]. Watanabe [15] not only has explained many situations involving large positive g shifts for $^6S_{5/2}$-state ions in covalent systems (and $^2S_{1/2}$ ions as well), but also has suggested the reason for the large cubic fine structure constant, a, which accompanies the large g shift. The explanation involves admixture into the d^5 ground configuration of a configuration with six d electrons and a hole on the ligands.

As we have shown, the spin-orbit interaction is very important in determining g factors. So far in this chapter we have used expressions for the spin-orbit interaction which apply to free atoms and ions, that is, to cases of spherical symmetry. We noted in Section 1–2 that in a crystal, since the symmetry is lower, the spin-orbit interaction no longer has its simple form, $\lambda\mathbf{L}\cdot\mathbf{S}$. For that matter angular momentum is of only approximate utility. The effects are exaggerated for covalent systems. Such modifications have been considered by several authors [6, 16].

The principal values for **D** are related to **g**, as predicted by Eq. (4-32). They are as follows:

$$D_{\alpha\alpha} = -\lambda^2 \sum_{n \neq 0} \frac{|\langle 0|L_\alpha|n\rangle|^2}{E_n - E_0}, \tag{4-35}$$

where α denotes a principal axis. The components of **D** have the form

$$D = -\frac{c}{2} \frac{\lambda^2}{\Delta E}, \tag{4-36}$$

where c, λ, and ΔE have the same values as in Eq. (4-34) for the corresponding g factor. In the usual definition of the elements of **D** we have

$$\sum_\alpha D_{\alpha\alpha} = 0. \tag{4-37}$$

Hence Eq. (4-36) should be modified to account for this. Nevertheless we see that relationships would exist between the elements of **D** and **g**.

Hyperfine structure arises from the electromagnetic interaction of the nucleus with its environment [17]. It is convenient to make a multipole expansion of the interaction of the nucleus with the electromagnetic field due to its surroundings. Aside from its charge or electric monopole moment, a nucleus may have a magnetic dipole moment, an electric quadrupole moment, and a magnetic octupole moment. The electric dipole moment, magnetic quadrupole moment, and so on are not observed, presumably because of parity invariance of the nucleus. Higher-order moments, if they occur, would produce only small effects.

The nuclear magnetic dipole moment interacts with the net local magnetic field. This includes any applied magnetic field, the magnetic field from the orbital motion of each electron, and the magnetic field produced by each electron's spin. The term in the Hamiltonian describing the interaction with an external field is given in Eq. (4-7). The same term occurs or is assumed to occur in most spin Hamiltonians.

The classical expression for the magnetic field at the nucleus arising from orbital motion is

$$\mathbf{H} = 2\pi \frac{\mathbf{r} \times \mathbf{i}}{r^2}, \tag{4-38}$$

where $\mathbf{i} = -(e/c)(\mathbf{v}/2\pi r)$. Thus we have

$$\mathbf{H} = -\frac{e}{c} \frac{\mathbf{r} \times \mathbf{v}}{r^3} = -\frac{eh}{mc} \frac{\mathbf{l}}{r^3} = -2\beta \frac{\mathbf{l}}{r^3}. \tag{4-39}$$

If we now replace **H** by the quantum-mechanical operator, we obtain

$$\mathbf{H} = -2\beta r^{-3}\mathbf{l} \tag{4-40}$$

or

$$\mathcal{H} = -g_n\beta_n\mathbf{H}\cdot\mathbf{I} = 2\beta g_n\beta_n r^{-3}\mathbf{l}\cdot\mathbf{I}. \tag{4-41}$$

For the interaction with the electron spin we use the dipole-dipole interaction:

$$\mathcal{H} = \frac{\boldsymbol{\mu}_n\cdot\boldsymbol{\mu}}{r^3} - 3\frac{(\boldsymbol{\mu}_n\cdot\mathbf{r})(\boldsymbol{\mu}\cdot\mathbf{r})}{r^5}, \tag{4-42}$$

where the electronic magnetic dipole moment operator is

$$\boldsymbol{\mu} = -g_e\beta\mathbf{s}, \tag{4-43}$$

and the nuclear magnetic moment operator is

$$\boldsymbol{\mu}_n = g_n\beta_n\mathbf{I}. \tag{4-44}$$

Thus we obtain

$$\mathcal{H} = -g_e\beta g_n\beta_n r^{-3}[\mathbf{I}\cdot\mathbf{s} - 3(\mathbf{I}\cdot\hat{\mathbf{r}})(\mathbf{s}\cdot\hat{\mathbf{r}})], \tag{4-45}$$

where $\hat{\mathbf{r}}$ is a unit vector in the direction of **r**. This interaction vanishes if the electron has a spherical charge density centered on the nucleus. In that case the integral over angular coordinates is zero. Nevertheless even then there is a hyperfine interaction.

All s electrons have a nonzero density at the nucleus, and this density is essentially constant throughout the small volume of the nucleus. Hence the nucleus is in a uniformly magnetized medium. This magnetization is

$$\mathbf{M} = -g_e\beta|\psi(0)|^2\mathbf{s}. \tag{4-46}$$

If we now calculate the field resulting from this magnetization and calculate the energy of a nuclear magnetic dipole in this field, we obtain the Fermi contact interaction [18]

$$\mathcal{H} = -\frac{8\pi}{3}\mathbf{M}\cdot\boldsymbol{\mu}_n = \frac{8\pi}{3}g_e\beta g_n\beta_n|\psi(0)|^2\mathbf{I}\cdot\mathbf{s}. \tag{4-47}$$

Equations (4-41), (4-45), and (4-47) involve individual electronic orbital and spin angular momenta. Adding the three equations, summing over all electrons, and integrating over r gives

$$\mathcal{H} = 2\beta g_n\beta_n\langle r^{-3}\rangle\mathbf{L}\cdot\mathbf{I} + g_e\beta g_n\beta_n\langle r^{-3}\rangle\xi[L(L+1)\mathbf{I}\cdot\mathbf{S} - \tfrac{3}{2}(\mathbf{L}\cdot\mathbf{I})(\mathbf{L}\cdot\mathbf{S})$$

$$- \tfrac{3}{2}(\mathbf{L}\cdot\mathbf{S})(\mathbf{L}\cdot\mathbf{I})] + \frac{8\pi}{3}g_e\beta g_n\beta_n|\psi(0)|^2\mathbf{I}\cdot\mathbf{S} \tag{4-48}$$

for the hyperfine interaction with nucleus of an atom or ion with a single open shell of electrons and a single *L-S* coupling term, where

$$\xi = \frac{2l+1-4S}{S(2l-1)(2l+3)(2L-1)} \tag{4-49}$$

and where core polarization has not been included [a serious deficiency for transition-group ions; see reference 19 and the discussion after Eq. (4-50)]. The unit vectors $\hat{\mathbf{r}}$ have been replaced everywhere by $\mathbf{L}$ in the spirit of the Wigner-Eckart theorem since matrix elements will be calculated within a manifold of states with fixed L.

This expression for the hyperfine interaction can then be incorporated into a second- or higher-order degenerate perturbation theory calculation to obtain the spin Hamiltonian constants in $\mathbf{A}$. The spin-orbit coupling is also required, as may be magnetic interactions among electrons. For the special case of an ion with an orbital singlet ground state with the first excited state so high in energy that it does not contribute, the hyperfine interaction with the nucleus of the ion is given by

$$\mathcal{H} = g_e\beta g_n\beta_n\langle r^{-3}\rangle\xi[L(L+1)\mathbf{I}\cdot\mathbf{S} - 3\langle L_z^2\rangle I_zS_z - 3\langle L_x^2\rangle I_xS_x - 3\langle L_y^2\rangle I_yS_y$$

$$- \tfrac{3}{2}\langle L_xL_y+L_yL_x\rangle(I_xS_y+I_yS_x) - \tfrac{3}{2}\langle L_yL_z+L_zL_y\rangle(I_yS_z+I_zS_y)$$

$$- \tfrac{3}{2}\langle L_zL_x+L_xL_z\rangle(I_zS_x+I_xS_z)] + \frac{8\pi}{3}g_e\beta g_n\beta_n|\psi(0)|^2\mathbf{I}\cdot\mathbf{S}. \tag{4-50}$$

This will then appear in the spin Hamiltonian. Note that only symmetric hyperfine tensor components result. The first term is present only if the free-ion orbital angular momentum is not zero and if the symmetry is lower than cubic. The second term is present only if the unfilled shell is an *s* shell (and hence $L=0$).

An interesting situation occurs if a state with $L=0$ arising from *p*, *d*, or *f* electrons is lowest, such as Mn^{2+} or Eu^{2+}. Our analysis would predict no hyperfine interaction, and yet one is observed. It arises because of the fact that $\Sigma_i|\psi_i(0)|^2\mathbf{s}_i$ is not zero. This can be regarded as a consequence of configuration interaction with configurations having unpaired *s* electrons, or equivalently as due to a difference in the spatial wave functions of electrons which differ only in their spin orientation. The latter phenomenon is termed core polarization and results naturally from an unrestricted Hartree-Fock calculation.

The analysis given above applies to a paramagnetic ion in a crystalline environment. We have in fact assumed that the electronic orbitals remain basically unaltered, and hence the angular momentum appears frequently throughout. The same interactions, however, exist for paramagnets which do not satisfy these conditions, such as those with multicenter orbitals or with hyperfine interaction with nuclei in the crystal. It may be necessary to generalize the spatial part of the operator in these cases.

The electric quadrupole interaction, which has been discussed in detail by Bleaney [20], can be written as

$$\mathcal{K} = \frac{e^2 Q}{2I(2I-1)} r^{-3}[I(I+1)-3(\hat{\mathbf{r}}\cdot\mathbf{I})^2] \qquad (4\text{-}51)$$

for a single electron. For an ion with one open shell and a single *L-S* coupling term the quadrupole interaction with the central nucleus results by application of the Wigner-Eckart theorem to Eq. (4-51), yielding

$$\mathcal{K} = \pm\frac{e^2 Q}{2I(2I-1)}\langle r^{-3}\rangle 2S\xi[3(\mathbf{L}\cdot\mathbf{I})^2+\tfrac{3}{2}\mathbf{L}\cdot\mathbf{I}-L(L+1)I(I+1)], \quad (4\text{-}52)$$

where ξ is given by Eq. (4-49) and the plus and minus signs refer to shells less than and more than half full, respectively. As with the magnetic dipole hyperfine interaction the term in Eq. (4-52) must be treated in perturbation theory in a manner similar to that used in Section 4–3. Again a simple case is that for an orbital singlet with all excited states so high in energy that they can be ignored. Then the quadrupole interaction is given by

$$\mathcal{K} = \pm\frac{e^2 Q}{2I(2I-1)}\langle r^{-3}\rangle 2S\xi[3\langle L_x^2\rangle I_x^2+3\langle L_y^2\rangle I_y^2+3\langle L_z^2\rangle I_z^2$$

$$+\tfrac{3}{2}\langle L_xL_y+L_yL_x\rangle(I_xI_y+I_yI_x)+\tfrac{3}{2}\langle L_yL_z+L_zL_y\rangle(I_yI_z+I_zI_y)$$

$$+\tfrac{3}{2}\langle L_zL_x+L_xL_z\rangle(I_zI_x+I_xI_z)-L(L+1)I(I+1)], \qquad (4\text{-}53)$$

and this is the appropriate operator in the spin Hamiltonian. If the symmetry is lower than cubic and $L\neq 0$, this term will be nonzero.

4–5 Supplemental Bibliography

There do not seem to be any references that give a detailed description of both the physical origin and the limitations of symmetry on the spin Hamiltonian. Listed below are documents which discuss at least one of these two aspects in some detail. The first three discuss the physical origin and the calculation of the spin Hamiltonian. Following these is a chronological listing of eleven journal references on the formulation of the spin Hamiltonian using symmetry arguments (usually group theory). Although the details differ, the treatments are fundamentally similar (if in fact a spin Hamiltonian is the end product and not some other—although equivalent—effective Hamiltonian).

1. A. Abragam and B. Bleaney, *Electron Paramagnetic Resonance of Transition Ions*, Oxford, New York, 1970.

2. J. W. Orton, *Electron Paramagnetic Resonance, an Introduction to Transition Group Ions in Crystals*, Gordon and Breach, New York, 1968.

3. B. Bleaney, "Hyperfine Structure and Electron Paramagnetic Resonance," in *Hyperfine Interactions* (A. J. Freeman and R. B. Frankel, eds.), Academic, New York, 1967, p. 1.

4. J. M. Luttinger, *Phys. Rev.* **102**, 1030 (1956). Although the subject of this paper is cyclotron resonance of holes in semiconductors, the method and some of the results apply directly to the spin Hamiltonian.

5. G. F. Koster and H. Statz, *Phys. Rev.* **113**, 445 (1959). The effective Hamiltonian that results from this analysis is not a spin Hamiltonian.

6. H. Statz and G. F. Koster, *Phys. Rev.* **115**, 1568 (1959). More on the method developed in reference 5.

7. J. S. Griffith, *Mol. Phys.* **3**, 79 (1960).

8. F. K. Kneubühl, *Phys. Kond. Mat.* **1**, 410 (1963).

9. W. J. C. Grant and M. W. P. Strandberg, *J. Phys. Chem. Solids* **25**, 635 (1964).

10. T. Ray, *Proc. Roy. Soc. (London)* **A277**, 76 (1964).

11. Huang Wu-Han, Lin Fu-Cheng, and Zhu Ji-Kang, *Proc. Phys. Soc.* **84**, 661 (1964).

12. F. K. Kneubühl, *Phys. Kond. Mat.* **4**, 50 (1965).

13. A. Bieri and F. K. Kneubühl, *Phys. Kond. Mat.* **4**, 230 (1965).

14. S. Geschwind, "Special Topics in Hyperfine Structure in EPR," in *Hyperfine Interactions* (A. J. Freeman and R. B. Frankel, eds.), Academic, New York, 1967, p. 251.

References Cited in Chapter 4

[1] See Section 8–3 of this book and the following: J. S. Griffith, *Phys. Rev.* **132**, 316 (1963); K. A. Müller, *Phys. Rev.* **171**, 350 (1968); S. Washimiya, K. Shinagawa, and S. Sugano, *Phys. Rev.* **B1**, 2976 (1970).
[2] E. Merzbacher, *Quantum Mechanics*, 2nd ed., Wiley, New York, 1970, p. 392.
[3] C. P. Slichter, *Principles of Magnetic Resonance*, Harper and Row, New York, 1963, p. 164; A. Abragam and B. Bleaney, *Electron Paramagnetic Resonance of Transition Ions*, Oxford, New York, 1970, p. 624; M. Tinkham, *Group Theory and Quantum Mechanics*, McGraw-Hill, New York, 1964, p. 126.
[4] G. F. Koster, J. O. Dimmock, R. G. Wheeler, and H. Statz, *Properties of the Thirty-Two Point Groups*, M.I.T., Cambridge, Mass., 1963.
[5] M. Tinkham, *Group Theory and Quantum Mechanics*, McGraw-Hill, New York, 1964, p. 54; G. Weinreich, *Solids: Elementary Theory for Advanced Students*, Wiley, New York, 1965, p. 20.

[6] F. S. Ham, *J. Phys. Chem. Solids* **24**, 1165 (1963).

[7] M. T. Hutchings, "Point-Charge Calculations of Energy Levels of Magnetic Ions in Crystalline Electric Fields," in *Solid State Physics*, (F. Seitz and D. Turnbull, eds.), Academic, New York, 1964, Vol. 16, p. 227; A. Abragam and B. Bleaney, *Electron Paramagnetic Resonance of Transition Ions*, Oxford, New York, 1970, p. 147.

[8] F. S. Ham, G. W. Ludwig, G. D. Watkins, and H. H. Woodbury, *Phys. Rev. Letters* **5**, 468 (1960).

[9] N. F. Ramsey, *Molecular Beams*, Oxford, 1956, p. 421.

[10] M. H. L. Pryce, *Proc. Phys. Soc. (London)* A**63**, 25 (1950).

[11] A. Abragam and M. H. L. Pryce, *Proc. Roy. Soc. (London)* A**205**, 135 (1951).

[12] E. Merzbacher, *Quantum Mechanics*, 2nd ed., Wiley, New York, 1970, p. 425; R. H. Dicke and J. P. Wittke, *Introduction to Quantum Mechanics*, Addison-Wesley, Reading, Mass., 1960, p. 231.

[13] D. H. Martin, *Magnetism in Solids*, Iliffe, London, 1967, p. 190.

[14] For a discussion of the third-order contributions to **g** see H. H. Tippins, *Phys. Rev.* **160**, 343 (1967).

[15] H. Watanabe, *J. Phys. Chem. Solids* **25**, 1471 (1964).

[16] C. P. Slichter, *Principles of Magnetic Resonance*, Harper and Row, New York, 1963, p. 195; F. K. Kneubühl, *Phys. Kond. Mat.* **1**, 410 (1963); A. A. Misetich and T. Buch, *J. Chem. Phys.* **41**, 2524 (1964).

[17] An excellent reference on hyperfine structure is *Hyperfine Interactions* (A. J. Freeman and R. B. Frankel, eds.), Academic, New York, 1967; especially the first article by B. Bleaney and the sixth by S. Geschwind.

[18] G. T. Rado, *Am. J. Phys.* **30**, 716 (1962).

[19] A. Abragam and B. Bleaney, *Electron Paramagnetic Resonance of Transition Ions*, Oxford, New York, 1970, p. 410.

[20] B. Bleaney, "Hyperfine Structure and Electron Paramagnetic Resonance," in *Hyperfine Interactions* (A. J. Freeman and R. B. Frankel, eds.), Academic, New York, 1967, p. 14.

CHAPTER 5

Electron Paramagnetic Resonance Spectra

Our purpose will now be to take the appropriate spin Hamiltonian, as obtained in Chapter 4, to solve for the energies and the intensities of the magnetic dipole transitions, and thus to deduce the nature of the electron paramagnetic resonance spectra that may occur. The detailed methods of solution are numerous, partly because a great variety is possible in spin Hamiltonians, and partly because different approximations are valid for different relative magnitudes of the parameters even for a unique spin Hamiltonian. We will usually employ a very quick and simple method, and normally we will not go beyond first order in perturbation calculations. The actual analysis of spectra will often require second- or third-order terms or even exact solutions. Obviously the results are then much more complicated, but only rarely is much of physical significance added. Therefore we will ignore these "real-situation" difficulties.

5–1 Zeeman Splitting

The second term in Eq. (4-2) is the most general form of the operator linear in **H** and **S**, what we may consider as the effective Zeeman interaction. At the outset we will ignore any possible skew-symmetric components of the g tensor but will otherwise consider a general case. The spin Hamiltonian

$$\mathcal{H} = \beta \mathbf{H} \cdot \mathbf{g} \cdot \mathbf{S} \tag{5-1}$$

is the inner product of the vector $\beta \mathbf{H} \cdot \mathbf{g}$ and the vector operator **S**. If we take the ζ axis to be in the direction of the vector $\beta \mathbf{H} \cdot \mathbf{g}$, then the spin Hamiltonian of Eq. (5-1) can be written as

$$\mathcal{H} = \beta |\mathbf{H} \cdot \mathbf{g}| S_\zeta . \tag{5-2}$$

The energy follows immediately and is

$$E = \beta |\mathbf{H} \cdot \mathbf{g}| M_S , \tag{5-3}$$

where M_S is the azimuthal or magnetic quantum number referred to the ζ axis and varies from $-S$ to S with unit intervals.

It is more conventional to rewrite Eq. (5-3) in terms of the three principal values of the g tensor (see Section 4–2) and the direction cosines of **H** with respect to the three principal axes. We denote the principal axes by x, y, and z and the direction cosines as l, m, and n, respectively. Thus, in terms of components along x, y, and z, we have

$$\mathbf{H} = (l, m, n)H, \tag{5-4}$$

$$\mathbf{g} = \begin{pmatrix} g_x & 0 & 0 \\ 0 & g_y & 0 \\ 0 & 0 & g_z \end{pmatrix}, \tag{5-5}$$

so that we obtain

$$\mathbf{H} \cdot \mathbf{g} = (g_x l, g_y m, g_z n)H, \tag{5-6}$$

and hence

$$E = \beta H \sqrt{g_x^2 l^2 + g_y^2 m^2 + g_z^2 n^2}\, M_S \equiv g\beta H M_S. \tag{5-7}$$

One of the advantages of Eq. (5-3) is that it is valid no matter what coordinate system is chosen to describe the components of **H** and **g**, thus leaving one free to choose the simplest alternative, as was done for Eq. (5-5). In this way some of the problems of tedious transformations are avoided.

As we indicated in many ways in Chapter 2, electron paramagnetic resonance occurs when an oscillating (or rotating) magnetic field induces transitions between the stationary states of the spin system (see especially Sections 2–3 and 5–4). Usually the direction of the oscillating magnetic field, $\mathbf{H}_1$, is perpendicular to the static field, or at least not parallel to it. For the present problem, using the Hamiltonian of Eq. (5-1) to describe the interaction with $\mathbf{H}_1$, ξ and η components of the spin would occur, not just the ζ component as in Eq. (5-2) for the static field [ξ, η, and ζ form a right-handed coordinate system with ζ defined by Eq. (5-2)]. The matrix elements of S_ξ and S_η are linearly related to those of S_+ and S_-, as we see in Appendix A, and thus we expect transitions between states differing in M_S by one unit. Setting this energy difference equal to $h\nu$, we have

$$h\nu = \Delta E = g\beta H \tag{5-8}$$

or

$$H = \frac{h\nu}{g\beta}. \tag{5-9}$$

But in contrast to the isotropic analog in Eq. (2-84), we have an anisotropic g factor,

$$g = \sqrt{g_x^2 l^2 + g_y^2 m^2 + g_z^2 n^2}. \tag{5-10}$$

As implied by Eq. (5-9), the most convenient way to obtain spectra is to hold the frequency v fixed and to vary the magnetic field, searching for the resonances. The anisotropy of the field in Eq. (5-9) at which the resonance is observed is related to the anisotropy of the g value.

For triclinic symmetry the g factor is as given by Eq. (5-10), and all three principal axes are unrelated to any axes of the crystal or the imperfection (there are no axes determined by symmetry). The form given in Eq. (5-10) is also appropriate for monoclinic and orthorhombic symmetry, although now some relationships will exist between the symmetry axes of the imperfections and the principal axes (see the discussion of the spin Hamiltonian in Section 4–2). For symmetries which are axial, hexagonal, tetragonal, or trigonal we have two identical principal values, denoted by $g_\perp$, and only one direction cosine is required, $\cos \theta$, where θ is the angle between the field and the axis of symmetry. The third principal value is

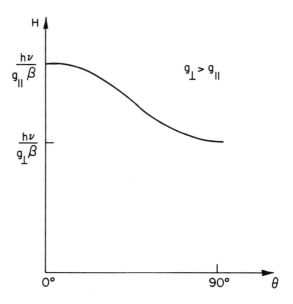

FIG. 5-1   The value of the magnetic field at resonance for a paramagnet with hexagonal, trigonal, tetragonal, or axial symmetry. The angle θ is the angle between the magnetic field and the axis. The particular case in which $g_\perp > g_\parallel$ is shown, and no terms other than the effective Zeeman interaction are included in the spin Hamiltonian.

denoted by $g_{\parallel}$, and the g factor can then be written as

$$g = \sqrt{g_{\parallel}^2 \cos^2 \theta + g_{\perp}^2 \sin^2 \theta}. \qquad (5\text{-}11)$$

In Figure 5-1 we show the expected angular dependence of the magnetic field at resonance for an ion described by Eqs. (5-9) and (5-11). In some cases the imperfection has a lower point symmetry than the crystalline site, and hence several equivalent orientations are possible (equivalent in the sense that symmetry operations carrying the perfect crystal into an identical crystal will carry these orientations into each other). If an imperfection has tetragonal or trigonal symmetry and occurs in a cubic crystal, several different but equivalent orientations of the symmetry axis exist. As an example we illustrate the result for an axial g factor in cubic symmetry where the axis is taken along one of the $\langle 100 \rangle$ cubic axes. Usually all three axes will be equally likely to be involved for any given imperfection, so that on averaging over a crystal one finds all three possible lines to be equal in intensity. This is illustrated by the angular dependence in Fig. 5-2, where the angle is measured between the field and one of the $\langle 100 \rangle$ axes and where the magnetic field is confined to a $\{110\}$ plane.

Finally, in cubic or spherical symmetry the g factor is isotropic, although certainly not necessarily equal to the free-electron value of 2.0023.

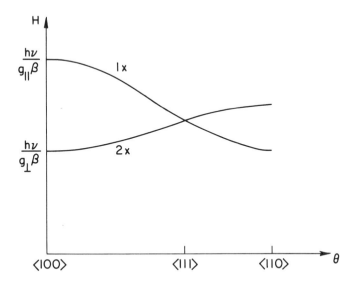

FIG. 5-2   The magnetic field at resonance for tetragonal paramagnets aligned along the fourfold axes in a cubic crystal. The field is in a $\{110\}$ plane. Two of the three superimposed spectra are coincident for such orientations and are indicated by $2\times$. The case in which $g_{\perp} > g_{\parallel}$ is shown.

Writing the spin Hamiltonian of Eq. (5-1) in the form of Eq. (5-2) has been an easy and elegant way to discuss the results so far in this section. It involves making a choice of the coordinate system such that the ζ axis is along $\mathbf{H} \cdot \mathbf{g}$. Three natural coordinate systems occur for this term in the spin Hamiltonian, and each of them is useful under certain circumstances. The other two coordinate systems are the principal axis system of the g tensor and one in which an axis is taken along $\mathbf{H}$ instead of $\mathbf{H} \cdot \mathbf{g}$. As already implied in Eq. (4-2), the principal axis system leads to a spin Hamiltonian of the form

$$\mathcal{H} = \beta(g_x H_x S_x + g_y H_y S_y + g_z H_z S_z), \tag{5-12}$$

which for axial symmetry is conveniently written as

$$\mathcal{H} = g_{\parallel}\beta H_z S_z + \tfrac{1}{2} g_{\perp}\beta(H_+ S_- + H_- S_+). \tag{5-13}$$

The quantities $H_{\pm}$ are defined analogously to $S_{\pm}$ (see Appendix A) as $H_{\pm} \equiv H_x \pm i H_y$, and z is the axis of symmetry.

The axes of the third natural coordinate system will be designated by indices 1, 2, and 3 with axis 3 taken as the direction of $\mathbf{H}$. If we carry out the required transformation from xyz to 123, we obtain for Eq. (5-13) (i.e., axial g tensor)

$$\mathcal{H} = \beta H[(g_{\parallel}\cos^2\theta + g_{\perp}\sin^2\theta)S_3 + \tfrac{1}{2}(g_{\parallel}-g_{\perp})\sin\theta\cos\theta(S_+ e^{-i\phi} + S_- e^{i\phi})], \tag{5-14}$$

where now $S_{\pm} = S_1 \pm i S_2$, and the particular value chosen for ϕ depends on the choice of axes 1 and 2. The angle θ is of course the angle of $\mathbf{H}$ with respect to the z axis.

Up until now in this section we have been considering only symmetric components of the g tensor. However, as we discussed in Section 4–2, symmetry allows skew-symmetric components in some cases, components which are zero according to the calculation of Section 4–3 but which could conceivably be nonzero for cases where the many approximations of Section 4–3 are not all applicable. Even with skew-symmetric components included, the analysis leading to Eqs. (5-2) and (5-3) is correct. The difference is that the g tensor of Eq. (5-5) can be written only as

$$\mathbf{g} = \begin{pmatrix} g_x & g_{xy} & g_{xz} \\ -g_{xy} & g_y & g_{yz} \\ -g_{xz} & -g_{yz} & g_z \end{pmatrix}, \tag{5-15}$$

where x, y, z are the principal axes for the symmetric components, and the three possible skew-symmetric components appear. The effect of this when $|\mathbf{H} \cdot \mathbf{g}|$ is calculated is to give the square root of a quadratic form in l, m, n but one not in its principal axis form. By a rotation of coordinates it is then possible to write this quadratic form in a principal axis system. The result will resemble Eq. (5-7) for the principal axis system of the symmetric components. Any axis determined by symmetry will be unchanged in this rotation of coordinates. Thus we may safely ignore the skew-symmetric components for the spin Hamiltonian of Eq. (5-1) since we cannot easily separate their existence from changes in the symmetric components and their principal axes. (For a possible way to observe them see [1].)

A rather different term proportional to H (i.e., an HS^3 term) is represented by the first part of Eq. (4-12). If such terms are small compared to HS terms, we may consider only the first-order effects. We will use an approach which will be worked out in more detail at the beginning of Section 5–2 for the simpler case of S^2 terms. Generally the part of the Hamiltonian which contains all HS^3 terms has the form

$$\mathcal{H} = \sum_{i,j,k,l} \beta u_{ijkl} H_i S_j S_k S_l, \tag{5-16}$$

where the indices $i, j, k,$ and l are summed over three Cartesian coordinates. In this form the particular coordinate system is unspecified. The first-order contribution comes from the term in this sum containing the spin irreducible tensor operator with $m = 0$, using a ζ axis along $\mathbf{H} \cdot \mathbf{g}$. If 3 is the label for the axis parallel to $\mathbf{H}$, then this first-order term is

$$\mathcal{H} = \tfrac{5}{2} \beta u_{3\zeta\zeta\zeta} H(S_\zeta^3 - \tfrac{3}{5} \mathbf{S}^2 S_\zeta + \tfrac{1}{5} S_\zeta). \tag{5-17}$$

The energy and magnetic field are then given to first order by [including Eq. (5-3)]

$$\begin{aligned} E &= \beta |\mathbf{H} \cdot \mathbf{g}| M_S + \tfrac{5}{2} \beta u_{3\zeta\zeta\zeta} H[M_S^3 - \tfrac{3}{5} S(S+1) M_S + \tfrac{1}{5} M_S] \\ H &= \frac{h\nu}{g\beta} \left\{ 1 - \frac{5}{2} \frac{u_{3\zeta\zeta\zeta}}{g} [3M_S^2 - 3M_S - \tfrac{3}{5} S(S+1) + \tfrac{6}{5}] \right\} \end{aligned} \tag{5-18}$$

for the $M_S \rightleftharpoons M_S - 1$ transition.

To be more specific we will consider the first term in Eq. (4-12). Since this applies in O_h, O, and T_d symmetry, the g factor is isotropic and axes 3 and ζ are identical. We may then write

$$u_{\zeta\zeta\zeta\zeta} = \frac{1}{H^4} \sum_{i,j,k,l} u_{ijkl} H_i H_j H_k H_l. \tag{5-19}$$

We can obtain the elements u_{ijkl} in terms of x, y, and z (the cubic axes) by inspection of the Hamiltonian of Eq. (4-12), which is rewritten as

$$\mathcal{H} = u\beta(H_x S_x^3 + H_y S_y^3 + H_z S_z^3 - \tfrac{3}{5} \mathbf{H} \cdot \mathbf{S} S^2 + \tfrac{1}{5} \mathbf{H} \cdot \mathbf{S}). \tag{5-20}$$

Keeping in mind that

$$\mathbf{H} \cdot \mathbf{SS}^2 = H_x S_x^3 + H_y S_y^3 + H_z S_z^3 + H_x S_x (S_y^2 + S_z^2)$$
$$+ H_y S_y (S_z^2 + S_x^2) + H_z S_z (S_x^2 + S_y^2), \tag{5-21}$$

we find

$$u_{ijkl} = \begin{cases} \frac{2}{5}u, & i = j = k = l, \\ -\frac{3}{5}u, & i = j \neq k = l. \end{cases} \tag{5-22}$$

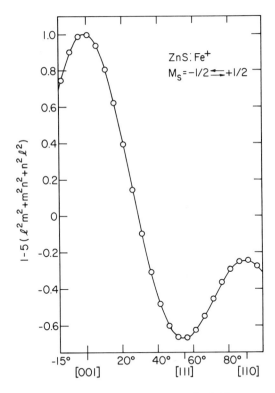

FIG. 5-3 The angular dependence of the magnetic field at resonance for Fe^+ in cubic ZnS [3]. The observed values of the field are shown by the circles, and the calculated angular dependence obtained from Eqs. (5-18) and (5-23) is given by the solid line. In order to convert from the relative scale of the ordinate to magnetic field, it is necessary to use the parameters $u = -0.00565(5)$ and $g = 2.2515(5)$ and to know the frequency. This angular dependence is typical of all cubic paramagnets containing in their spin Hamiltonians measurable terms of the type HS^3.

Combining this with $\mathbf{H} = H(l, m, n)$ expressed in the cubic axis system, we obtain from Eq. (5-19)

$$u_{\zeta\zeta\zeta\zeta} = \tfrac{2}{5}u(l^4 + m^4 + n^4) - \tfrac{6}{5}u(l^2m^2 + m^2n^2 + n^2l^2)$$

$$= \tfrac{2}{5}u[1 - 5(l^2m^2 + m^2n^2 + n^2l^2)]. \tag{5-23}$$

Substituting Eq. (5-23) into Eq. (5-18) gives the result observed for O_h and T_d symmetry [2]. An example, Fe^+ in ZnS, is shown in Fig. 5-3 [3]. This angular dependence is encountered again in the case of quartic fine structure [see Eq. (5-52)].

It is possible to obtain exact solutions for the energies if the Hamiltonian has the form we have just analyzed, that is,

$$\mathcal{H} = g\beta\mathbf{H}\cdot\mathbf{S} + u\beta\{H_xS_x^3 + H_yS_y^3 + H_zS_z^3 - \tfrac{1}{5}[3S(S+1) - 1]\mathbf{H}\cdot\mathbf{S}\}. \tag{5-24}$$

The resultant equations are rather complicated, particularly if expressed in terms of the parameters g and u [4].

5–2 Fine Structure

The Zeeman interaction considered in Section 5–1 is the essential part of the Hamiltonian of a paramagnet. However, the structure which can occur, and which is classified as fine or hyperfine, provides much of the richness of the observed spectra and thus makes electron paramagnetic resonance a powerful tool in many fields of study. The fine structure arises from the operators which do not involve $\mathbf{H}$ or $\mathbf{I}$; therefore they are the operators of the type S^b.

The simplest case of fine structure that we can consider is that of a spin Hamiltonian consisting of the first two terms of Eq. (4-2):

$$\mathcal{H} = \beta\mathbf{H}\cdot\mathbf{g}\cdot\mathbf{S} + \mathbf{S}\cdot\mathbf{D}\cdot\mathbf{S}. \tag{5-25}$$

This problem is already quite complicated, but simpler behavior occurs for the two limiting cases, one in which the first term dominates and the other in which the second term dominates. We will consider first the case of a small second term, thus leading to a small zero-field splitting [5].

As discussed in conjunction with Eq. (4-2), the tensor $\mathbf{D}$ has only five independent components. Thus we may expand the second term in Eq. (5-25) to give

$$\mathbf{S}\cdot\mathbf{D}\cdot\mathbf{S} = D_{xx}S_x^2 + D_{yy}S_y^2 + D_{zz}S_z^2 + D_{xy}(S_xS_y + S_yS_x) + D_{yz}(S_yS_z + S_zS_y)$$

$$+ D_{zx}(S_zS_x + S_xS_z), \tag{5-26}$$

where we have already eliminated all skew-symmetric terms. To eliminate a parameter using $S_x^2 + S_y^2 + S_z^2 = \mathbf{S}^2$, we would do better to write

Eq. (5-26) in terms of $\mathbf{S}^2$, $3S_z^2 - \mathbf{S}^2$, and $S_x^2 - S_y^2$ rather than of S_x^2, S_y^2, and S_z^2. Doing this, we obtain

$$\mathbf{S} \cdot \mathbf{D} \cdot \mathbf{S} = \tfrac{1}{3}(D_{xx} + D_{yy} + D_{zz})\mathbf{S}^2 + \tfrac{1}{2}D_{zz}(3S_z^2 - \mathbf{S}^2)$$

$$- \tfrac{1}{6}(D_{xx} + D_{yy} + D_{zz})(3S_z^2 - \mathbf{S}^2) + \tfrac{1}{2}(D_{xx} - D_{yy})(S_x^2 - S_y^2)$$

$$+ D_{xy}(S_x S_y + S_y S_x) + D_{yz}(S_y S_z + S_z S_y) + D_{zx}(S_z S_x + S_x S_z). \quad (5\text{-}27)$$

Elimination of the constant $\mathbf{S}^2$ term is accomplished by setting the trace of $\mathbf{D}$ to zero, a result independent of the choice of coordinates,

$$D_{xx} + D_{yy} + D_{zz} = 0. \quad (5\text{-}28)$$

The only term remaining that is diagonal, using $|M_S\rangle$ as a basis with z as the axis of quantization, is $\tfrac{1}{2}D_{zz}(3S_z^2 - \mathbf{S}^2)$.

Applying the ideas in the previous paragraph to the solution of the eigenvalue problem for Eq. (5-25) when the second term is small involves using $\mathbf{H} \cdot \mathbf{g}$ as the ζ axis (the z axis of the previous paragraph). Thus to first order we consider that the Hamiltonian of Eq. (5-25) becomes

$$\mathcal{H} = \beta|\mathbf{H} \cdot \mathbf{g}|S_\zeta + \frac{\mathbf{H} \cdot \mathbf{g} \cdot \mathbf{D} \cdot \mathbf{g} \cdot \mathbf{H}}{|\mathbf{H} \cdot \mathbf{g}|^2} \tfrac{1}{2}(3S_\zeta^2 - \mathbf{S}^2), \quad (5\text{-}29)$$

where we have included the explicit expression for $D_{\zeta\zeta}$ in terms of $\mathbf{H}$, $\mathbf{g}$, and $\mathbf{D}$. The energy is given by

$$E = \beta|\mathbf{H} \cdot \mathbf{g}|M_S + \frac{\mathbf{H} \cdot \mathbf{g} \cdot \mathbf{D} \cdot \mathbf{g} \cdot \mathbf{H}}{|\mathbf{H} \cdot \mathbf{g}|^2} \tfrac{1}{2}[3M_S^2 - S(S+1)]. \quad (5\text{-}30)$$

That the fine structure does produce structure in an otherwise simple spectrum (a single line) is evident when the energy differences and the magnetic fields at resonance are calculated:

$$h\nu = \Delta E = E(M_S) - E(M_S - 1) = g\beta H + \frac{3}{2}\frac{\mathbf{H} \cdot \mathbf{g} \cdot \mathbf{D} \cdot \mathbf{g} \cdot \mathbf{H}}{g^2 H^2}(2M_S - 1),$$

$$(5\text{-}31)$$

$$H = \frac{h\nu}{g\beta} - \frac{3}{2}\frac{\mathbf{H} \cdot \mathbf{g} \cdot \mathbf{D} \cdot \mathbf{g} \cdot \mathbf{H}}{g\beta g^2 H^2}(2M_S - 1).$$

For $S = \tfrac{1}{2}$, M_S must be $\tfrac{1}{2}$ and no contribution occurs from the fine structure, as we had anticipated in Chapter 4. For $S \geq 1$, however, there will be $2S$ equally spaced lines (equally spaced because we have included only the first order in perturbation theory).

The spacing in first order depends on $\mathbf{g}$ and $\mathbf{D}$ and on the orientation of $\mathbf{H}$ with respect to the paramagnet. For the case of axial, hexagonal, tetragonal, or trigonal symmetry there is only one independent element of **D**. If we ignore any possible skew-symmetric components of **g**, we find

$$\mathbf{g} = \begin{pmatrix} g_\perp & 0 & 0 \\ 0 & g_\perp & 0 \\ 0 & 0 & g_\| \end{pmatrix},$$

$$\mathbf{H} = H(\sin\theta, 0, \cos\theta),$$

$$\mathbf{H} \cdot \mathbf{g} = H(g_\perp \sin\theta, 0, g_\| \cos\theta), \qquad (5\text{-}32)$$

$$\mathbf{D} = \begin{pmatrix} -\tfrac{1}{3}D & 0 & 0 \\ 0 & -\tfrac{1}{3}D & 0 \\ 0 & 0 & \tfrac{2}{3}D \end{pmatrix},$$

$$\frac{\mathbf{H} \cdot \mathbf{g} \cdot \mathbf{D} \cdot \mathbf{g} \cdot \mathbf{H}}{g^2 H^2} = \tfrac{1}{3}D \, \frac{3g_\|^2 \cos^2\theta - g^2}{g^2}.$$

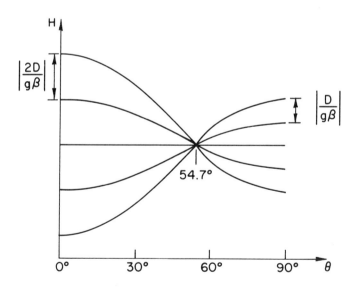

FIG. 5-4   The predicted angular dependence of the fine structure resulting from terms quadratic in spin components in first order of perturbation theory for a paramagnet with $S = \tfrac{5}{2}$ for the case of axial, hexagonal, tetragonal, or trigonal symmetry. The g factor is assumed isotropic. The angle between the field and the axis is θ.

The choice of the elements of **D** is made in such a way that the parameter D has its conventional value. Thus Eq. (5-31) for the field becomes

$$H = \frac{h\nu}{g\beta} - \frac{1}{2}\frac{D}{g\beta}\frac{3g_\parallel^2 \cos^2\theta - g^2}{g^2}(2M_S - 1). \tag{5-33}$$

The splitting between the fine structure lines is therefore given by (still in first order)

$$\Delta H = \left|\frac{D}{g\beta}\frac{3g_\parallel^2 \cos^2\theta - g^2}{g^2}\right|. \tag{5-34}$$

Since g depends on angle [see Eq. (5-11)], the angular variation of the first-order fine structure splitting is somewhat complicated. Frequently spectra requiring such a description have a very nearly isotropic g factor. In this case the angular dependence results from $3\cos^2\theta - 1$, and the predicted first-order spectrum with $S = \frac{5}{2}$ (as for Mn^{2+} or Fe^{3+}) is given in Fig. 5-4. An actual case, which includes moderate higher-order effects, is shown in Fig. 5-5 [6].

A still more complicated result occurs if the symmetry is orthorhombic. The equivalent of Eq. (5-32) is then

$$\mathbf{g} = \begin{pmatrix} g_x & 0 & 0 \\ 0 & g_y & 0 \\ 0 & 0 & g_z \end{pmatrix},$$

$$\mathbf{H} = H(l, m, n),$$

$$\frac{\mathbf{H}\cdot\mathbf{g}}{gH} = \frac{1}{g}(g_x l, g_y m, g_z n), \tag{5-35}$$

$$\mathbf{D} = \begin{pmatrix} -\frac{1}{3}D + E & 0 & 0 \\ 0 & -\frac{1}{3}D - E & 0 \\ 0 & 0 & \frac{2}{3}D \end{pmatrix},$$

$$\frac{\mathbf{H}\cdot\mathbf{g}\cdot\mathbf{D}\cdot\mathbf{g}\cdot\mathbf{H}}{g^2 H^2} = \frac{1}{g^2}\left[\frac{1}{3}D(-g_x^2 l^2 - g_y^2 m^2 + 2g_z^2 n^2) + E(g_x^2 l^2 - g_y^2 m^2)\right].$$

The g factor is anisotropic [see Eq. (5-10)]. The parameter E is also introduced in a conventional way. (Although the symbol E is used both for the

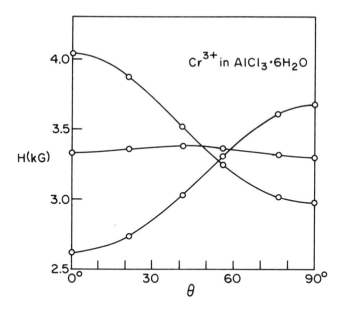

FIG. 5-5   The observed angular dependence of the fine structure for Cr^{3+} in $AlCl_3 \cdot 6H_2O$ [6]. In addition to the fact that $S = \frac{3}{2}$ in this case, the difference between this spectrum and that in Fig. 5-4 is caused by the higher-order effects which occur when D is not very small in relation to $g\beta H$.

energy and for a parameter in the spin Hamiltonian, the two can be distinguished by the context.) Considering again the limit of isotropic g factors, we obtain

$$\frac{\mathbf{H} \cdot \mathbf{g} \cdot \mathbf{D} \cdot \mathbf{g} \cdot \mathbf{H}}{g^2 H^2} = \tfrac{1}{3} D(3n^2 - 1) + E(l^2 - m^2). \tag{5-36}$$

In the case of monoclinic symmetry both $\mathbf{g}$ and $\mathbf{D}$ can be expressed in terms of principal axes. However, the principal axes are not the same for the two tensors. Two different but equivalent expressions result from basing the calculations on the two different sets of principal axes. Employing the principal axes for $\mathbf{D}$ to determine all components, but using x, y, z as the three principal axes of $\mathbf{g}$, we may write

$$\mathbf{g} = \begin{pmatrix} g_x \cos^2\theta + g_y \sin^2\theta & -(g_x - g_y)\sin\theta\cos\theta & 0 \\ -(g_x - g_y)\sin\theta\cos\theta & g_x \sin^2\theta + g_y \cos^2\theta & 0 \\ 0 & 0 & g_z \end{pmatrix},$$

$$\mathbf{H} = H(l, m, n),$$

$$\mathbf{D} = \begin{pmatrix} -\tfrac{1}{3}D+E & 0 & 0 \\ 0 & -\tfrac{1}{3}D-E & 0 \\ 0 & 0 & \tfrac{2}{3}D \end{pmatrix}, \qquad (5\text{-}37)$$

$$\frac{\mathbf{H}\cdot\mathbf{g}\cdot\mathbf{D}\cdot\mathbf{g}\cdot\mathbf{H}}{g^2 H^2}$$

$$= \frac{1}{g^2}\{(-\tfrac{1}{3}D+E)[lg_x\cos^2\theta + lg_y\sin^2\theta + m(g_x-g_y)\sin\theta\cos\theta]^2$$

$$+ (-\tfrac{1}{3}D-E)[l(g_x-g_y)\sin\theta\cos\theta + mg_x\sin^2\theta + mg_y\cos^2\theta]^2$$

$$+ \tfrac{2}{3}Dn^2 g_z^2\},$$

where θ is the angle between the sets of two axes, which differ for $\mathbf{g}$ and $\mathbf{D}$ in such a way that the x coordinate axis lies between the first two principal axes for $\mathbf{D}$. In the limit that $\theta \to 0$, the result in Eq. (5-37) is the same as for orthorhombic symmetry [Eq. (5-35)].

Consider next the solution of the problem of Eq. (5-25) for the case in which the second term is the larger. In fact let us first consider the case for which $H = 0$. ere the Hamiltonian is

$$\mathcal{H} = D[S_z^2 - \tfrac{1}{3}S(S+1)] + E(S_x^2 - S_y^2) = D[S_z^2 - \tfrac{1}{3}S(S+1)] + \tfrac{1}{2}E(S_+^2 + S_-^2).$$
$$(5\text{-}38)$$

Even if the parameter $E = 0$, there will be at most a degeneracy between $\pm M_S$; if $E \neq 0$, only Kramers degeneracy remains. Thus one obtains zero-field splitting associated with quadratic fine structure.

For simplicity we will consider only symmetries for which the parameter E is zero (higher than orthorhombic) when we analyze the effects of nonzero magnetic field:

$$\mathcal{H} = \beta[g_{\parallel}H_z S_z + \tfrac{1}{2}g_{\perp}(H_+ S_- + H_- S_+)] + D[S_z^2 - \tfrac{1}{3}S(S+1)]. \quad (5\text{-}39)$$

The magnetic field has the effect of lifting the twofold degeneracy for $\pm M_S$. Thus we need only solve these two-by-two problems to get the first-order result. The energy for $M_S = 0$ is

$$E = -\tfrac{1}{3}S(S+1)D. \qquad (5\text{-}40)$$

For $M_S = \pm\tfrac{1}{2}$ the energy matrix to be diagonalized is

$$\mathcal{H}_{ij} = \begin{pmatrix} D[\tfrac{1}{4}-\tfrac{1}{3}S(S+1)]+\tfrac{1}{2}g_{\parallel}\beta H_z & \tfrac{1}{2}g_{\perp}\beta H_-\sqrt{S(S+1)+\tfrac{1}{4}} \\ \tfrac{1}{2}g_{\perp}\beta H_+\sqrt{S(S+1)+\tfrac{1}{4}} & D[\tfrac{1}{4}-\tfrac{1}{3}S(S+1)]-\tfrac{1}{2}g_{\parallel}\beta H_z \end{pmatrix}, (5\text{-}41)$$

which has eigenvalues

$$E = D[\tfrac{1}{4} - \tfrac{1}{3}S(S+1)] \pm \tfrac{1}{2}\beta H\sqrt{g_{\parallel}^2 \cos^2\theta + [g_{\perp}(S+\tfrac{1}{2})]^2 \sin^2\theta}. \quad (5\text{-}42)$$

The angle θ is the angle between $\mathbf{H}$ and z. Except for the energy shift common to both levels, the energies have the same form as for an axial g factor and a spin of $\tfrac{1}{2}$ [see Eqs. (5-7) and (5-11)]. We can thus describe the first-order effect of the Zeeman interaction when D dominates by saying that the Kramers doublet with $M_S = \pm\tfrac{1}{2}$ has an effective spin and effective g values given by

$$S' = \tfrac{1}{2},$$
$$g'_{\parallel} = g_{\parallel}, \qquad g'_{\perp} = g_{\perp}(S+\tfrac{1}{2}). \qquad (5\text{-}43)$$

In this way we are replacing the spin Hamiltonian, which is itself an effective Hamiltonian, by another effective Hamiltonian corresponding to the primed spin and g factors. It is because of Eq. (5-43) that line positions corresponding to g values which vary from 2 to 4 or 2 to 6 are fairly common (i.e., for $S = \tfrac{3}{2}$ and $\tfrac{5}{2}$, respectively).

For $|M_S| > \tfrac{1}{2}$ the energy matrix is

$$\mathcal{H}_{ij} = \begin{pmatrix} D[M_S^2 - \tfrac{1}{3}S(S+1)] + g_{\parallel}\beta H_z M_S & 0 \\ 0 & D[M_S^2 - \tfrac{1}{3}S(S+1)] - g_{\parallel}\beta H_z M_S \end{pmatrix}$$

$$(5\text{-}44)$$

with eigenvalues

$$E = D[M_S^2 - \tfrac{1}{3}S(S+1)] \pm M_S g_{\parallel}\beta H \cos\theta. \qquad (5\text{-}45)$$

Again an effective spin and effective g values describe the energy difference [7]:

$$S' = \tfrac{1}{2},$$
$$g'_{\parallel} = 2M_S g_{\parallel}, \qquad g'_{\perp} = 0. \qquad (5\text{-}46)$$

It is appropriate at this point to note that no magnetic resonance transitions within this doublet are present if $g_{\perp} = 0$ (or generally if $g_{\perp} = 0$ for $S = \tfrac{1}{2}$). The reason can be seen easily if one realizes that the spin is always along z and that no transverse component of $\mathbf{H} \cdot \mathbf{g}$ can exist to cause the transitions (see Section 5-4).

The somewhat more complicated case obtained by letting $D = 0$ but making E large in Eq. (5-38) has been discussed, as well as cases intermediate between these limits [8].

In addition to the quadratic spin operators already discussed, both fourth- and sixth-order operators exist and play particularly important roles in the commonly observed S-state impurity ions, Mn^{2+}, Fe^{3+}, Eu^{2+}, and Gd^{3+}. Quite generally we may write the quartic spin operator as

$$\mathcal{H} = \sum_{i,j,k,l} a_{ijkl} S_i S_j S_k S_l, \qquad (5\text{-}47)$$

an equation similar to Eq. (5-16). If we assume that the Zeeman interaction is large compared to the terms in Eq. (5-47), a good approximation to the energy can again be obtained by the first-order contribution. If ζ is again along $\mathbf{H} \cdot \mathbf{g}$, then

$$\mathcal{H} = \tfrac{3}{8}\tfrac{5}{}a_{\zeta\zeta\zeta\zeta}[S_\zeta^4 - \tfrac{6}{7}S(S+1)S_\zeta^2 + \tfrac{5}{7}S_\zeta^2 + \tfrac{3}{35}S^4 - \tfrac{6}{35}S^2], \qquad (5\text{-}48)$$

where only the part diagonal in M_S is shown. The energy is thus (again including the Zeeman interaction)

$$E = \beta|\mathbf{H} \cdot \mathbf{g}|M_S + \tfrac{35}{8}a_{\zeta\zeta\zeta\zeta}[M_S^4 - \tfrac{6}{7}S(S+1)M_S^2 + \tfrac{5}{7}M_S^2$$

$$+ \tfrac{3}{35}S^2(S+1)^2 - \tfrac{6}{35}S(S+1)]. \qquad (5\text{-}49)$$

The results for cubic symmetry can be analyzed using Eq. (5-50) [the sum of Eq. (4-8) and the first term in Eq. (4-5)]:

$$\mathcal{H} = g\beta\mathbf{H} \cdot \mathbf{S} + \tfrac{1}{6}a[S_x^4 + S_y^4 + S_z^4 - \tfrac{1}{5}S(S+1)(3S^2+3S-1)], \qquad (5\text{-}50)$$

where x, y, and z are the cubic axes. Obtaining the elements a_{ijkl} by comparison of Eq. (5-50) with Eq. (5-47) gives

$$a_{ijkl} = \begin{cases} \tfrac{1}{15}a, & i=j=k=l, \\ -\tfrac{1}{10}a, & i=j \neq k=l, \end{cases} \qquad (5\text{-}51)$$

and all others are zero. Thus we obtain

$$a_{\zeta\zeta\zeta\zeta} = \frac{1}{H^4}\sum_{i,j,k,l} a_{ijkl}H_iH_jH_kH_l = \tfrac{1}{15}a(l^4+m^4+n^4) - \tfrac{1}{5}a(l^2m^2+m^2n^2+n^2l^2)$$

$$= \frac{a}{15}[1 - 5(l^2m^2+m^2n^2+n^2l^2)], \qquad (5\text{-}52)$$

the same angular dependence obtained in Eq. (5-23).

To examine the result in more detail let us consider $S = \tfrac{5}{2}$, the case for ions having a $3d^5$ configuration in the weak crystal-field limit (see Tables 3-2 and 3-3). Combining Eqs. (5-49) and (5-52), we obtain

$$E = g\beta H M_S + \frac{a}{120}[1 - 5(l^2m^2+m^2n^2+n^2l^2)]\left(35M_S^4 - \frac{475}{2}M_S^2 + \frac{2835}{16}\right).$$

$$(5\text{-}53)$$

The transitions corresponding to $\Delta M_S = \pm 1$ are the most intense ones by approximately a factor of $g\beta H/a$ and occur at

$$hv = \Delta E = E(M_S) - E(M_S - 1)$$

$$= g\beta H + \frac{a}{120}[1 - 5(l^2m^2 + m^2n^2 + n^2l^2)]$$

$$\times \left(140M_S^3 - 210M_S^2 - 335M_S + \frac{405}{2}\right). \qquad (5\text{-}54)$$

The results for the five allowed $\Delta M_S = \pm 1$ transitions are thus:

$M_S = \tfrac{5}{2} \rightleftharpoons M_S = \tfrac{3}{2}:$ $hv = g\beta H + 2a[1 - 5(l^2m^2 + m^2n^2 + n^2l^2)],$

$M_S = \tfrac{3}{2} \rightleftharpoons M_S = \tfrac{1}{2}:$ $hv = g\beta H - \tfrac{3}{2}a[1 - 5(l^2m^2 + m^2n^2 + n^2l^2)],$

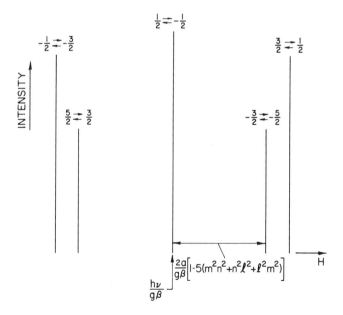

FIG. 5-6   The fine structure resulting from terms quartic in spin components in first order of perturbation theory for $S = \tfrac{5}{2}$ in cubic symmetry. The height of the lines is proportional to the intensity of the various transitions, assuming $g\beta H \ll kT$. The sign of a/g can be determined by observing the changes in relative intensity which occur at liquid-helium temperatures.

$$M_S = \tfrac{1}{2} \rightleftharpoons M_S = -\tfrac{1}{2}: \qquad h\nu = g\beta H, \tag{5-55}$$

$$M_S = -\tfrac{1}{2} \rightleftharpoons M_S = -\tfrac{3}{2}: \quad h\nu = g\beta H + \tfrac{5}{2}a[1 - 5(l^2 m^2 + m^2 n^2 + n^2 l^2)],$$

$$M_S = -\tfrac{3}{2} \rightleftharpoons M_S = -\tfrac{5}{2}: \quad h\nu = g\beta H - 2a[1 - 5(l^2 m^2 + m^2 n^2 + n^2 l^2)].$$

If we neglect the mixing of states from the fine structure, the relative intensities of the five lines are given [as we showed in Eq. (2-83)] by

$$I \propto S(S+1) - M_S(M_S - 1), \tag{5-56}$$

where M_S is the larger of the two magnetic quantum numbers. The ratios of the intensities for $S = \tfrac{5}{2}$ are $5:8:9:8:5$. Thus the spectrum looks like that in Fig. 5-6. The angular dependence of the spectrum of Fig. 5-6 is shown for a $\{110\}$ plane in Fig. 5-7. In Fig. 5-8 we show an actual example, that of Fe^{3+} in GaAs, which therefore includes higher-order effects [9].

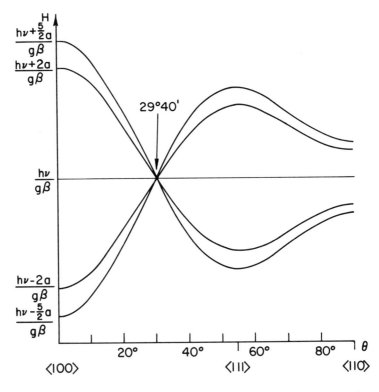

Fig. 5-7 The angular dependence of the fine structure of Fig. 5-6 for the magnetic field in a $\{110\}$ plane. Only first-order effects are included.

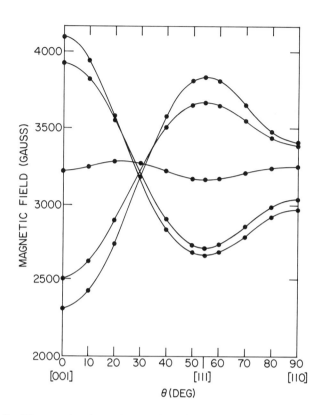

FIG. 5-8   The angular dependence of the intense lines observed for Fe^{3+} in GaAs [9]. This case is analogous to that of Fig. 5-7 except that contributions from higher orders of perturbation theory than first order are evident.

5–3 Hyperfine Structure

The operators in the spin Hamiltonian which contain components of **I** contribute to the hyperfine structure (HFS). Hyperfine structure is present because there are interactions with nuclear spins. Thus it is frequently possible to identify some of the important elements present in a paramagnet by the characteristics of their isotopes with nonzero nuclear spin. However, we can learn much more about a paramagnetic entity from a careful study of its HFS than just the identity of some of the atoms.

Let us begin by considering Eq. (4-2) again and choosing the second and third terms as the only significant ones:

$$\mathcal{H} = \beta \mathbf{H} \cdot \mathbf{g} \cdot \mathbf{S} + \mathbf{S} \cdot \mathbf{A} \cdot \mathbf{I}. \tag{5-57}$$

This approximation is valid if no fine structure occurs and if the bilinear term in $\mathbf{S}$ and $\mathbf{I}$ produces a larger effect on the energy levels than any other terms involving $\mathbf{I}$. This bilinear term is frequently referred to as the hyperfine interaction even though, strictly speaking, other terms may also contribute to the HFS. If we consider the case for which the first term in Eq. (5-57) is much larger than the second one, we may write

$$\mathcal{H} = \beta |\mathbf{H} \cdot \mathbf{g}| S_\zeta + S_\zeta \frac{\mathbf{H} \cdot \mathbf{g} \cdot \mathbf{A} \cdot \mathbf{I}}{|\mathbf{g} \cdot \mathbf{H}|}, \tag{5-58}$$

where we have ignored terms which contribute only in second order. We can now pick a coordinate system with one axis, ζ', along $\mathbf{H} \cdot \mathbf{g} \cdot \mathbf{A}$ and write $\mathcal{H}$ to first order as

$$\mathcal{H} = g\beta H S_\zeta + \frac{|\mathbf{H} \cdot \mathbf{g} \cdot \mathbf{A}|}{gH} S_\zeta I_{\zeta'}. \tag{5-59}$$

The energy is expressed to first order by

$$E = g\beta H M_S + K M_S M_I, \tag{5-60}$$

where g is given by Eq. (5-10), and K is defined by

$$K \equiv \frac{1}{gH} |\mathbf{H} \cdot \mathbf{g} \cdot \mathbf{A}|. \tag{5-61}$$

It is straightforward to work out the expression for K using a convenient coordinate system, although the result may be somewhat complicated for triclinic and monoclinic symmetry because $\mathbf{g}$ and $\mathbf{A}$ need not have the same principal axis system for their symmetric components.

Consider first orthorhombic symmetry and evaluate K by expressing the tensors in terms of the three orthorhombic axes. Thus we have

$$\mathbf{H} = (l, m, n)H,$$

$$\mathbf{g} = \begin{pmatrix} g_x & 0 & 0 \\ 0 & g_y & 0 \\ 0 & 0 & g_z \end{pmatrix},$$

$$\mathbf{A} = \begin{pmatrix} A_x & 0 & 0 \\ 0 & A_y & 0 \\ 0 & 0 & A_z \end{pmatrix}, \tag{5-62}$$

and g is given by Eq. (5-10). It then follows that

$$\mathbf{H} \cdot \mathbf{g} \cdot \mathbf{A} = (A_x g_x l, A_y g_y m, A_z g_z n)H \tag{5-63}$$

and

$$K = \frac{1}{g}[A_x^2 g_x^2 l^2 + A_y^2 g_y^2 m^2 + A_z^2 g_z^2 n^2]^{1/2}. \tag{5-64}$$

To first order we can write the expression for the magnetic field at which the resonance occurs from Eq. (5-60),

$$h\nu = g\beta H + KM_I,$$

$$H = \frac{h\nu}{g\beta} - \frac{K}{g\beta}M_I, \tag{5-65}$$

where again the transitions have $\Delta M_S = \pm 1$ since $g\beta HM_S$ is the largest term present in the energy. Thus the spectrum consists of $2I+1$ equally spaced lines (since we are considering only first-order effects). The spacing between these hyperfine lines varies with the angle that the field makes with the symmetry axes. This spacing is

$$\Delta H = \frac{K}{g\beta}, \tag{5-66}$$

where both K and g vary with the orientation of the magnetic field.

We can now deduce the behavior for axial, trigonal, tetragonal, and hexagonal symmetry by particularizing Eq. (5-64) to axial g and A tensors

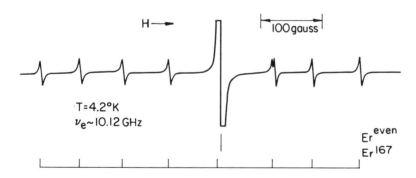

FIG. 5-9 The EPR spectrum of cubic Er^{3+} in $SrCl_2$, observed at 4.2°K and 10 GHz [10]. The strong central line results from the erbium isotopes with $I = 0$, whereas the seven weaker lines result from the isotope ^{167}Er, which has a 22.82% natural abundance and $I = \frac{7}{2}$. The center of the hyperfine pattern is shifted downward in field because of second-order effects in a perturbation treatment. This causes one of the expected eight lines to be obscured. The line near the ^{167}Er hyperfine line third down from high field is not part of this spectrum.

(we will consider only symmetric g and A tensors as well). In this case

$$K = \frac{1}{g}[A^2 g_{\parallel}^2 \cos^2 \theta + B^2 g_{\perp}^2 \sin^2 \theta]^{1/2}, \qquad (5\text{-}67)$$

where g is given by Eq. (5-11), A is the principal value of **A** along the axis, and B is the principal value perpendicular to it. The final particularization to cubic or spherical symmetry gives

$$K = A, \qquad (5\text{-}68)$$

where A is the common diagonal element of **A**.

In Figs. 5-9 and 5-10 we show examples of HFS with the characteristic uniformly spaced (nearly) lines. Both cases, Er^{3+} and Yb^{3+}, consist of several isotopes with different I and g_n, including $I = 0$. The presence of second-order effects can be seen in the displacement of the center of the HFS from the single line for $I = 0$ [10].

Although the hyperfine interaction $\mathbf{S} \cdot \mathbf{A} \cdot \mathbf{I}$ produces most of the effects associated with hyperfine structure, one more term is always present. This term is the interaction of the nuclear magnetic dipole moment with the magnetic field. In its most general form [see Eq. (4-2)] it can be written as

$$\mathcal{H} = -\beta_n \mathbf{H} \cdot \mathbf{g}_n \cdot \mathbf{I} \qquad (5\text{-}69)$$

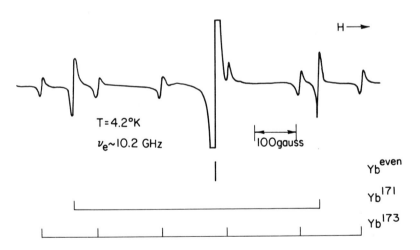

FIG. 5-10   The spectrum of cubic Yb^{3+} in $SrCl_2$, observed at 4.2°K and 10 GHz [10]. In addition to the strong line resulting from the isotopes with $I = 0$, the spectra produced by ^{171}Yb with $I = \frac{1}{2}$ and a 14.27% natural abundance and by ^{173}Yb with $I = \frac{5}{2}$ and a natural abundance of 16.08% are evident. Second-order effects shift the center of the hyperfine patterns down in field.

in exact analogy to all other bilinear terms in the spin Hamiltonian. In the absence of any effects due to the electronic paramagnetism Eq. (5-69) will take on the form [see Eq. (4-7)]

$$\mathscr{H} = -g_n \beta_n \mathbf{H} \cdot \mathbf{I}. \tag{5-70}$$

Let us add the term in Eq. (5-70) to the spin Hamiltonian of Eq. (5-57) and solve for the results in two limiting cases: $g\beta H \gg A \gg g_n\beta_n H$ and $g\beta H \gg g_n\beta_n H \gg A$. [We could use the general expression of Eq. (5-69) instead of the simpler isotropic interaction of Eq. (5-70). However, the former is encountered only infrequently, so we will use the simpler form.]

For the first limiting case, $g\beta H \gg A \gg g_n\beta_n H$, the energy is given by Eq. (5-60), neglecting terms of the order of $A^2/g\beta H$ and $g_n\beta_n H$ and smaller. In this we have chosen to quantize the nuclear spin along $\mathbf{H} \cdot \mathbf{g} \cdot \mathbf{A}$. Thus the diagonal part of Eq. (5-70) is

$$\mathscr{H} = -g_n \beta_n \frac{\mathbf{H} \cdot \mathbf{g} \cdot \mathbf{A} \cdot \mathbf{H}}{|\mathbf{H} \cdot \mathbf{g} \cdot \mathbf{A}|} I_{\zeta'}. \tag{5-71}$$

The energy is now, neglecting terms of the order of $A^2/g\beta H$ and $(g_n\beta_n H)^2/A$,

$$E = g\beta H M_S + K M_S M_I - g_n\beta_n \frac{\mathbf{H} \cdot \mathbf{g} \cdot \mathbf{A} \cdot \mathbf{H}}{KgH} M_I, \tag{5-72}$$

where g and K are defined by Eqs. (5-10) and (5-61), respectively. The particular form that Eq. (5-72) takes for orthorhombic symmetry is

$$E = g\beta H M_S + K M_S M_I - g_n\beta_n H \frac{A_x g_x l^2 + A_y g_y m^2 + A_z g_z n^2}{Kg} M_I, \tag{5-73}$$

where g is still given by Eq. (5-10), and K is given by Eq. (5-64). The result for axial, trigonal, tetragonal, or hexagonal symmetry and symmetric tensors only is

$$E = g\beta H M_S + K M_S M_I - g_n\beta_n H \frac{A g_\parallel \cos^2\theta + B g_\perp \sin^2\theta}{Kg} M_I, \tag{5-74}$$

where g is given by Eq. (5-11) and K by Eq. (5-67). Finally, for cubic symmetry the result is

$$E = g\beta H M_S + A M_S M_I - g_n\beta_n H M_I, \tag{5-75}$$

where g and A are now just the single isotropic constants allowed.

In the other limit, $g\beta H \gg g_n\beta_n H \gg A$, the largest term involving $\mathbf{I}$ is diagonalized if the components of $\mathbf{I}$ along and normal to $\mathbf{H}$ are used. We have previously labeled this coordinate system as 123, where the 3 axis is along **H**. The spin Hamiltonian can now be written as

$$\mathcal{H} = g\beta H S_\zeta - g_n\beta_n H I_3 + \frac{\mathbf{H}\cdot\mathbf{g}\cdot\mathbf{A}\cdot\mathbf{H}}{gH^2}S_\zeta I_3, \qquad (5\text{-}76)$$

where terms involving S_ξ, S_η, I_1, and I_2 are not shown since they contribute only in a higher order of perturbation theory. We see that the numerator of the last term in the spin Hamiltonian is the same as that in Eq. (5-71). Thus the results follow immediately from Eqs. (5-72) to (5-75). As an example, in orthorhombic symmetry the energy is

$$E = g\beta H M_S - g_n\beta_n H M_I + \frac{A_x g_x l^2 + A_y g_y m^2 + A_z g_z n^2}{g}M_S M_I, \quad (5\text{-}77)$$

where g is given by Eq. (5-10).

A somewhat more complicated behavior results if in fact $g_n\beta_n H$ and A are comparable. Although we will not attempt a detailed analysis, a few qualitative remarks may be useful. If $g\beta H$ is still the dominant term, the spin Hamiltonian can be written approximately as

$$\mathcal{H} = g\beta H S_\zeta + \left(\frac{\mathbf{H}\cdot\mathbf{g}\cdot\mathbf{A}}{gH}S_\zeta - g_n\beta_n\mathbf{H}\right)\cdot\mathbf{I}. \qquad (5\text{-}78)$$

We might infer that the results would follow in a similar way if we simply use the vector in parentheses as the third coordinate axis for writing the components of **I**. However, this vector depends on the value of M_S, and therefore the eigenfunctions for the nuclear spin will vary with M_S. Generally this means that the nuclear spin eigenfunctions for different values of M_S are not orthogonal and no selection rule involving M_I exists. The positions of the transitions are somewhat complicated, but straightforward, consequences of analyzing Eq. (5-78) [11].

Another term which often contributes to the hyperfine structure is the quadrupole interaction,

$$\mathcal{H} = \mathbf{I}\cdot\mathbf{Q}\cdot\mathbf{I}, \qquad (5\text{-}79)$$

the last term in Eq. (4-2). It can be handled similarly to the fine structure of Section 5-2 if we consider the limiting case $g\beta H \gg A \gg Q$. By analogy to Eq. (5-29) the first-order term is

$$\mathcal{H} = \frac{\mathbf{H}\cdot\mathbf{g}\cdot\mathbf{A}\cdot\mathbf{Q}\cdot\mathbf{A}\cdot\mathbf{g}\cdot\mathbf{H}}{g^2 K^2 H^2}\tfrac{3}{2}(I_\zeta^2 - \tfrac{1}{3}\mathbf{I}^2). \qquad (5\text{-}80)$$

In the limit of symmetric tensors and axial, hexagonal, tetragonal, or trigonal symmetry, the result is

$$\mathcal{H} = \tfrac{1}{2}Q[I_\zeta^2 - \tfrac{1}{3}I(I+1)]\left(3\frac{A^2 g_\parallel^2}{K^2 g^2}\cos^2\theta - 1\right). \qquad (5\text{-}81)$$

However, since this does not depend on M_S, there is no first-order effect of the quadrupole interaction on EPR spectra. The quadrupole effects usually discussed in the literature are second-order phenomena [12].

Although we developed the spin Hamiltonian in Chapter 4 assuming that only one nuclear spin is involved and that it is located at the symmetry point, we can and frequently do include interactions with many nuclei. These additional terms are merely added to the spin Hamiltonian, the symmetry of each term being appropriate for the location of the nucleus in question. As an example let us consider the case of a cubic paramagnetic entity described by the spin Hamiltonian

$$\mathcal{H} = g\beta \mathbf{H} \cdot \mathbf{S} + \sum_i \mathbf{S} \cdot \mathbf{A}_i \cdot \mathbf{I}_i. \tag{5-82}$$

The index i is assumed to run from 1 to 6, and the $\mathbf{I}_i$ are the nuclear spin operators for six nearest-neighbor nuclei along the positive and negative cubic axes (see Fig. 3-12). This is the superhyperfine interaction with the nearest neighbors in the case of an octahedrally coordinated paramagnetic ion. Although the paramagnet is cubic (i.e., its wave function and the significant terms in the potential energy have cubic symmetry), the coupling tensors for the superhyperfine interaction have tetragonal symmetry. Each tetragonal axis passes through the nucleus in question and through the center of the paramagnet, that is, there are three different mutually perpendicular tetragonal axes. The problem may be solved in a now familiar way by writing that part of Eq. (5-82) which will yield the first-order contribution:

$$\mathcal{H} = g\beta H S_\zeta + \sum_i \frac{|\mathbf{H} \cdot \mathbf{A}_i|}{H} I_{i\zeta_i'} S_\zeta. \tag{5-83}$$

The energy eigenvalues are

$$E = g\beta H M_S + \sum_i \frac{|\mathbf{H} \cdot \mathbf{A}_i|}{H} M_S m_i \qquad (-I_i \leq m_i \leq I_i). \tag{5-84}$$

Equation (5-84) would apply for nuclei at sites of any symmetry. For our present case we have for six identical isotopes (using components in terms of the cubic axes)

$$\mathbf{H} = H(l, m, n),$$

$$\mathbf{A}_i = \begin{pmatrix} A & 0 & 0 \\ 0 & B & 0 \\ 0 & 0 & B \end{pmatrix} \qquad (i = 1, 4),$$

$$\mathbf{A}_i = \begin{pmatrix} B & 0 & 0 \\ 0 & A & 0 \\ 0 & 0 & B \end{pmatrix} \quad (i = 2, 5), \tag{5-85}$$

$$\mathbf{A}_i = \begin{pmatrix} B & 0 & 0 \\ 0 & B & 0 \\ 0 & 0 & A \end{pmatrix} \quad (i = 3, 6).$$

Substituting in Eq. (5-84), we obtain

$$\begin{aligned} E = g\beta H M_S &+ \sqrt{A^2 l^2 + B^2(1 - l^2)}\, M_S(m_1 + m_4) \\ &+ \sqrt{A^2 m^2 + B^2(1 - m^2)}\, M_S(m_2 + m_5) \\ &+ \sqrt{A^2 n^2 + B^2(1 - n^2)}\, M_S(m_3 + m_6), \end{aligned} \tag{5-86}$$

from which we can obtain in the usual way the expression for the locations of the allowed $\Delta M_S = \pm 1$, $\Delta m_i = 0$ transitions:

$$\begin{aligned} H = \frac{h\nu}{g\beta} &- \frac{1}{g\beta}\sqrt{A^2 l^2 + B^2(1 - l^2)}\,(m_1 + m_4) \\ &- \frac{1}{g\beta}\sqrt{A^2 m^2 + B^2(1 - m^2)}\,(m_2 + m_5) \\ &- \frac{1}{g\beta}\sqrt{A^2 n^2 + B^2(1 - n^2)}\,(m_3 + m_6). \end{aligned} \tag{5-87}$$

For a general direction the three square roots will be unequal. If we fix m_2, m_3, m_5, and m_6, we can investigate the influence of m_1 and m_4 on the spectrum. The lowest-field line that will then result occurs when m_1 and m_4 have their maximum values, I. As a result $m_1 + m_4 = 2I$. The next higher line will occur for $m_1 + m_4 = 2I - 1$. This can be accomplished in two ways, $m_1 = I$ and $m_4 = I - 1$ or $m_1 = I - 1$ and $m_4 = I$. In effect there are two resonance lines at identical values of the field, leading to an observed line twice the intensity of the lowest-field line. In a similar manner the third line has three times the intensity of the lowest line, the fourth line is four times larger, and so on. The process ends when $m_1 + m_4 = 0$ and the line is larger by a factor of $2I + 1$. The rest of the spectrum is symmetrical about $m_1 + m_4 = 0$. The predicted behavior for $I = \frac{1}{2}$, 1, and $\frac{3}{2}$ is shown in Fig. 5-11.

A similar argument could be given for each value of m_2, m_3, m_5, and m_6, and the contributions of $m_2 + m_5$ and $m_3 + m_6$ can be analyzed as we have treated $m_1 + m_4$. To determine the whole spectrum we can

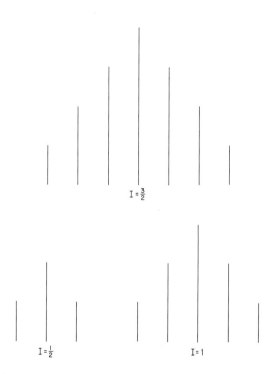

FIG. 5-11   The spectra of paramagnets which have hyperfine interactions with two identical nuclei for which $I = \frac{1}{2}$, 1, and $\frac{3}{2}$. Only contributions which are first order in perturbation theory are included. The relative intensities of the transitions are proportional to the heights of the lines. The intensities for the different I values relative to each other have no significance.

start with the single line for no hyperfine structure, split it in the way typical of $m_1 + m_4$, split each of the resulting lines in the way typical of $m_2 + m_5$, and finally split each resulting line as appropriate for $m_3 + m_6$. This process and the result is indicated for $I = \frac{1}{2}$ in Fig. 5-12, where each splitting is taken as four times smaller than the previous one (this simplifies the appearance of the resultant).

However, if the magnetic field makes the same angle with two or three of the cubic axes, then two or three of the splittings are equal and the number of observed lines decreases. To show what happens let us consider $I = \frac{1}{2}$ and the field along a $\langle 111 \rangle$ direction (the cube body diagonal, $l = m = n = 1/\sqrt{3}$). Then the transitions occur at

$$H = \frac{h\nu}{g\beta} - \frac{1}{g\beta} \sqrt{\tfrac{1}{3}A^2 + \tfrac{2}{3}B^2} \sum_{i=1}^{6} m_i. \qquad (5\text{-}88)$$

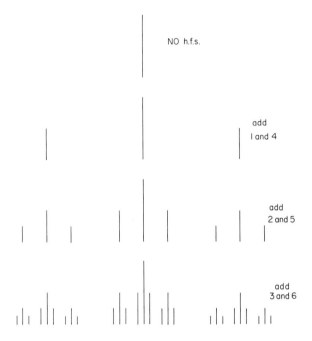

FIG. 5-12   The spectrum of a cubic paramagnet interacting with six equivalent nuclei with $I = \frac{1}{2}$ located on the cubic axes. The hyperfine coupling tensor and the direction of the magnetic field are taken so that the hyperfine splittings for the pairs of nuclei are in the ratio $1 : \frac{1}{4} : \frac{1}{16}$. The four patterns show the various stages of the spectrum as hyperfine structure is added, ending finally with the full pattern for all six nuclei. The relative intensities within the spectrum at any stage are indicated by the heights of the lines. The total intensity should not change, although it is shown twice as large for each stage as it is for the next less elaborate stage. Only first-order effects are included.

If all m_i are $\frac{1}{2}$, then $\Sigma_{i=1}^{6} m_i = 3$ and the lowest-field line occurs at

$$H = \frac{h\nu}{g\beta} - \frac{3}{g\beta} \sqrt{\tfrac{1}{3}A^2 + \tfrac{2}{3}B^2}. \tag{5-89}$$

The next higher line results from $\Sigma_{i=1}^{6} m_i = 2$. This can occur if one of the six m_i is $-\frac{1}{2}$. Thus six lines are superimposed, and the intensity will be 6 times as great as for the lowest line. The third line is then 15 times more intense since there are 15 different permutations of $\frac{1}{2}, \frac{1}{2} \frac{1}{2}, \frac{1}{2}, -\frac{1}{2}, -\frac{1}{2}$. The result is the spectrum shown in Fig. 5-13 (the center line is 20 times as intense as the outer lines).

Let us ask a general question: If N nuclei of spin I produce identical hyperfine splittings, what will the first-order spectrum look like? The answer is that it will consist of $2NI+1$ equally spaced lines with intensities given by

$$I \propto p_N(M_I) = \frac{1}{(2I+1)^N} \sum_{j=0}^{k} (-1)^j \binom{N}{j} \binom{NI-M_I-j(2I+1)+N-1}{N-1}, \quad (5\text{-}90)$$

where

$$M_I = \sum_{i=1}^{N} m_i, \ k \text{ is the largest integer less than or equal to } (NI - M_I)/(2I+1),$$

and

$$\binom{a}{b}$$

is a binomial coefficient.

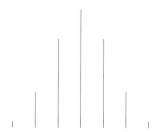

FIG. 5-13   The spectrum of a cubic paramagnet interacting with six equivalent nuclei for which $I = \frac{1}{2}$ and which are located on the cubic axes. The magnetic field is along a $\langle 111 \rangle$ direction making the same angle with each of the axes from the center of the cubic symmetry to the nuclei. This produces identical hyperfine splittings for all six nuclei, in contrast with the case in Fig. 5-12. Only first order in perturbation theory is employed. The relative intensities are indicated by the heights of the lines.

A table of $(2I+1)^N p_N(M_I)$ for the range of N and I of most utility is given in Appendix C. In Fig. 5-14 we show an example in which eight nuclei with $I = \frac{1}{2}$ are equivalent, that of interstitial hydrogen atoms in CaF_2 [13].

If two paramagnetic entities differ only in regard to the particular isotopes involved, they are usually considered to be identical and lead to identical EPR spectra save for the hyperfine structure (for small but

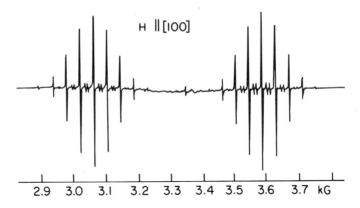

FIG. 5-14 The EPR spectrum of cubic interstitial atomic hydrogen in CaF_2 [13]. The principal splitting into two patterns is a consequence of the hyperfine interaction with the hydrogen nucleus for which $I = \frac{1}{2}$. The two symmetric patterns arise from the hyperfine interaction with eight equivalent ^{19}F nuclei for which $I = \frac{1}{2}$. The splittings are identical for all eight with the field in a $\langle 100 \rangle$ direction, yielding the nine lines in each pattern with intensities in the ratio 1:8:28:56:70:56:28:8:1. The part of the spectrum consisting of two weak lines between every pair of strong lines is a consequence of the competition between the nuclear Zeeman interaction and the anisotropic ^{19}F hyperfine interaction.

measurable exceptions see reference 14). Thus, to describe the observed spectrum for a system containing several isotopes, we must add the spectra obtained for each different possible choice of isotopes weighted by factors determined by the relative abundance of the isotopes. To illustrate this situation in its simplest form we consider the hyperfine interaction with a single nucleus with two isotopes, one with $I = 0$ and fractional abundance $1 - \alpha$, the other with $I = \frac{1}{2}$ and fractional abundance α. The resultant spectrum is one with three equally spaced lines (to first order) with relative intensities $\frac{1}{2}\alpha$, $1 - \alpha$, $\frac{1}{2}\alpha$. Figure 5-15(a) illustrates this case for the full range of α.

The interpretation of this spectrum or similar spectra is quite straight-forward and provides more information than a spectrum with only one isotope with nuclear spin (α, the two values of the nuclear spins, and the ratios of their magnetic moments obtained from the hyperfine interactions frequently provide a unique identification of the nucleus involved). The examples of HFS provided by Figs. 5-9 and 5-10 show this very convincingly. However, if we consider two identical nuclei rather than one, the results are more complicated. For the isotopes used above we would need to add the spectrum for two nuclei having $I = \frac{1}{2}$ and relative

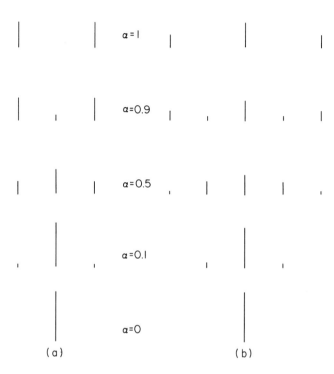

FIG. 5-15 The spectrum for a paramagnet, showing first-order hyperfine structure resulting from the interaction with (a) one nucleus and (b) two identical nuclei. The nuclei consist of isotopes with $I = 0$ and one isotope with $I = \frac{1}{2}$ and natural abundance α.

weighting α^2, the spectrum for one nucleus with $I = \frac{1}{2}$ and one with $I = 0$ with relative weighting $2\alpha(1 - \alpha)$, and the spectrum for two nuclei having $I = 0$ with relative weighting $(1 - \alpha)^2$. The results for two nuclei as described above are shown in Fig. 5-15(b) for the full range of values for α. We see that for small values of α the results for one nucleus and two nuclei are qualitatively similar. This is so because, compared to the case of all nuclei having $I = 0$, the next most probable occurrence is for one nucleus to have $I = \frac{1}{2}$. Because of the possibility of this occurring in either of two nuclear sites, the probability and therefore the intensity are twice as large for two nuclei as for a single nucleus.

To generalize somewhat, let us consider the problem of an isotope with spin I and fractional abundance α. We will consider only the case in which all other isotopes of this element have $I = 0$ and fractional abundance $1 - \alpha$. If there is a total of N_0 nuclear sites for which the HFS would be identical, then the probability that exactly N of these will contain the isotope with nonzero spin is

$$p(N) = \alpha^N (1-\alpha)^{N_0-N} \binom{N_0}{N}. \qquad (5\text{-}91)$$

For each value of N we have a certain spectrum, the observed spectrum being then the superposition of these spectra weighted by $p(N)$. Since both $p(N)$ and $p_N(M_I)$ are normalized, we can combine them to give the fractional intensity of the line corresponding to M_I:

$$I \propto p(M_I) = \sum_{N=0}^{N_0} p(N) p_N(M_I)$$

$$= (1-\alpha)^{N_0} \sum_{N=0}^{N_0} \left[\frac{\alpha}{(2I+1)(1-\alpha)} \right]^N \binom{N_0}{N} \sum_{j=0}^{k} (-1)^j$$

$$\binom{N}{j} \binom{NI - M_I - j(2I+1) + N - 1}{N-1}. \qquad (5\text{-}92)$$

where k was defined just after Eq. (5-90). An example of this is shown in Fig. 5-16 for F centers in MgO [15]. The spectrum which results if two isotopes have nonzero nuclear spin is much more complicated since it does not in general consist of uniformly spaced lines.

So far we have considered only cases for which the hyperfine interaction is weak compared with the electronic Zeeman interaction. Hyperfine splittings are normally about 0.1 cm^{-1} or less. Electron paramagnetic resonance experiments are most commonly performed with $h\nu$ between 0.3 cm^{-1} and 1.2 cm^{-1}. In these cases it is reasonable to consider the hyperfine interaction small. However, some experiments are performed at lower frequencies, and occasional hyperfine interactions are larger (see Section 10–2). Thus it is important to develop an understanding of hyperfine structure under a wider range of experimental conditions.

Let us consider the spin Hamiltonian of Eq. (5-57), augmented by including the term in Eq. (5-70). This problem in general does not have simple algebraic solutions. However, if we particularize to cubic or spherical symmetry, the spin Hamiltonian is

$$\mathcal{H} = g\beta \mathbf{H} \cdot \mathbf{S} + A\mathbf{S} \cdot \mathbf{I} - g_n \beta_n \mathbf{H} \cdot \mathbf{I}, \qquad (5\text{-}93)$$

which for $S = \frac{1}{2}$ can be solved in closed form. Let us rewrite Eq. (5-93),

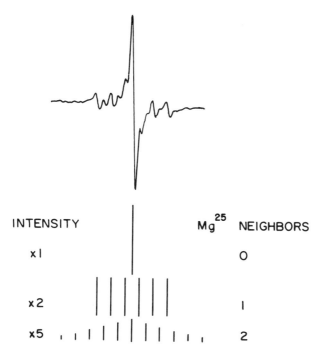

FIG. 5-16   The EPR spectrum for F centers in MgO [15]. The F center is an electron trapped at a negative-ion vacancy. Hyperfine structure is observed with ^{25}Mg nuclei located on any of the six equivalent Mg sites surrounding the oxygen vacancy. Since ^{25}Mg has a natural abundance of 10.05% and the remaining isotopes have $I = 0$, we expect a strong line surrounded by the spectrum resulting from the interaction with a single ^{25}Mg. In this pattern are still weaker lines arising from the interaction with two ^{25}Mg nuclei. The probability that three or more of the six nearest Mg sites will be occupied by ^{25}Mg nuclei is so low that they make no contribution to the observed spectra.

taking as the ζ axis the direction of $\mathbf{H}$ (actually $\mathbf{H} \cdot \mathbf{g}$ but $\mathbf{g}$ is isotropic),

$$\mathcal{H} = g\beta H S_\zeta + A S_\zeta I_\zeta - g_n \beta_n H I_\zeta + \tfrac{1}{2} A (S_+ I_- + S_- I_+). \tag{5-94}$$

This operator has matrix elements only between the states $M_S = \tfrac{1}{2}, M_I - 1$, and $M_S = -\tfrac{1}{2}, M_I$. Thus its exact solution simply involves diagonalizing a 2×2 matrix, which is

$$\mathcal{H}_{ij} = \begin{pmatrix} \tfrac{1}{2}g\beta H - g_n\beta_n H(M_I - 1) + \tfrac{1}{2}A(M_I - 1) & \tfrac{1}{2}A\sqrt{I(I+1) - M_I(M_I - 1)} \\ \tfrac{1}{2}A\sqrt{I(I+1) - M_I(M_I - 1)} & -\tfrac{1}{2}g\beta H - g_n\beta_n H M_I - \tfrac{1}{2}A M_I \end{pmatrix}.$$

$$\tag{5-95}$$

The solution to this eigenvalue problem is (the Breit-Rabi formula)

$$E = -\tfrac{1}{4}A - g_n\beta_n H(M_I - \tfrac{1}{2})$$
$$\pm \tfrac{1}{2}\{(g\beta H + g_n\beta_n H)^2 + A(g\beta H + g_n\beta_n H)(2M_I - 1) + A^2[I(I+1) + \tfrac{1}{4}]\}^{1/2}.$$

$$(5\text{-}96)$$

In zero magnetic field there are only two levels with energies of $\tfrac{1}{2}AI$ and $-\tfrac{1}{2}A(I+1)$. These energy levels are the $F = I + \tfrac{1}{2}$ and $F = I - \tfrac{1}{2}$ levels, respectively, where $\mathbf{F} = \mathbf{S} + \mathbf{I}$. As a function of field the energy levels are as shown in Fig. 5-17 for $I = \tfrac{1}{2}$ and $I = 1$ (neglecting the nuclear Zeeman interaction). The states are often labeled in terms of their high-field quantum numbers even though considerable mixing occurs at low fields. In the limit of very high magnetic fields ($g\beta H \gg A$), if we expand the square root and keep only the terms in $g\beta H$, A, and $g_n\beta_n H$, the results are the same as we encountered for Eq. (5-75). There will, however, be smaller terms of higher order. If we expand the square root and keep terms as small as $A^3/(g\beta H)^2$ and $(A^2/g\beta H)(g_n\beta_n/g\beta)$, we may write the energy of the levels whose high-field quantum numbers are $M_S = \pm\tfrac{1}{2}$, M_I as

$$E = \pm\tfrac{1}{2}g\beta H \pm \tfrac{1}{2}AM_I - g_n\beta_n HM_I \pm \frac{1}{4}\frac{A^2}{g\beta H}[I(I+1) - M_I(M_I \pm 1)]$$

$$\mp \frac{1}{8}\frac{A^3}{(g\beta H)^2}(2M_I \pm 1)[I(I+1) - M_I(M_I \pm 1)]$$

$$\mp \frac{1}{4}\frac{A^2}{g\beta H}\frac{g_n\beta_n}{g\beta}[I(I+1) - M_I(M_I \pm 1)].$$

$$(5\text{-}97)$$

In obtaining Eq. (5-97) we must remember that Eq. (5-96) refers to a different pair of states. If we now set the energy difference for the strong $M_S = \tfrac{1}{2} \rightleftharpoons M_S = -\tfrac{1}{2}$, $\Delta M_I = 0$ transitions equal to $h\nu$, we can solve for the magnetic field at resonance,

$$H = \frac{h\nu}{g\beta} - \frac{A}{g\beta}M_I - \frac{1}{2}\frac{A}{g\beta}\frac{A}{h\nu}[I(I+1) - M_I^2] - \frac{1}{4}\frac{A}{g\beta}\frac{A^2}{(h\nu)^2}M_I$$

$$+ \frac{1}{2}\frac{A}{g\beta}\frac{A}{h\nu}\frac{g_n\beta_n}{g\beta}[I(I+1) - M_I^2].$$

$$(5\text{-}98)$$

In replacing the $g\beta H$ in the denominator of Eq. (5-97) by quantities independent of field we may use $h\nu$ for the highest-order terms but we must use $g\beta H = h\nu - AM_I$ for the next to the highest, continuing the process as far as necessary and finally expanding the denominator in a power series in $A/g\beta H$ or $g_n\beta_n/g\beta$. Equations (5-97) and (5-98) could have been obtained directly from a perturbation solution of the spin Hamiltonian of Eq. (5-94). The energy results from introducing the specific matrix elements into the usual expression,

$$E = E_0 + \langle 0|\mathcal{H}_1|0\rangle + \sum_{n \neq 0} \frac{|\langle 0|\mathcal{H}_1|n\rangle|^2}{E_0 - E_n} + \sum_{m,n \neq 0} \frac{\langle 0|\mathcal{H}_1|m\rangle\langle m|\mathcal{H}_1|n\rangle\langle n|\mathcal{H}_1|0\rangle}{(E_0 - E_m)(E_0 - E_n)}$$

$$- \sum_{n \neq 0} \frac{|\langle 0|\mathcal{H}_1|n\rangle|^2\langle 0|\mathcal{H}_1|0\rangle}{(E_0 - E_n)^2} + \cdots, \tag{5-99}$$

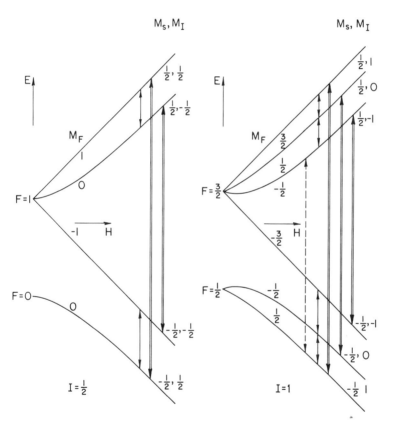

FIG. 5-17   The energy levels of paramagnets with $S = \frac{1}{2}$, $I = \frac{1}{2}$ and $S = \frac{1}{2}$, $I = 1$ on the left and the right, respectively. The Zeeman and hyperfine interactions are taken to be isotropic, g and A are taken as positive, and the nuclear Zeeman interaction is neglected. The states are labeled by their high-field quantum numbers on the right of each diagram and by the total angular momentum, F, on the left. Transitions allowed in the high-field limit are indicated by double lines. Those allowed in first order at low field or via the nuclear Zeeman interaction are shown by a single line. The dotted line denotes a transition allowed in second order only.

where

$$E_0 \equiv \langle M_S, M_I | \mathcal{H}_0 | M_S, M_I \rangle, \qquad |M_S, M_I\rangle \equiv |M_S\rangle |M_I\rangle,$$

$$E_n \equiv \langle M'_S, M'_I | \mathcal{H}_0 | M'_S, M'_I \rangle,$$

$$\langle 0 | \mathcal{H}_1 | 0 \rangle \equiv \langle M_S, M_I | \mathcal{H}_1 | M_S, M_I \rangle, \qquad (5\text{-}100)$$

$$\langle m | \mathcal{H}_1 | n \rangle \equiv \langle M''_S, M''_I | \mathcal{H}_1 | M'_S, M'_I \rangle,$$

$$\sum_{n \neq 0} \equiv \sum_{\substack{M'_S, M'_I \\ M'_S, M'_I \neq M_S, M_I}},$$

and where $\mathcal{H}_0$ is the unperturbed spin Hamiltonian, and $\mathcal{H}_1$ is the perturbing part. For the problem just considered a convenient way to proceed is to take everything with only diagonal elements as contributing to $\mathcal{H}_0$. Thus we have

$$\mathcal{H}_0 = g\beta H S_\zeta + A S_\zeta I_\zeta - g_n \beta_n H I_\zeta,$$

$$\mathcal{H}_1 = \tfrac{1}{2} A(S_+ I_- + S_- I_+). \qquad (5\text{-}101)$$

This choice is practical because $\mathcal{H}_1$ only has matrix elements between states differing in energy by about $g\beta H$. Although the process may be much more difficult than our application above, perturbation theory can be used to give additional terms for almost all of the expressions in this chapter. We have stopped at first order except in our discussion of the levels described by the Breit-Rabi formula (see also App. B). It is usually necessary, however, to consider second- or higher-order terms in analyzing EPR spectra quantitatively. For example, by reference to Eq. (5-100) we see that to first order the hyperfine lines are uniformly spaced and that the center of the spectrum occurs exactly at $h\nu/g\beta$. But if we also include the second-order term, the lines are not uniformly spaced and we cannot identify $h\nu/g\beta$ with the field at the center of all or part of the spectrum. This is illustrated in Fig. 5-18, assuming that all parameters are positive.

At the end of Section 5-1 we discussed the terms like HS^3 in cubic symmetry. As we noted in Eq. (4-12), there are also $S^3 I$ terms. The analysis proceeds in a similar manner for both.

For some experiments, such as ENDOR (see Sections 5-4 and 11-4), one is interested in $\Delta M_S = 0$, $\Delta M_I = \pm 1$ transitions. It is then possible to eliminate the electronic spin operators, in a manner similar to that used in Section 4-3 to obtain the spin Hamiltonian, and thus to derive a nuclear spin Hamiltonian (one for each electronic state) involving nuclear spin operators only.

Near the end of Section 5-1 we showed that the skew-symmetric components of **g** allowed by some point symmetries lead to behavior of the

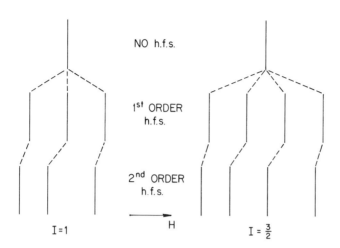

FIG. 5-18   The effect of second-order contributions to the hyperfine structure. The cases considered are for $I = 1$ and $I = \frac{3}{2}$. The hyperfine interaction is isotropic.

energy which can be obtained from symmetric components alone. The same point symmetries that allow **g** to have nonzero skew-symmetric components allow similar components for **A**. For hyperfine structure also, no effect arises from skew-symmetric components which could not result from a suitable set of symmetric components consistent with symmetry.

5–4 The Intensities of Magnetic Resonance Transitions

As we indicated in Chapter 2, magnetic resonance transitions are produced by applying an oscillating magnetic field to the paramagnetic substance. The oscillating field is usually, but not always, perpendicular to the static magnetic field (which on rare occasions is omitted). As in Section 2–3, we may assume that a small perturbing Hamiltonian, $\mathcal{K}_1$, describes the interaction of the paramagnetic entity with the oscillating magnetic field. If we assume further that $\mathcal{K}_1 = \mathcal{K}_1' \cos \omega t$, then the transition probability or rate is given by [see Eq. (2-80) for an analogous expression]

$$w_{ij} = \frac{1}{\hbar^2} |\langle j | \mathcal{K}_1' | i \rangle|^2 g(v), \qquad (5\text{-}102)$$

where $g(v)$ is a normalized shape function which is assumed common to all transitions (an assumption that is valid only for the simplest cases).

The intensity of this transition is proportional to w_{ij} and to parameters which depend on the experimental equipment. For simplicity we will define a parameter which is a relative measure of the intensity:

$$I_{ij} \equiv |\langle j|\mathcal{K}_1'|i\rangle|^2 . \tag{5-103}$$

Of course if line widths and shapes vary from transition to transition, it will be necessary to allow for this in making comparisons of I_{ij} with experimental results.

Providing that all relaxation times (they will be introduced later in Chapter 8) are long compared to the period $2\pi/\omega$, we describe the interaction with the oscillating field by the same Hamiltonian and spin Hamiltonian that we used for the interaction with the static magnetic field. Thus all terms in the spin Hamiltonian involving **H** should be used. Although in principal we should add terms like HS^3 and others, we can usually obtain accurate results from HS and HI terms alone. Thus we have

$$\mathcal{K}_1' = \beta \mathbf{H}_1 \cdot \mathbf{g} \cdot \mathbf{S} - g_n \beta_n \mathbf{H}_1 \cdot \mathbf{I}, \tag{5-104}$$

where $\mathbf{H}_1 \cos \omega t$ is the oscillating magnetic field. We have chosen the most common and simplest form for the HI term. Substituting in Eq. (5-103), we obtain

$$I_{ij} = \beta^2 |\langle j|\mathbf{H}_1 \cdot \mathbf{g} \cdot \mathbf{S}|i\rangle|^2 + g_n^2 \beta_n^2 |\langle j|\mathbf{H}_1 \cdot \mathbf{I}|i\rangle|^2$$
$$- 4 g_n \beta_n \beta \, \Re e \left\{ \langle j|\mathbf{H}_1 \cdot \mathbf{g} \cdot \mathbf{S}|i\rangle \langle j|\mathbf{H}_1 \cdot \mathbf{I}|i\rangle^* \right\} . \tag{5-105}$$

For almost all paramagnets the first term will dominate when it is nonzero. However, for transitions such that the first term is zero, the second may produce transitions. The third term does not play a role since it is zero if the first one is zero and negligible otherwise. We may regard transitions produced by the first term as EPR transitions and those produced by the second term as NMR transitions.

In most of the cases discussed in this chapter the term $\beta \mathbf{H} \cdot \mathbf{g} \cdot \mathbf{S}$ is the largest term in the spin Hamiltonian. We choose ζ along $\mathbf{H} \cdot \mathbf{g}$ and write the eigenfunctions in terms of this coordinate system. Then, unless $\mathbf{H}_1$ is parallel to $\mathbf{H}$ or unless two principal values of the g tensor are zero, we expect to find S_+ and S_- in $\beta \mathbf{H}_1 \cdot \mathbf{g} \cdot \mathbf{S}$. This then results in transitions for which $\Delta M_S = \pm 1$. To the approximation that the eigenfunctions are determined completely by $\beta \mathbf{H} \cdot \mathbf{g} \cdot \mathbf{S}$ to be $|M_S\rangle$, these are the only allowed transitions. We can readily calculate the expression for I_{ij} by writing the components of **H** and **g** in terms of the principal axis system for **g**:

$$\mathcal{K} = \beta \mathbf{H} \cdot \mathbf{g} \cdot \mathbf{S},$$

$$\mathcal{K}_1' = \beta \mathbf{H}_1 \cdot \mathbf{g} \cdot \mathbf{S},$$

$$\mathbf{H} = H(l, m, n),$$

$$\mathbf{H}_1 = H_1(l_1, m_1, n_1),\qquad(5\text{-}106)$$

$$\mathbf{g} = \begin{pmatrix} g_x & 0 & 0 \\ 0 & g_y & 0 \\ 0 & 0 & g_z \end{pmatrix}.$$

Unit vectors in the direction of $\mathbf{H} \cdot \mathbf{g}$ and $\mathbf{H}_1 \cdot \mathbf{g}$ are

$$\mathbf{k} = \frac{\mathbf{H} \cdot \mathbf{g}}{gH} = \frac{1}{g}(g_x l, g_y m, g_z n),$$

$$(5\text{-}107)$$

$$\mathbf{k}_1 = \frac{\mathbf{H}_1 \cdot \mathbf{g}}{g_1 H_1} = \frac{1}{g_1}(g_x l_1, g_y m_1, g_z n_1),$$

where

$$g = \sqrt{g_x^2 l^2 + g_y^2 m^2 + g_z^2 n^2},$$

$$(5\text{-}108)$$

$$g_1 = \sqrt{g_x^2 l_1^2 + g_y^2 m_1^2 + g_z^2 n_1^2}.$$

The spin operator in $\mathcal{K}_1'$, which is the component of $\mathbf{S}$ along $\mathbf{k}_1$, can be expressed as a component along $\mathbf{k}$ and a component along $\mathbf{i}$, a unit vector normal to $\mathbf{k}$ but in the $\mathbf{k}$-$\mathbf{k}_1$ plane. The geometry is shown in Fig. 5-19.

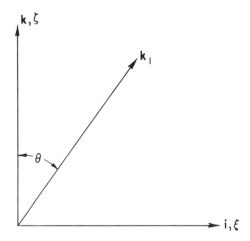

FIG. 5-19   The axes employed in calculating the intensities of EPR transitions. The ζ axis is the direction along which the spin is quantized. The time-dependent Hamiltonian has only a component of the spin along $\mathbf{k}_1$. This component is expressed in terms of components along $\mathbf{k}$ and $\mathbf{i}$, where $\mathbf{i}$ is an axis normal to $\mathbf{k}$ and in the $\mathbf{k}$-$\mathbf{k}_1$ plane.

In terms of ξ and ζ axes we may write $\mathcal{H}_1'$ as

$$\mathcal{H}_1' = g_1\beta H_1(S_\zeta \cos\theta + S_\xi \sin\theta). \tag{5-109}$$

Since the time-independent Hamiltonian, $\mathcal{H} = \beta \mathbf{H}\cdot\mathbf{g}\cdot\mathbf{S}$, in the $\xi\eta\zeta$ coordinate system has only an S_ζ component present, the eigenstates are $|M_S\rangle$. Then only $S_\xi = \frac{1}{2}(S_+ + S_-)$ produces matrix elements between the stationary states. Thus the relative intensities are given by

$$I_{M_S M_S'} = (g_1\beta H_1)^2 \sin^2\theta |\langle M_S'|\tfrac{1}{2}(S_+ + S_-)|M_S\rangle|^2. \tag{5-110}$$

The value of $\cos\theta$ can be obtained from Eq. (5-107) since it is the scalar product of $\mathbf{k}$ and $\mathbf{k}_1$,

$$\cos\theta = \mathbf{k}\cdot\mathbf{k}_1 = \frac{1}{gg_1}(g_x^2 ll_1 + g_y^2 mm_1 + g_z^2 nn_1). \tag{5-111}$$

From Eq. (5-111) we may calculate $\sin^2\theta$ to insert in Eq. (5-110):

$$\sin^2\theta = 1 - \cos^2\theta = \frac{1}{g^2 g_1^2}[g_y^2 g_z^2(mn_1 - m_1 n)^2 + g_z^2 g_x^2(nl_1 - n_1 l)^2$$

$$+ g_x^2 g_y^2(lm_1 - l_1 m)^2] \equiv \frac{g_t^4}{g^2 g_1^2}. \tag{5-112}$$

This allows us to write I_{ij} as

$$I_{M_S M_S'} = \frac{g_t^4}{g^2}\beta^2 H_1^2 |\langle M_S'|\tfrac{1}{2}(S_+ + S_-)|M_S\rangle|^2, \tag{5-113}$$

or, substituting in the matrix elements of S_+ and S_-, we obtain

$$I_{M_S, M_S\pm 1} = \frac{1}{4}\frac{g_t^4}{g^2}\beta^2 H_1^2[S(S+1) - M_S(M_S\pm 1)]. \tag{5-114}$$

By examining Eqs. (5-112) and (5-114) we can see many of the important properties of the intensities for systems which have a spin Hamiltonian consisting solely of the electronic Zeeman interaction or which are dominated by such a term. We note that g_1, the g factor corresponding to the orientation of $\mathbf{H}_1$, does not appear as such. If two of the three principal values of the g tensor are zero, say $g_\perp = 0$, then $\sin\theta$ and g_t are zero and hence so is I_{ij}. Thus, for example, the $M_S = \pm\frac{3}{2}$ or $M_S = \pm\frac{5}{2}$ Kramers doublets arising from a spin of $\frac{5}{2}$ with a large axial quadratic fine structure and described by Eqs. (5-45) and (5-46) will have no transitions, whether described by $S = \frac{5}{2}$ or $S' = \frac{1}{2}$, since in the latter case $g_\perp = 0$. Equation (5-112) shows that $\sin\theta$ and g_t are zero if $\mathbf{H}_1$ is parallel to $\mathbf{H}$

(or antiparallel). In general this means that any component of $\mathbf{H}_1$ which is parallel to $\mathbf{H}$ is ineffective in causing transitions. Hence the maximum intensity results if $\mathbf{H}_1$ and $\mathbf{H}$ are perpendicular. For a given $\mathbf{H}$ there will be a particular direction for $\mathbf{H}_1$ normal to $\mathbf{H}$ at which the intensity is maximum. Finally we note the characteristic dependence of I_{ij} on M_S that occurs for $S > 1$. The result is essentially the same as in Eq. (2-83) and as used in Eq. (5-56) to explain the intensities of the fine structure lines for a spin of $\frac{5}{2}$ in cubic symmetry. Bleaney has discussed an informative special case [16].

By going to second-order time-dependent perturbation theory we can calculate the transition rate corresponding to simultaneous absorption of two quanta for the case in which the single quantum transition is forbidden. The expression for the transition rate is

$$w_{ij} = \frac{1}{\hbar^4} \frac{|\langle j|\mathcal{JC}_1'|n\rangle|^2|\langle n|\mathcal{JC}_1'|i\rangle|^2}{(\omega_{ni} - \frac{1}{2}\omega_{ji})^2} g(2\nu), \qquad (5\text{-}115)$$

the analog of Eq. (5-102). We have assumed that only one other state, labeled n, is important in determining w_{ij}. Examination of the denominator in Eq. (5-115) indicates that the transition probability will be small unless level n is nearly midway between levels i and j. Such transitions have been observed for Mn^{2+} in MgO [17] and especially for $S = 1$ systems in cubic symmetry, such as Ni^{2+} in MgO [18] and V^{3+} in ZnS [19].

In Sections 5–1 to 5–3 we frequently discussed paramagnets described by a spin Hamiltonian dominated by $\beta\mathbf{H}\cdot\mathbf{g}\cdot\mathbf{S}$ but also containing other terms such as fine and hyperfine structure terms. As long as these other terms are small, the allowed transitions will have relative intensities given approximately by Eq. (5-114). However, weaker "forbidden" transitions can also occur. These are nonzero because the eigenstates are not pure $|M_S\rangle$ with ζ along $\mathbf{H}\cdot\mathbf{g}$. For example, the quadratic fine structure terms will generally mix in $|M_S \pm 1\rangle$ and $|M_S \pm 2\rangle$ with an amplitude of the order of $D/g\beta H$. Other functions are also mixed in but with even smaller amplitudes $[D^2/(g\beta H)^2$ or higher order]. Thus we expect transitions corresponding to $\Delta M_S = \pm 2, \pm 3$ (using high-field quantum numbers) but having relative intensities of the order of $D^2/(g\beta H)^2$ times the value in Eq. (5-114).

For hyperfine structure the results are somewhat more complicated because of the increase in the number of states by a factor of $2I + 1$ (in the case of a single isotope with a nuclear spin of I). If we ignore the weak, low-frequency NMR transitions caused by the second term of Eq. (5-105), and if $\beta\mathbf{H}\cdot\mathbf{g}\cdot\mathbf{S}$ is still the dominant term in the spin Hamiltonian, then the allowed transitions are $\Delta M_S = \pm 1$, $\Delta M_I = 0$ transitions. However, the presence of the term $\mathbf{S}\cdot\mathbf{A}\cdot\mathbf{I}$ [see Eq. (5-57) and its solution] causes the eigenstates not to be precisely $|M_S, M_I\rangle$, where M_S refers to $\mathbf{H}\cdot\mathbf{g}$ as the ζ axis, and M_I to $\mathbf{H} \cdot \mathbf{g} \cdot \mathbf{A}$ as the ζ' axis. Admixtures with amplitudes of approximately $A/g\beta H$ occur for the functions $|M_S \pm 1, M_I\rangle$, $|M_S \pm 1, M_I \pm 1\rangle$, and $|M_S \pm 1, M_I \mp 1\rangle$. This results in "forbidden" transitions whose intensity is lower by about $A^2/(g\beta H)^2$ than the value given by Eq. (5-114). These "forbidden" transitions have selection rules (for the quantum numbers of the major contribution, the high-field quantum numbers) of $\Delta M_S = \pm 2$ and $\Delta M_I = 0, \pm 1$. In order to observe "forbidden" transitions with $\Delta M_S = \pm 1$ there must be another term involving the nuclear spin to compete with the hyperfine interaction. One of these is the quadrupole interaction term of Eq. (5-79), and another is $-g_n\beta_n\mathbf{H} \cdot \mathbf{I}$, as mentioned in discussing Eq. (5-78). If we consider the spin Hamiltonian of Eq. (5-93) in the opposite extreme for which the hyperfine term is largest, there will be transitions for all states such that $\Delta M_F = \pm 1$. These transitions are shown on Fig. 5-17.

Since the fine and hyperfine structure terms in the spin Hamiltonian may mix some of the functions $|M_S \pm 1\rangle$, and so forth into a state dominated by $|M_S\rangle$, it is possible to produce weak transitions with $\mathbf{H}_1$ parallel to $\mathbf{H}$. There are paramagnetic entities for which these are the only observable transitions [20].

We have noted that the second term in Eq. (5-105) may produce NMR transitions. If the transitions in question happen to be between levels resulting from the hyperfine interaction of a paramagnet with some nucleus, they can be very useful in characterizing and understanding the paramagnet. Unfortunately these transitions are very weak because I_{ij} is quadratic in $\beta_n/\beta \sim 10^{-3}$ and also because ΔE is considerably less than the value for the usual microwave EPR experiment [see Eq. (2-95)]. However, such transitions can be observed by their effect on the much stronger EPR transitions. This technique, known as ENDOR (Electron Nuclear Double Resonance), will be discussed further in Section 11-4.

Here let us merely illustrate some features of ENDOR spectra by considering a paramagnet described by Eq. (5-72) plus the energy resulting from Eq. (5-80). The energy is

$$E = g\beta H M_S + K M_S M_I - g_n\beta_n \frac{\mathbf{H} \cdot \mathbf{g} \cdot \mathbf{A} \cdot \mathbf{H}}{KgH} M_I$$

$$+ \frac{\mathbf{H} \cdot \mathbf{g} \cdot \mathbf{A} \cdot \mathbf{Q} \cdot \mathbf{A} \cdot \mathbf{g} \cdot \mathbf{H}}{g^2 K^2 H^2} \tfrac{3}{2}[(M_I^2 - \tfrac{1}{3}I(I+1)]. \tag{5-116}$$

The ENDOR transitions correspond to $\Delta M_S = 0$ and $\Delta M_I = \pm 1$. Thus we have for the $M_I \rightleftharpoons M_I - 1$ transition

$$\Delta E = K M_S - g_n\beta_n \frac{\mathbf{H} \cdot \mathbf{g} \cdot \mathbf{A} \cdot \mathbf{H}}{KgH} + \frac{\mathbf{H} \cdot \mathbf{g} \cdot \mathbf{A} \cdot \mathbf{Q} \cdot \mathbf{A} \cdot \mathbf{g} \cdot \mathbf{H}}{g^2 K^2 H^2} \tfrac{3}{2}(2M_I - 1).$$

$$\tag{5-117}$$

Because the transitions are observed through their influence on the electron paramagnetic resonance, ENDOR spectra are obtained at fixed field by varying the frequency (usually in the range of 1 MHz to a few hundred megahertz). Hence Eq. (5-117) when divided by h gives the experimentally determined parameter.

5–5 Supplemental Bibliography

Solutions of the many eigenvalue problems arising from spin Hamiltonians are usually scattered through the literature. Nevertheless some pertinent references exist, and two are listed below.

1. A. Abragam and B. Bleaney, *Electron Paramagnetic Resonance of Transition Ions*, Oxford, New York, 1970. Probably the most complete treatment of the subject.

2. J. W. Orton, *Electron Paramagnetic Resonance*, Gordon and Breach, New York, 1968.

References Cited in Chapter 5

[1] F. K. Kneubühl, *Phys. Kond. Mat.* **1**, 410 (1963).
[2] F. S. Ham, G. W. Ludwig, G. D. Watkins, and H. H. Woodbury, *Phys. Rev. Letters* **5**, 468 (1960).
[3] W. C. Holton, J. Schneider, and T. L. Estle, *Phys. Rev.* **133**, A1638 (1964).
[4] B. Bleaney, *Proc. Phys. Soc.* **73**, 939 (1959); Y .Ayant, E. Belorizky, and J. Rosset, *J. Phys. Rad.* **23**, 201 (1962); A. Abragam and B. Bleaney, *Electron Paramagnetic Resonance of Transition Ions*, Oxford, New York, 1970, p. 725.
[5] The approach we use is described by W. Jung and G. S. Newell, *Phys. Rev.* **132**, 648 (1963).
[6] G. Emch and R. Lacroix, *Helv. Phys. Acta* **33**, 1021 (1960).
[7] For non-Kramers doublets (integral M_S) a preferable approach is given by K. A. Müller, *Phys. Rev.* **171**, 350 (1968). See also Section 8–3 of this book.
[8] T. Castner, Jr., G. S. Newell, W. C. Holton, and C. P. Slichter, *J. Chem. Phys.* **32**, 668 (1960); W. C. Holton, M. de Wit, T. L. Estle, B. Dischler, and J. Schneider, *Phys. Rev.* **169**, 359 (1968).
[9] M. de Wit and T. L. Estle, *Phys. Rev.* **132**, 195 (1963).
[10] L. A. Boatner, R. W. Reynolds, and M. M. Abraham, *J. Chem. Phys.* **49**, 745 (1968).
[11] A. Abragam and B. Bleaney, *Electron Paramagnetic Resonance of Transition Ions*, Oxford, New York, 1970, p. 195; H. H. Woodbury and G. W. Ludwig, *Phys. Rev.* **124**, 1083 (1961).
[12] A. Abragam and B. Bleaney, *Electron Paramagnetic Resonance of Transition Ions*, Oxford, New York, 1970, p. 181.
[13] J. L. Hall and R. T. Schumacher, *Phys. Rev.* **127**, 1892 (1962).
[14] S. A. Marshall, J. A. Hodges, and R. A. Serway, *Phys. Rev.* **133**, A1427 (1964); O. F. Schirmer, *J. Phys. Chem. Solids* **29**, 1407 (1968).
[15] J. E. Wertz, P. Auzins, R. A. Weeks, and R. H. Silsbee, *Phys. Rev.* **107**, 1535 (1957).

[16] B. Bleaney, *Proc. Phys. Soc.* **75**, 621 (1960). See also A. Abragam and B. Bleaney, *Electron Paramagnetic Resonance of Transition Ions*, Oxford, New York, 1970, p. 135.

[17] P. P. Sorokin, I. L. Gelles, and W. V. Smith, *Phys. Rev.* **112**, 1513 (1958).

[18] J. W. Orton, P. Auzins, and J. E. Wertz, *Phys. Rev. Letters* **4**, 128 (1960).

[19] W. C. Holton, J. Schneider, and T. L. Estle, *Phys. Rev.* **133**, A1638 (1964).

[20] T. L. Estle, G. K. Walters, and M. de Wit in *Paramagnetic Resonance* (W. Low, ed.), Academic, New York, 1963, Vol. I, p. 144.

CHAPTER 6

Interactions

The difference between isolated and therefore noninteracting paramagnetic species, such as those discussed in Chapters 1 through 5, and interacting magnetic dipoles can be as great as the difference between paramagnetism and ferromagnetism. Thus a study of materials which have a magnetically ordered state at low temperatures provides information on interactions and phenomena resulting from interactions. For this purpose the reader is referred to one of the excellent books on magnetism [1]. Our purpose is more specialized: we wish to study some of the effects of interactions on paramagnetism and specifically on electron paramagnetic resonance in nonmetals.

6–1 The Nature of Interactions; Exchange

When two magnetic dipoles are close together, their interaction is strong enough that it must be taken into account (being close enough varies with the system but is usually a few atomic radii or less). There is, of course, always the magnetic dipole-dipole interaction, which can be written as

$$\mathcal{H}_{jk} = \frac{\mu_j \cdot \mu_k}{r_{jk}^3} - 3\frac{(\mu_j \cdot r_{jk})(\mu_k \cdot r_{jk})}{r_{jk}^5}, \tag{6-1}$$

where j and k are the indices specifying the two interacting dipoles, and $\mu_j = -g_j\beta S_j$, or a generalization thereof. This magnetic interaction is relatively weak for point dipoles separated by distances on an atomic scale. The magnetic field equivalent to a typical point dipole-dipole interaction is $\beta/r^3 = 1159$ G for $r = 2$Å. Such a weak interaction could produce an ordered magnetic state, such as ferromagnetism, only at temperatures below $1\,°K$. The occurrence of transition temperatures larger by more than two orders of magnitude shows that another, much stronger interaction exists. This interaction is called the exchange interaction, and its strength arises from its electrostatic origin.

The exchange interaction is an equivalent way of describing certain spin-dependent splittings arising from Coulomb interactions and the Pauli exclusion principle. The simpler cases arise for two electrons; the simplest is the helium atom, where exchange is equivalent to Hund's first rule (see Section 3–2). Let us consider here the somewhat more complicated case of the H_2 molecule since it resembles more closely the problem of interacting magnetic dipoles. The solution of the hydrogen molecule is a standard textbook topic [2] which, in its simplest form, can be accomplished in either of two ways, by the molecular orbital method or the Heitler-London method. The molecular orbital method ignores or minimizes considerations of correlation, whereas the Heitler-London method makes extreme allowance for correlation. However, if configuration interaction is included, the two methods are equivalent. We will choose the Heitler-London method since to a first approximation we will assume that the two interacting paramagnetic species are localized.

If we define $a(1)$ as a $1s$ atomic orbital about nucleus (proton) a which is occupied by electron 1, and if $a(2)$, $b(1)$, and $b(2)$ are defined by analogy (see Fig. 6-1), then the lowest two states of the two-electron system are linear combinations of $a(1)b(2)$ and $a(2)b(1)$. We have assumed that the electrostatic repulsion between electrons will prevent the two electrons from occupying orbitals on the same atom (the Heitler-London approximation or method). The overlap integral, α, is given by

$$\alpha \equiv \int a(i)b(i)\,d\tau_i, \tag{6-2}$$

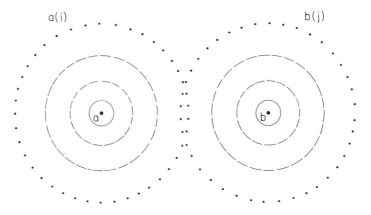

FIG. 6-1 Hydrogenic $1s$ orbitals used in describing the hydrogen molecule by the Heitler-London method. The function $a(i)$ is a $1s$ hydrogen orbital on proton a when occupied by electron i. The circles are constant probability contours in a plane containing the two protons. The ratio of the probabilities for the various contours is $1:0.5:0.2:0.05:0.01$ for the center, the solid circle, the two dashed circles, and the dotted circle, respectively. Any power of these numbers could also be used with a change in scale. With the scale implied, the separation of the nuclei is much larger than the equilibrium spacing.

where the $\int d\tau_i$ is the integral over all space for the coordinates of the ith electron. By using symmetry we can see that the eigenstates are either symmetric or antisymmetric under electron interchange. These are, respectively,

$$\psi_{\pm} = \frac{1}{\sqrt{2(1 \pm \alpha^2)}} [a(2)b(1) \pm a(1)b(2)], \tag{6-3}$$

where we have used normalized functions throughout. The Pauli principle requires that the total wave function be antisymmetric under electron interchange. Since the spatial function ψ_+ is symmetric, it must multiply an antisymmetric spin function, and vice versa for ψ_-. Four possible spin functions can be obtained for two electrons. They are the three triplet functions

$$|\tfrac{1}{2}\rangle_1 |\tfrac{1}{2}\rangle_2, \qquad \frac{1}{\sqrt{2}} [|\tfrac{1}{2}\rangle_1 |-\tfrac{1}{2}\rangle_2 + |\tfrac{1}{2}\rangle_2 |-\tfrac{1}{2}\rangle_1], \qquad |-\tfrac{1}{2}\rangle_1 |-\tfrac{1}{2}\rangle_2,$$

which are symmetric under electron interchange, and one antisymmetric singlet:

$$\frac{1}{\sqrt{2}} [|\tfrac{1}{2}\rangle_1 |-\tfrac{1}{2}\rangle_2 - |\tfrac{1}{2}\rangle_2 |-\tfrac{1}{2}\rangle_1].$$

Thus ψ_+ is the spatial part of a singlet state, and ψ_- corresponds to a triplet.

The energies of these states are

$$E_{\pm} = \frac{1}{2(1 \pm \alpha^2)} \langle a(2)b(1) \pm a(1)b(2) | \mathcal{H} | a(2)b(1) \pm a(1)b(2) \rangle$$

$$= \frac{1}{1 \pm \alpha^2} \{ \langle a(2)b(1) | \mathcal{H} | a(2)b(1) \rangle \pm \langle a(2)b(1) | \mathcal{H} | a(1)b(2) \rangle \}. \tag{6-4}$$

The Hamiltonian of the whole system is given by

$$\mathcal{H} = T_1 + T_2 + V_{a1} + V_{a2} + V_{b1} + V_{b2} + V_{12}, \tag{6-5}$$

where T_i is the kinetic energy of the ith electron, and V_{a1} is the potential energy for the electrostatic interaction between the nucleus a and the 1st electron. If the energy of the 1s atomic orbital is given by E_0, then

$$\langle a(2)b(1) | \mathcal{H} | a(2)b(1) \rangle = 2E_0 + Q \tag{6-6}$$

and

$$\langle a(2)b(1) | \mathcal{H} | a(1)b(2) \rangle = 2\alpha^2 E_0 + J', \tag{6-7}$$

where

$$Q = \langle a(2)b(1)|V_{12}+V_{1a}+V_{2b}|a(2)b(1)\rangle \tag{6-8}$$

and

$$J' = \langle a(2)b(1)|V_{12}+V_{1b}+V_{2a}|a(1)b(2)\rangle. \tag{6-9}$$

The quantities Q and J', referred to as the Coulomb and exchange integrals, respectively, can perhaps be better understood from the expressions

$$Q = \int \rho_a(2)\rho_b(1)\frac{e^2}{r_{12}}d\tau_1\,d\tau_2 - 2\int \rho_b(1)\frac{e^2}{r_{1a}}d\tau_1,$$

$$J' = \int \rho_{ab}(1)\rho_{ab}(2)\frac{e^2}{r_{12}}d\tau_1\,d\tau_2 - 2\alpha\int \rho_{ab}(1)\frac{e^2}{r_{1b}}d\tau_1, \tag{6-10}$$

where $\rho_a(i) = [a(i)]^2$ and $\rho_{ab}(i) = a(i)b(i)$ (since the functions may be taken to be real). The Coulomb integral consists of the electrostatic interactions previously ignored in computing the orbital energies. This term would be unaltered in a classical (point electron) treatment. The exchange integral is strictly a quantum phenomenon and depends on the existence of overlap between $a(i)$ and $b(i)$, that is, $\rho_{ab}(i) \neq 0$ somewhere.

Returning to the energy, we obtain

$$E_{\pm} = 2E_0 + \frac{Q \pm J'}{1 \pm \alpha^2}. \tag{6-11}$$

Thus we find the triplet state to be lower than the singlet state by

$$\Delta E = \frac{2(J' - \alpha^2 Q)}{1 - \alpha^4}. \tag{6-12}$$

This energy difference turns out to be negative (i.e., the singlet is lowest) for the hydrogen molecule.

This energy splitting, which may be said to be the result of exchange, can be shown to be equivalent to the splitting produced by the Heisenberg Hamiltonian:

$$\mathcal{H}_{12} = -2J\mathbf{S}_1\cdot\mathbf{S}_2. \tag{6-13}$$

We can show by analogy with Section 1-2 that

$$\mathcal{H}_{12} = -J(\mathbf{S}^2 - \mathbf{S}_1^2 - \mathbf{S}_2^2), \tag{6-14}$$

so that the energy is

$$E = -J[S(S+1) - \tfrac{3}{2}] \tag{6-15}$$

and the triplet is lower in energy than the singlet by an amount $2J$. Thus, if

$$J = \frac{J' - \alpha^2 Q}{1 - \alpha^4}, \qquad (6\text{-}16)$$

the two are equivalent. The quantity J is called the exchange constant.

We have considered a simple example of direct exchange, an exchange interaction which results from the direct overlap of the atomic orbitals on the two interacting paramagnets. It is possible to have indirect exchange as well. The type of indirect exchange with which we will be most concerned, called superexchange, occurs between two magnetic ions when their wave functions have negligible overlap but when one or more intermediate diamagnetic ions overlaps both magnetic ions.

Frequently both direct and indirect exchange can be written in terms of Heisenberg Hamiltonians, even for more complicated systems and values of spin larger than $\frac{1}{2}$. However, we can obtain the exact form that such an interaction operator must take in terms of spin operators in the same manner that we obtained the spin Hamiltonian in Section 4-2. To do this for two interacting paramagnets the interaction must couple the lowest manifold of states (the spin) on the two paramagnetic species. In such a calculation we obtain no information concerning the values of the parameters in the Hamiltonian or the mechanisms causing the interaction.

If we examine Table 4-2, realizing that the symmetry of two interacting paramagnetic species must be lower than cubic, we see that two or more bilinear forms are required for an operator linear in the components of S_1 and also of S_2. Thus for the symmetries D_{6h}, D_6, C_{6v}, D_{3h}, D_{4h}, D_4, C_{4v}, D_{2d}, D_{3d}, D_3, C_{3v}, $D_{\infty h}$, $C_{\infty v}$ we can write the most general bilinear interaction as

$$\mathcal{H}_{12} = -2J S_1 \cdot S_2 + K(2S_{1z}S_{2z} - S_{1x}S_{2x} - S_{1y}S_{2y}), \qquad (6\text{-}17)$$

where z is the axis of rotational symmetry. The first term has the isotropic Heisenberg form, whereas the second term has the same angular dependence as the dipolar interaction and is sometimes called the pseudodipolar interaction. In fact, if $K = -g_1 g_2 \beta^2 / r_{12}^3$, the pseudodipolar term is identical in form with that for dipolar interaction given in Eq. (6-1) when the g factors are isotropic.

However, many symmetries listed in Table 4-2 require more than two independent bilinear terms in general. All of those requiring three, except for orthorhombic, have an additional skew-symmetric term allowed. This term may be written as

$$\mathcal{H}_{12} \propto -\frac{1}{2i}(S_{1+}S_{2-} - S_{1-}S_{2+}) = S_{1x}S_{2y} - S_{1y}S_{2x} = (S_1 \times S_2)_z \qquad (6\text{-}18)$$

where x and y may have any orientation normal to z as long as they form with z a right-handed Cartesian coordinate system. The last term in Eq. (6-18) is possibly more familiar and is referred to as the Dzyaloshinski-Moriya or asymmetric exchange interaction [3].

For very low symmetry there may be as many as nine independent bilinear interaction operators. Three of these are skew symmetric, and three represent the principal values of the symmetric part. The remaining three are the parameters required to specify the principal axes of the symmetric part. These results are essentially the same as for operators linear in the components of **H** and **S** (see Section 4–2).

If the spins are greater than $\frac{1}{2}$, it is necessary in principle to introduce still higher powers of the spin components in the interaction operators. We are thus led to biquadratic, linear-cubic, and other similar forms of operators. Again examining Table 4-2, we see that we always require at least three independent biquadratic operators. If the z axis is taken as the symmetry axis, these would be

$$\mathcal{K}_{12} = K_1 S_{1z}^2 S_{2z}^2 + K_2[(S_{1z}S_{1-} + S_{1-}S_{1z})(S_{2z}S_{2+} + S_{2+}S_{2z})$$

$$+ (S_{1z}S_{1+} + S_{1+}S_{1z})(S_{2z}S_{2-} + S_{2-}S_{2z})] + K_3\, S_{1+}^2 S_{2-}^2 + S_{1-}^2 S_{2+}^2).$$

$$(6\text{-}19)$$

Sometimes the isotropic form,

$$\mathcal{K}_{12} = -j(\mathbf{S}_1 \cdot \mathbf{S}_2)^2, \tag{6-20}$$

is found to be sufficient [4].

As we shall see in Section 6–3, two interacting paramagnets can sometimes be studied by electron paramagnetic resonance. Such studies should permit the determination of the parameters in the proper two-spin interaction Hamiltonian which we have been discussing. Occasionally a group of three or more interacting dipoles is observed, and certainly in magnetic materials which have ordered states (ferro-, antiferro-, and ferrimagnetism) a large number of mutually interacting spins must be considered. More than two interacting paramagnets leads to interaction terms involving simultaneously three or more spins [5]. There is also a change in the coefficients of the pair interaction terms. In addition to these consequences of additional interactions, if there is any change in symmetry it must be allowed for. Finally, even if the symmetry is the same, the nonmagnetic part of the environment has changed.

6–2 The Effects of Interactions; Electron Paramagnetic Resonance Line Shape

We now ask how the introduction of interactions modifies the description of electron paramagnetic resonance given in Chapters 1 through 5, a description based primarily on a collection of isolated paramagnetic entities. There are several answers to this question. For very dilute paramagnetic impurities in an otherwise diamagnetic solid it is possible to have no readily observable effects from interactions. Although the concentration below which interactions may be ignored varies with the solid and the paramagnetic entity, they can usually be disregarded below concentrations of 100 parts per million.

If the concentration of impurities is high or if a crystal containing paramagnetic constituents at rather large spacings is considered, we find two related phenomena caused by interactions. First, energy can be transferred from one paramagnetic entity to another. This requires that the lifetime associated with this transfer be shorter than the spin-lattice relaxation time, T_1. This new relaxation time, called the spin-spin relaxation time, T_2, was introduced in Eq. (2-24) phenomenologically. The second effect is that interactions produce a line breadth greater than that from T_1 lifetime broadening. Let us consider the latter effect, using the method of moments to obtain some insight into line widths and shapes.

We shall assume that the interactions arise from isotropic exchange [Eq. (6-13)] and from the magnetic dipole-dipole interaction [Eq. (6-1)] and that the paramagnets are ions regularly arranged in a crystal. To develop a real theory of the width requires more than a simple vector summation of the magnetic fields of the dipoles at neighboring lattices sites. Each of the ions is equivalent (or, in more complicated lattices, there are a few species of equivalent ions), and we are required to treat an assembly of a large number of interacting ions. This is a many-body problem which was essentially solved in 1948 by Van Vleck [6]. In this calculation, Van Vleck showed that broadening resulted from the dipolar interaction but that exchange caused a line narrowing.

Neglecting hyperfine and fine structure and assuming an isotropic g factor for a single paramagnetic species, we can write the Hamiltonian for interacting dipoles as

$$\mathcal{H} = \mathcal{H}_Z + \mathcal{H}_d + \mathcal{H}_e,$$

$$\mathcal{H}_Z = \sum_{j=1}^{N} g\beta \mathbf{H} \cdot \mathbf{S}_j,$$

$$\mathcal{H}_d = \sum_{(jk)} g^2\beta^2 r_{jk}^{-3}[\mathbf{S}_j \cdot \mathbf{S}_k - 3(\mathbf{S}_j \cdot \hat{\mathbf{r}}_{jk})(\mathbf{S}_k \cdot \hat{\mathbf{r}}_{jk})], \qquad (6\text{-}21)$$

$$\mathcal{H}_e = -\sum_{(jk)} 2J_{jk}\mathbf{S}_j \cdot \mathbf{S}_k.$$

The sum $\Sigma_{(jk)}$ is over all pairs of the indices of the dipoles. The vector $\hat{\mathbf{r}}_{jk}$ is a unit vector in the direction of $\mathbf{r}_{jk}$, that is, $\hat{\mathbf{r}}_{jk} = \mathbf{r}_{jk}/r_{jk}$. Taking z to be along $\mathbf{H}$, we find that the eigenfunctions of $\mathcal{H}_Z + \mathcal{H}_e$ are also eigenfunctions of $S_z = \Sigma_{j=1}^{N} S_{jz}$. This means that EPR transitions correspond to $\Delta M = \pm 1$, where M is the eigenvalue of S_z. Therefore, if $\mathcal{H}_Z$ is the largest term in the Hamiltonian $\mathcal{K}_z + \mathcal{K}_e$, the only transitions that occur in first-order time-dependent perturbation theory (see Section 5–4) are near $v = g\beta H/h$. Including $\mathcal{K}_d$ modifies this result somewhat. If we define θ_{jk} as the angle between $\mathbf{r}_{jk}$ and $\mathbf{H}$, we can write $\mathcal{K}_d$ in terms of operators with simple matrix elements:

$$\mathbf{S}_j \cdot \mathbf{S}_k - 3(\mathbf{S}_j \cdot \hat{\mathbf{r}}_{jk})(\mathbf{S}_k \cdot \hat{\mathbf{r}}_{jk})$$

$$= -\tfrac{1}{2}(3\cos^2\theta_{jk} - 1)(3S_{jz}S_{kz} - \mathbf{S}_j \cdot \mathbf{S}_k)$$

$$- \tfrac{3}{2}\sin\theta_{jk}\cos\theta_{kj}(S_{jz}S_{k+} + S_{j+}S_{kz} + S_{jz}S_{k-} + S_{j-}S_{kz})$$

$$- \tfrac{3}{4}\sin^2\theta_{jk}(S_{j+}S_{k+} + S_{j-}S_{k-}). \tag{6-22}$$

The second and third terms in Eq. (6-22) mix states with $\Delta M = \pm 1$ and $\Delta M = \pm 2$, respectively. If it is assumed that $\mathcal{K}_d$ is a perturbation to $\mathcal{K}_z$, this admixture is of the order of $\beta^2 r_0^{-3}/\beta H$, where r_0 is the distance to the closest dipole. We thus find weak EPR transitions for which $\Delta M = 0$, ± 2, ± 3 with intensities relative to the strong $\Delta M = \pm 1$ transition of $\beta^2/H^2 r_0^6$ [7]. In addition, there are transitions at still higher frequencies (i.e., $|\Delta M| > 3$) which are even weaker. Our interest lies in describing the line width and the shape of the strong $\Delta M = \pm 1$ transition. We must recognize the existence of these weak lines, however, in order to correctly calculate the desired quantities.

Think of the Hamiltonian of N interacting dipoles given by Eq. (6-21) as having been diagonalized. Let n stand for the set of quantum numbers of the various eigenstates. The magnetic resonance near $v = g\beta H/h$ is then regarded as an envelope of sharp lines, each of which corresponds to the excess of absorption over emission, owing to the Boltzmann population excess in the lower state, for a transition between a state n and a state n' (see Fig. 6-2). For $\mathbf{H}_1$ normal to $\mathbf{H}$, the intensity of each of these lines is

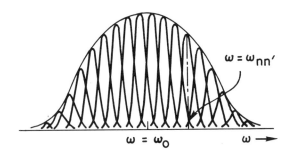

FIG. 6-2 Illustration of the way in which individual sharp transitions between states of the complete Hamiltonian, with dipolar interactions, make up the total absorption line.

proportional to $|\langle n'|S_x|n\rangle|^2$ [see Eq. (5-110)]. The mean-square frequency, or second moment of the resonance, is found by weighting $\omega_{nn'}^2$ for each line with its intensity,

$$\langle\omega^2\rangle = \frac{\sum\limits_{n,n'} \omega_{nn'}^2 |\langle n'|S_x|n\rangle|^2}{\sum\limits_{n,n'} |\langle n'|S_x|n\rangle|^2}, \tag{6-23}$$

where $\omega_{nn'} \equiv (E_n - E_{n'})/\hbar$, and where the high-temperature approximation is made, that is, $g\beta H \ll kT$ (do not confuse the symbol $\langle\rangle$ as employed above with its use for expectation value, as introduced in Chapter 2). We are assuming that T_1 is long enough that the individual transitions shown in Fig. 6-2 are so narrow that they make a negligible contribution to the second moment. We have then integrated over all ω to obtain the average in Eq. (6-23). Van Vleck's success in the calculation is possible because he can express Eq. (6-23) as the trace or diagonal sum of a matrix, which sum can be calculated in any convenient representation because of the well-known property that the trace of a matrix is independent of representation. The denominator of Eq. (6-23) is clearly the diagonal sum of a matrix product. The numerator is

$$\hbar^{-2} \sum_{n,n'} [\langle n|\mathcal{H}|n\rangle - \langle n'|\mathcal{H}|n'\rangle]^2 \langle n|S_x|n'\rangle \langle n'|S_x|n\rangle$$

$$= -\hbar^{-2}\, \mathrm{tr}\, [\mathcal{H}S_x - S_x\mathcal{H}]^2 \tag{6-24}$$

as can perhaps be seen most readily by identifying each term in the expression

$$\mathrm{tr}\, [\mathcal{H}S_x\mathcal{H}S_x - S_x\mathcal{H}^2 S_x - \mathcal{H}S_x^2\mathcal{H} + S_x\mathcal{H}S_x\mathcal{H}]$$

with one in the left-hand member of Eq. (6-24). The resulting expression is

$$\langle\omega^2\rangle = -\frac{\mathrm{tr}\, [\mathcal{H}S_x - S_x\mathcal{H}]^2}{\hbar^2\, \mathrm{tr}\, S_x^2} = -\frac{\mathrm{tr}\, [\mathcal{H}, S_x]^2}{\hbar^2\, \mathrm{tr}\, S_x^2}. \tag{6-25}$$

Equation (6-25) is, in fact, only a special case of the general expression [8]

$$\hbar^{2k}\langle\omega^{2k}\rangle = (-1)^k \frac{\mathrm{tr}\, [\mathcal{H}, [\mathcal{H}, \cdots [\mathcal{H}, S_x] \cdots]]^2}{\mathrm{tr}\, S_x^2}, \tag{6-26}$$

$$\langle\omega^{2k}\rangle = \frac{\mathrm{tr}\, [(d/dt)^k S_x]^2}{\mathrm{tr}\, S_x^2},$$

where k is an integer ≥ 1 and there are k commutator brackets. The time derivative is of course the Heisenberg time derivative of the operator.

Returning to Eq. (6-25), we note before we proceed with the calculation that the exchange interaction in Eq. (6-21) contributes nothing to $\langle \omega^2 \rangle$ because $S_x = \Sigma_j S_{jx}$ commutes with it. This can be seen by direct evaluation of the commutators or, most simply, by noting that S_x generates infinitesimal rotations about the x axis and that $\mathbf{S}_j \cdot \mathbf{S}_k$, a scalar product of two vectors, is invariant under such rotations. It is thus apparent that *exchange interactions contribute nothing to the mean-square frequency.*

Before proceeding to evaluate Eq. (6-25), we must make an essential simplification. We are calculating the mean-square width or second moment of the *main line* near $\omega_0 = g\beta H/\hbar$ and are not interested in the subsidiary lines discussed after Eq. (6-22). These lines, although weaker, are weighted heavily by large frequency displacements from the center of the main line, and they would contribute appreciably to the second moment measured from the center of the main line. We define $\Omega \equiv \omega - \omega_0$. Then the second moment about the line center will be denoted as μ_Ω^2:

$$\mu_\Omega^2 = \langle \Omega^2 \rangle = \langle (\omega - \omega_0)^2 \rangle. \tag{6-27}$$

To eliminate the subsidiary lines, Van Vleck therefore proceeds to truncation of the Hamiltonian, that is, removal of the off-diagonal parts of $\mathcal{JC}_d$ which produce the mixing that leads to the lines at 0, $2\omega_0$, and $3\omega_0$:

$$\mathcal{JC}_{\text{trunc}} = \sum_{j=1}^{N} g\beta H S_{jz} - g^2\beta^2 \sum_{(jk)} r_{jk}^{-3} \tfrac{1}{2}(3\cos^2\theta_{jk} - 1)(3S_{jz}S_{kz} - \mathbf{S}_j \cdot \mathbf{S}_k)$$

$$- 2\sum_{(jk)} J_{jk}\mathbf{S}_j \cdot \mathbf{S}_k. \tag{6-28}$$

Evaluating the required commutators and taking the necessary traces is straightforward if the familiar representation in which each S_{jz} is diagonal is used. We illustrate the nature of the calculation by treating only $\mathcal{JC}_z$, which we anticipate should certainly correspond to a δ-function line at $\omega_0 = g\beta H/\hbar$, inasmuch as no interactions are then present to broaden the resonance. We thus must evaluate the commutator and its square,

$$\left[\sum_j S_{jz}, \sum_k S_{kx}\right] = \sum_j [S_{jz}, S_{jx}] = i\sum_j S_{jy},$$

$$\left(i\sum_j S_{jy}\right)^2 = -\sum_{j,k} S_{jy}S_{ky}, \tag{6-29}$$

and then take the trace. Now it is readily seen that, within its own manifold, $(\text{tr})_j S_{jy} = (\text{tr})_j S_{jz} = (\text{tr})_j S_{jx} = 0$. Hence the only important terms in Eq. (6-29) are those with $j = k$:

$$\text{tr}\,[\mathcal{JC}_z, S_x]^2 = -g^2\beta^2 H^2\,\text{tr}\left(\sum_{j=1}^{N} S_{jy}^2\right). \tag{6-30}$$

Now S_{jy} is diagonal in the magnetic quantum numbers of the $N-1$ dipoles other than dipole j. Thus the matrix element of S_{jy} is

$$\langle m_1 m_2 \cdots m_j \cdots m_N | S_{jy} | m_1' m_2' \cdots m_j' \cdots m_N' \rangle$$

$$= \delta_{m_1 m_1'} \delta_{m_2 m_2'} \cdots \langle m_j | S_{jy} | m_j' \rangle \cdots \delta_{m_N m_N'}. \tag{6-31}$$

Within the m_j manifold alone,

$$(\text{tr})_j S_{jy}^2 = \tfrac{1}{3} S(S+1)(2S+1). \tag{6-32}$$

If we now observe that

$$\text{tr } 1 = \sum_{m_1 = -S}^{S} \sum_{m_2 = -S}^{S} \cdots \sum_{m_N = -S}^{S} 1 = (2S+1)^N, \tag{6-33}$$

it readily follows from Eqs. (6-31) and (6-32) that

$$\text{tr } S_{jy}^2 = \tfrac{1}{3} S(S+1)(2S+1)^N, \tag{6-34}$$

and hence that

$$\text{tr } [\mathcal{K}_z S_x - S_x \mathcal{K}_z]^2 = -g^2 \beta^2 H^2 \left(\frac{N}{3}\right) S(S+1)(2S+1)^N. \tag{6-35}$$

The denominator in Eq. (6-25) is similarly $\tfrac{1}{3} N S(S+1)(2S+1)^N$, so that we obtain

$$\langle \omega^2 \rangle = \frac{g^2 \beta^2 H^2}{\hbar^2} = \omega_0^2, \tag{6-36}$$

as expected.

Van Vleck [6] carries through the calculation of dipolar broadening as included in Eq. (6-28) and finds

$$\hbar^2 \langle \omega^2 \rangle = g^2 \beta^2 H^2 + \tfrac{3}{4} S(S+1) \sum_j g^4 \beta^4 r_{jk}^{-6} (3 \cos^2 \theta_{jk} - 1)^2. \tag{6-37}$$

Here the site k upon which the sum is based is a typical interior ion site of the crystal. As we noted earlier, exchange does not influence the second moment.

We can give Eq. (6-37) more meaning in situations where the resonance is narrow compared to ω_0 by noting that the symmetry of possible m_j values in essence assures a symmetrical line at ω_0. Then, recalling our definition, Eq. (6-27), and generalizing the notation μ_Ω^n as the nth moment, we conclude from the symmetry of the line that $\mu_\Omega^1 = 0$. Then

$$\langle \omega^2 \rangle = \langle (\omega_0 + \Omega)^2 \rangle = \omega_0^2 + \mu_\Omega^2,$$

$$\mu_\Omega^2 = \langle \omega^2 \rangle - \omega_0^2 \tag{6-38}$$

$$= \tfrac{3}{4} S(S+1) \hbar^{-2} \sum_j g^4 \beta^4 r_{jk}^{-6} (3 \cos^2 \theta_{jk} - 1)^2.$$

The result in Eq. (6-38) implies that the line width is proportional to the dipolar energy, $g^2\beta^2/r_0^3$, divided by $\hbar$. The failure of exchange to influence Eq. (6-38) at all, however, appears as something of a surprise, since exchange is expected to influence line shape. This mystery will be cleared up in what follows.

On re-examination of the previous paragraphs we observe that

$$\hbar^2\langle\Omega^2\rangle = \frac{-\text{tr }[\mathcal{H}_d, S_x]^2}{\text{tr }S_x^2} \tag{6-39}$$

where we suppose that the relevant part of $\mathcal{H}_d$ after truncation is used. Although it was permissible to drop $\mathcal{H}_e$ from Eq. (6-39) because $[\mathcal{H}_e, S_x]=0$, $\mathcal{H}_e$ cannot be dropped from the fourth-moment calculation because it does not commute with $[\mathcal{H}_d, S_x]$. To an order-of-magnitude approximation, we can write Eq. (6-26), for $k = 2$, in a form similar to Eq. (6-39):

$$\hbar^4\langle\Omega^4\rangle \approx \frac{\text{tr }[\mathcal{H}_e+\mathcal{H}_d, [\mathcal{H}_d, S_x]]^2}{\text{tr }S_x^2}. \tag{6-40}$$

Equation (6-40) is not precisely an equality because, recalling that odd moments vanish for a symmetrical line,

$$\langle(\omega_0+\Omega)^4\rangle = \omega_0^4+6\omega_0^2\langle\Omega^2\rangle+\langle\Omega^4\rangle = \omega_0^4+6\omega_0^2\mu_\Omega^2+\mu_\Omega^4, \tag{6-41}$$

and the cross term is not included in Eq. (6-40).

The fourth-moment calculation is too long to include here. Examination of Van Vleck's result [6] quickly reveals how $\hbar^4\mu_\Omega^4$ depends on the magnitude of exchange couplings. If J is the exchange constant and $E_d^2 \approx g^4\beta^4 r_0^{-6}$, where r_0 is the nearest dipole distance, then

$$\hbar^4\mu_\Omega^4 \approx J^2E_d^2+E_d^4 \tag{6-42}$$

follows from Van Vleck's result or even from inspection of Eq. (6-40). In the same approximation Eq. (6-38) states that

$$\hbar^2\mu_\Omega^2 \approx E_d^2. \tag{6-43}$$

First we consider Eqs. (6-42) and (6-43) when no exchange interaction is present. Then it follows that

$$(\hbar^2\mu_\Omega^2)^2 \approx \hbar^4\mu_\Omega^4, \tag{6-44}$$

and this, coupled with Eq. (6-43), is characteristic of a simple absorption curve confined to a frequency interval of order $E_d/\hbar$ at ω_0. For example, a Gaussian curve of width $E_d/\hbar$ would have this property. In fact, it is readily shown that the ratio $(\mu_\Omega^4)^{1/4}/(\mu_\Omega^2)^{1/2}$ is 1.32 for a Gaussian and 1.16 for a rectangular curve.

It is evident, however, that the presence of a J larger than E_d has the effect of greatly increasing μ_Ω^4 while leaving μ_Ω^2 totally unaffected. Here is the indication of the exchange-narrowing phenomenon. Figure 6-3 sketches first a Gaussian curve, which might not differ greatly from the line shape existing under the influence of dipolar broadening alone. If exchange were added to the same lattice of ions, however, the line would have to alter in such a way as to increase μ_Ω^4 while preserving μ_Ω^2 and its intensity, μ_Ω^0.

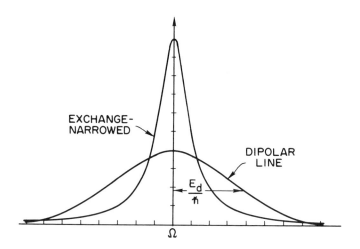

FIG. 6-3 Comparison of resonance line shapes for two identical lattices of paramagnetic ions, except that one lattice has exchange and the other does not.

The key to the requisite change in shape lies in the great influence of the wings of the line on

$$\mu_\Omega^n = \int_{-\infty}^{\infty} \Omega^n F(\Omega)\, d\Omega, \qquad (6\text{-}45)$$

where we here use an expression for the moment in terms of the line shape function, $F(\Omega)$, which is equivalent to Eqs. (6-23) and (6-38) for second moments. If one takes intensity out of the line at points near $\Omega \approx E_d/\hbar$, then he can put some of it in the wings, increasing μ_Ω^4 until the second moment is nearly restored, and throw whatever remains into a sharp peak near $\Omega = 0$, which will contribute very little to μ_Ω^2 or to μ_Ω^4. Of course, the resulting line will have an enhanced μ_Ω^4 because Ω^4 weighs the wings more heavily than does Ω^2. Figure 6-3 sketches the qualitative change in line shape, which will be regarded experimentally as a narrowing of the line.

When $J \gg E_d$, the resonance has essentially a Lorentzian shape (see Fig. 2-19) with a cutoff at $\Omega \sim \pm J/\hbar$ [9]. Using Eq. (2-59), we can obtain an expression for $F(\Omega)$ for a Lorentzian line (assuming no saturation):

$$F(\Omega) = \frac{T_2}{\pi} \frac{1}{1 + T_2^2 \Omega^2}. \tag{6-46}$$

Substituting this in Eq. (6-45) and integrating out to the cutoff frequency, we obtain

$$\mu_\Omega^n = \frac{T_2}{\pi} \int_{-J/\hbar}^{J/\hbar} \frac{\Omega^n}{1 + T_2^2 \Omega^2} d\Omega$$

$$\approx \frac{(2/\pi)(J/\hbar)^{n-1}}{(n-1)T_2}, \tag{6-47}$$

where 1 is neglected in relation to $T_2^2 \Omega^2$ in the integrand, and n is taken as even to obtain the approximate result. If we consider the second moment, we have

$$\mu_\Omega^2 \approx \frac{(2/\pi)(J/\hbar)}{T_2}. \tag{6-48}$$

In Eq. (6-43) we have an alternative expression for μ_Ω^2, that is,

$$\mu_\Omega^2 \approx \left(\frac{E_d}{\hbar}\right)^2. \tag{6-49}$$

Combining Eqs. (6-48) and (6-49), we may obtain an expression for $1/T_2$:

$$\frac{1}{T_2} \approx \frac{(\pi/2)(E_d/\hbar)^2}{J/\hbar}, \tag{6-50}$$

which from Eq. (2-61) is the half-width in angular frequency.

Defining $\omega_d \equiv \hbar^{-1} E_d$, $\omega_e \equiv \hbar^{-1} J$, we obtain from Eq. (6-50) that

$$\frac{1}{T_2} = \Delta\omega_{1/2} = \frac{(\pi/2)\omega_d^2}{\omega_e}. \tag{6-51}$$

This is a result quite similar to extreme motional narrowing of a magnetic resonance line for a liquid, with $1/\omega_e$ here replacing τ_c, the correlation time for molecular motion in the liquid [10]. Exchange narrowing can be viewed as a physically similar phenomenon, wherein the portion $J[S_{j+}S_{k-} + S_{j-}S_{k+}]$ of $2J\mathbf{S}_j \cdot \mathbf{S}_k$ is thought of as flipping neighboring oppositely oriented spins at a rate $J/\hbar$, thereby leading to an effective migration of spin orientation through the lattice.

Crystalline materials which exhibit extreme exchange narrowing are the crystalline organic radicals [11], examples of the chemical formulas of which are given in Fig. 6-4. These crystals are molecular or Van der Waals crystals, with a typical molecular weight near perhaps 400. The molecule is paramagnetic by virtue of an unused valence, leaving the molecule with an unpaired electron. The most common of these materials is DPPH,

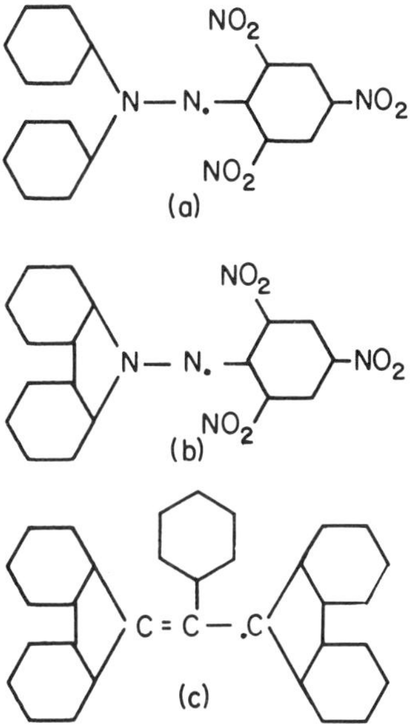

FIG. 6-4   Schematic structures of some organic radical molecules that form relatively stable molecular crystals under ordinary conditions of temperature and pressure: (a) diphenyl picryl hydrazyl (DPPH), (b) picryl amino carbazyl, (c) bisdiphenylene phenyl allyl.

diphenyl picryl hydrazyl (see Fig. 6-4). It is reasonably stable in air at ordinary temperatures and has a sharp resonance line which is quite exchange-narrowed. The calculated root-mean-square width in the absence of exchange narrowing would be about 100 G, or 300 MHz. The observed resonance width [12] is near 3 G, or about 10 MHz, corresponding to $T_2 = 2.4 \times 10^{-8}$ sec. Converting to angular frequencies as required by Eq. (6-51), we estimate that $\omega_e = 2\pi(20{,}000 \text{ MHz}) = J/\hbar$. From this we find $J/k \approx 1\,°\text{K}$, which is a magnitude of J confirmed by specific heat measurements [13].

Two interesting conclusions can be drawn from the results on DPPH and similar materials. First, exchange narrowing is pronounced, giving in fact as little as 1% of the dipolar width that would be present without exchange. Second, the model seems to check quantitatively with $\omega_e \approx J/\hbar$. Indeed, the line shape in these materials is, to a very good approximation, Lorentzian.

The question may be asked how there can be exchange interaction between DPPH molecules when it is simply an unpaired electron of a central nitrogen atom that provides the magnetic properties. The answer is that the wave function of the unpaired electron is highly "delocalized," that is, spread out widely over the molecular skeleton and even beyond its limits, making overlap possible. This is known from the measurable isotropic hyperfine couplings to nuclei throughout the entire molecular structure [14]. These hyperfine splittings can be rendered measurable if the free-radical molecules are dissolved in dilute liquid solution so that exchange effects are removed and rapid tumbling averages away anisotropic hyperfine effects.

6–3 The Effects of Interactions; Strongly Interacting Pairs

In Section 6–2 we considered a large number of mutually interacting paramagnets. Interactions also exist between a few well-defined and well-localized paramagnetic entities with splittings as large as 100 cm^{-1} or more. Thus, if concentration and crystal structure allow such strong interactions between a few paramagnets, we face a rather different problem, one in which the electron paramagnetic resonance spectra, not just the line shapes, are changed. This can result because the crystal structure allows two paramagnetic ions to be much closer to each other than to any other ions. More commonly, however, pairs or triples of ions occur close to each other but far from all others in crystals containing a small concentration of paramagnetic species. The spectrum for these interacting paramagnets results from the solution of the Hamiltonian consisting of the two separate spin Hamiltonians (allowing for any possible modifications in symmetry and in the parameters) plus the interaction Hamiltonian, as discussed in Section 6–1. Since the possible variations of this problem are large, we will not attempt a thorough discussion but will let a few simple examples illustrate the behavior.

Of the several bilinear operators introduced in Section 6–1 to describe the interaction between pairs of paramagnetic species, the isotropic (Heisenberg) form usually dominates,

$$\mathcal{H}_{12} = -2J\mathbf{S}_1 \cdot \mathbf{S}_2. \tag{6-52}$$

The reason is that, if spin-dependent terms in the actual Hamiltonian can be neglected in determining the exchange, then the total spin is a good quantum number. The largest spin-dependent term is usually the spin-orbit interaction, which ordinarily makes only a small contribution to the properties of iron-group ions with orbital singlet ground states (the well-known quenching of the orbital angular momentum is an example). In such cases the skew-symmetric terms in the bilinear interaction (if allowed by symmetry) should be first order in λ, and the symmetric anisotropic terms should be second order [15].

If the bilinear term in Eq. (6-52) is the dominant one, the two (effective) spins couple to give values of S in the range

$$|S_1 - S_2| \leq S \leq S_1 + S_2. \tag{6-53}$$

Neglecting all other terms in the Hamiltonian (they are presumably smaller), we obtain the energies [see Section 1–2 and Eq. (6-14) for the method]

$$E = -J[S(S+1) - S_1(S_1+1) - S_2(S_2+1)]. \tag{6-54}$$

Calculating the difference in energy between adjacent levels, we obtain

$$E(S) - E(S-1) = 2JS. \tag{6-55}$$

Thus the spacing between levels is proportional to the larger of the values of S, an analog of the Landé interval rule of atomic spectra [16].

A manifold of states corresponding to a given total spin is degenerate by our considerations above, but it will in fact be split by other terms in the Hamiltonian. We will assume that this splitting is small compared to J. In this case we need consider only that part of the Hamiltonian which produces matrix elements between states with the same S. The terms producing matrix elements between states of different S will contribute only in higher orders of perturbation theory. We may express this by writing down a separate spin Hamiltonian for each value of S according to our prescription of Chapter 4. This gives unrelated descriptions for all values of S. It is of more interest to use a description in terms of the individual spin Hamiltonians of the paramagnets and the spin Hamiltonian describing the interactions. Thus we wish to express the spin Hamiltonians written in terms of S by using the parameters describing the spin Hamiltonian in terms of S_1 and S_2.

Within a manifold of states of given S the operators in terms of S_1 and S_2 may be written in terms of operators involving S by using the Wigner-Eckart theorem. The process of finding these relationships requires in general rather tedious calculations involving the properties of tensor operators and n-j symbols. For the interested reader the books by Edmonds [17], Messiah [18], and Judd [19] and the tables of Rotenberg *et al.* [20] are recommended.

If we consider for simplicity only terms quadratic or lower in powers of the components of S_1 and S_2 and assume identical paramagnetic species, we then have two types of terms. One type (I) involves either components of S_1 or of S_2 but not both. The other type (II) always involves both components of S_1 and of S_2. The Wigner-Eckart theorem can be applied to both types with the results

$$\langle S, M'|T_{lm}^I|S, M\rangle = \alpha_l \langle S, M'|S_{lm}|S, M\rangle, \qquad T_{lm}^I \to \alpha_l S_{lm},$$

$$\langle S, M'|T_{lm}^{II}|S, M\rangle = \beta_l \langle S, M'|S_{lm}|S, M\rangle, \qquad T_{lm}^{II} \to \beta_l S_{lm}, \tag{6-56}$$

where Tables 6-1 and 6-2 list the various values of α_l, β_l, T_{lm}^i, and S_{lm} (recall that $S_1 = S_2$). We note immediately that no interaction operators described by $l = 1$ will produce any first-order contributions to the energy. These are the skew-symmetric (or Dzyaloshinski-Moriya) exchange terms.

Table 6-1

l	0	1	2
α_l	$\dfrac{S_1(S_1+1)}{S(S+1)}$	$\frac{1}{2}$	$\dfrac{3S(S+1)-4S_1(S_1+1)-3}{2(2S-1)(2S+3)}$
β_l	$\dfrac{S(S+1)-2S_1(S_1+1)}{2S(S+1)}$	0	$\dfrac{S(S+1)+4S_1(S_1+1)}{2(2S-1)(2S+3)}$

Table 6-2

l	m	S_{lm}	T_{lm}^I (and Similarly for S_2)	T_{lm}^{II}
0	0	$-\dfrac{2}{\sqrt{3}}\mathbf{S}^2$	$-\dfrac{2}{\sqrt{3}}\mathbf{S}_1^2$	$-\dfrac{2}{\sqrt{3}}\mathbf{S}_1\cdot\mathbf{S}_2$
1	-1	S_-	S_{1-}	$S_{1z}S_{2-}-S_{1-}S_{2z}$
1	0	$\sqrt{2}S_z$	$\sqrt{2}S_{1z}$	$\dfrac{1}{\sqrt{2}}(S_{1-}S_{2+}-S_{1+}S_{2-})$
1	1	$-S_+$	$-S_{1+}$	$S_{1z}S_{2+}-S_{1+}S_{2z}$
2	-2	S_-^2	S_{1-}^2	$S_{1-}S_{2-}$
2	-1	$S_zS_-+S_-S_z$	$S_{1z}S_{1-}+S_{1-}S_{1z}$	$S_{1z}S_{2-}+S_{1-}S_{2z}$
2	0	$\sqrt{\frac{2}{3}}(3S_z^2-\mathbf{S}^2)$	$\sqrt{\frac{2}{3}}(3S_{1z}^2-\mathbf{S}_1^2)$	$\sqrt{\frac{2}{3}}(3S_{1z}S_{2z}-\mathbf{S}_1\cdot\mathbf{S}_2)$
2	1	$-(S_zS_++S_+S_z)$	$-(S_{1z}S_{1+}+S_{1+}S_{1z})$	$-(S_{1z}S_{2+}+S_{1+}S_{2z})$
2	2	S_+^2	S_{1+}^2	$S_{1+}S_{2+}$

The results summarized in Tables 6-1 and 6-2 can be generalized to include higher l values, dissimilar paramagnets, biquadratic and more complicated interactions, and terms off-diagonal in S. Such generalization complicates the problem considerably, however, and therefore will not be considered. It should be understood that the treatment leading to these results is convenient (especially when off-diagonal matrix elements are small compared to J) but not necessary.

Let us now consider the effect of interactions between two identical paramagnetic ions, each with a hyperfine interaction with its own nucleus. If we assume only an isotropic exchange interaction, then the spin Hamiltonian is

$$\mathcal{H} = \sum_{i=1}^{2} \mathcal{H}_i -- 2J\mathbf{S}_1 \cdot \mathbf{S}_2, \tag{6-57}$$

where

$$\mathcal{H}_i = \beta \mathbf{H} \cdot \mathbf{g} \cdot \mathbf{S}_i + \mathbf{S} \cdot \mathbf{A} \cdot \mathbf{I}_i. \tag{6-58}$$

If we now write down a spin Hamiltonian valid within a manifold of states with constant S, using Eq. (6-56) and Tables 6-1 and 6-2, we obtain

$$\mathcal{H} = \beta \mathbf{H} \cdot \mathbf{g} \cdot \mathbf{S} + \tfrac{1}{2}\mathbf{S} \cdot \mathbf{A} \cdot \sum_{i} \mathbf{I}_i - J[S(S+1) - 2S_1(S_1+1)]. \tag{6-59}$$

For a given value of S the splitting of these states is the same as for the original paramagnetic center except that now the hyperfine interaction is with two nuclei, not one nucleus, and the interaction is only half as large (S is of course not generally equal to S_1). The results are similar to those in Fig. 5-11 and in the corresponding text of Chapter 5. This case may be viewed as one in which the exchange causes the magnetic electron to be delocalized. The electrons now divide their time equally between the two nuclei and thus interact only half as much with a given nucleus. This has been demonstrated for the case of shallow donors (phosphorus, arsenic, antimony) in silicon [21]. For example an isolated phosphorus donor has a two-line hyperfine structure arising from the interaction with the ^{31}P nucleus, which has a 100% natural abundance, that is, it is the only stable isotope. If two donors are interacting strongly enough, a line appears half way between the two lines produced by the isolated ^{31}P. This extra line is the only line from the pair which can be resolved. It is also possible to observe the effect for three or four interacting donors. In the case of donors $\mathbf{g}$ and $\mathbf{A}$ are isotropic, $S_i = \tfrac{1}{2}$, and an appreciable intensity of the spectra from interacting donors is obtained by having a sufficiently large concentration of donors so that interactions are quite probable.

As another example let us consider the general interaction of two $S_i = \tfrac{1}{2}$ paramagnetic species with no hyperfine interaction. Then we have the spin Hamiltonian

$$\mathcal{H} = \sum_{i=1}^{2} \mathcal{H}_i - 2J\mathbf{S}_1 \cdot \mathbf{S}_2 + K(3S_{1z}S_{2z} - \mathbf{S}_1 \cdot \mathbf{S}_2) + K'(S_{1x}S_{2x} - S_{1y}S_{2y}) + \mathcal{H}_{ss}$$

(6-60)

with

$$\mathcal{H}_i = \beta\mathbf{H} \cdot \mathbf{g} \cdot \mathbf{S}_i \qquad\qquad (6\text{-}61)$$

and $\mathcal{H}_{ss}$ the skew-symmetric interaction terms. Using Tables 6-1 and 6-2, we obtain

$$\mathcal{H} = \beta\mathbf{H} \cdot \mathbf{g} \cdot \mathbf{S} + \tfrac{1}{3}D[3S_z^2 - S(S+1)] + E(S_x^2 - S_y^2) - J[S(S+1) - \tfrac{3}{2}], \qquad (6\text{-}62)$$

where

$$\tfrac{1}{3}D = \beta_2 K, \qquad E = \beta_2 K',$$

$$\beta_2 = \frac{S(S+1)+3}{2(2S-1)(2S+3)} = \begin{cases} -\tfrac{1}{2}, & S = 0, \\[2mm] \tfrac{1}{3}, & S = 1, \end{cases} \qquad (6\text{-}63)$$

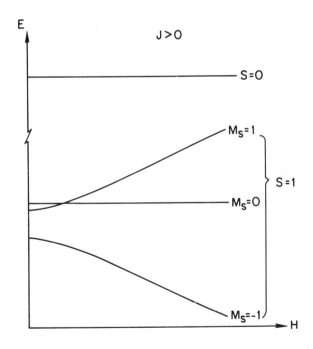

FIG. 6-5 The energy level diagram for the most general interaction of two paramagnets with $S_i = \tfrac{1}{2}$. The exchange constant, J, is taken as positive and much larger than the Zeeman splitting of the triplet. The direction of the field is chosen so that $\mathbf{H} \cdot \mathbf{g}$ is parallel to the z axis.

and where x, y, and z are principal axes of the exchange interaction. The $S = 0$ state is not influenced by $\mathbf{H}$ or the anisotropic exchange in first order. The $S = 1$ state is split in a manner identical to that for fine structure consistent with the symmetry of the interacting pair and its surroundings. The energy level diagram for $\mathbf{H} \cdot \mathbf{g}$ parallel to z is shown in Fig. 6-5.

6–4 Supplemental Bibliography

No general references to all of the topics covered in this chapter seem adequate. Therefore we will list references for four distinct topics: exchange, interaction spin Hamiltonians, method of moments, and electron paramagnetic resonance of interacting pairs.

I. Exchange

1. D. H. Martin, *Magnetism in Solids*, Iliffe, London, 1967, Chapters 5 and 6.

2. P. W. Anderson, "Exchange in Insulators: Superexchange, Direct Exchange, and Double Exchange," in *Magnetism* (G. T. Rado and H. Suhl, eds.), Academic, New York, 1963, Vol. I, p. 25.

3. C. Herring, "Direct Exchange between Well-Separated Atoms," in *Magnetism* (G. T. Rado and H. Suhl, eds.), Academic, New York, 1966, Vol. IIB, p. 1. Also a reference on interaction spin Hamiltonians.

II. Interaction Spin Hamiltonians

1. C. Herring, cited as reference 3 under topic I.

2. K. W. H. Stevens, "Spin Hamiltonians," in *Magnetism* (G. T. Rado and H. Suhl, eds.), Academic, New York, 1963, Vol. I, p. 17.

3. H. P. Baltes, J. F. Moser, and F. K. Kneubühl, *J. Phys. Chem. Solids* **28**, 2635 (1967).

III. Method of Moments

1. C. P. Slichter, *Principles of Magnetic Resonance*, Harper and Row, New York, 1963, p. 45.

2. A. Abragam, *The Principles of Nuclear Magnetism*, Oxford, New York, 1961, p. 97.

IV. Electron Paramagnetic Resonance of Interacting Pairs

1. J. Owen, *J. Appl. Phys.*, Suppl., **32**, 213S (1961).

2. J. Owen, *J. Appl. Phys.*, Suppl., **33**, 355 (1962).

References Cited in Chapter 6

[1] D. H. Martin, *Magnetism in Solids*, Iliffe, London, 1967; D. C. Mattis, *The Theory of Magnetism*, Harper and Row, New York, 1965; G. T. Rado and H. Suhl, eds., *Magnetism*, Academic, New York, 1963.

[2] D. H. Martin, *Magnetism in Solids*, Iliffe, London, 1967, p. 274.

[3] I. Dzyaloshinski, *J. Phys. Chem. Solids* **4**, 241 (1958); T. Moriya, *Phys. Rev.* **120**, 91 (1960); P. Erdös, *J. Phys. Chem. Solids* **27**, 1705 (1966).

[4] E. A. Harris and J. Owen, *Phys. Rev. Letters* **11**, 9 (1963).

[5] C. Herring, "Direct Exchange between Well-Separated Atoms," in *Magnetism* (G. T. Rado and H. Suhl, eds.), Academic, New York, 1966, Vol. IIB, p. 160.

[6] J. H. Van Vleck, *Phys. Rev.* **74**, 1168 (1948).

[7] For the discussion of a simple example see C. P. Slichter, *Principles of Magnetic Resonance*, Harper and Row, New York, 1963, p. 46.

[8] A. Abragam, *The Principles of Nuclear Magnetism*, Oxford, New York, 1961, p. 108.

[9] A. Abragam, *The Principles of Nuclear Magnetism*, Oxford, New York, 1961, p. 107.

[10] A. Abragam, *The Principles of Nuclear Magnetism*, Oxford, New York, 1961, p. 424.

[11] For more information on organic radicals see D. J. E. Ingram, *Free Radicals*, Academic, New York, 1958; M. Bersohn and J. C. Baird, *An Introduction to Electron Paramagnetic Resonance*, Benjamin, New York, 1966.

[12] J. P. Goldsborough, M. Mandel, and G. E. Pake, *Phys. Rev. Letters*, **4**, 13 (1960).

[13] J. P. Goldsborough, M. Mandel, and G. E. Pake, Proceedings of the VII International Conference on Low Temperature Physics, Un. of Toronto Press, 1960, p. 235; A. M. Prokhorov and V. B. Fedorov, Sov. Phys. — J.E.T.P. **16**, 1489 (1963).

[14] G. E. Pake, S. I. Weissman, and J. Townsend, *Discussions Faraday Soc.* **19**, 147 (1955).

[15] T. Moriya, *Phys. Rev.* **120**, 91 (1960).

[16] M. Tinkham, *Group Theory and Quantum Mechanics*, McGraw-Hill, New York, 1964, p. 184.

[17] A. R. Edmonds, *Angular Momentum in Quantum Mechanics*, Princeton University Press, Princeton, N.J., 1957.

[18] A. Messiah, *Quantum Mechanics*, North Holland, Amsterdam, 1962, Vol. 2, p. 1075.

[19] B. R. Judd, *Operator Techniques in Atomic Spectroscopy*, McGraw-Hill, New York, 1963.

[20] M. Rotenberg, R. Bivins, N. Metropolis, and J. K. Wooten, Jr., *The 3-j and 6-j Symbols*, Technology Press, Cambridge, 1959.

[21] G. W. Ludwig and H. H. Woodbury, "Electron Spin Resonance in Semiconductors" in *Solid State Physics* (F. Seitz and D. Turnbull, eds.), Academic, New York, 1962, Vol. 13, p. 247.

CHAPTER 7

Effects of Stress and Electric Fields

Electron paramagnetic resonance spectra will generally change if additional external fields, either elastic or electric, are applied. These changes may facilitate the analysis of the field-free spectra, although they are rarely used in this way. More frequently the information derived by applying fields is complementary to that obtained from the field-free spectra and is useful in explaining other phenomena, most particularly spin-lattice relaxation, the subject of Chapter 8.

7–1 The Spin Hamiltonian Description

In Section 4–2 we developed the concept of the spin Hamiltonian as an effective Hamiltonian operating within the ground manifold of states. We wrote the terms in the spin Hamiltonian entirely as products of components of the axial vectors **S**, **H**, and **I**. Table 4-2 gave the number of such terms allowed by symmetry. The actual form could, in many cases, be obtained by inspection. If this were difficult, it would be necessary to use group theory to couple the components properly, an approach beyond the scope of this book.

We will now describe the effects of stress and electric field in a similar way, that is, by introducing additional terms in the spin Hamiltonian. We will include terms linear in the stress tensor and the electric field vector and occasionally even more complicated terms (although we work with stress throughout, the form of the results is unchanged if strain is used instead). Table 7-1 gives the number of terms linear in the stress (T) or electric field ($\mathcal{E}$) and either quadratic or bilinear in the axial vectors. This table is analogous to Table 4-2 for the field-free terms in the spin Hamiltonian. There can be additional terms containing higher powers of the components of the axial vectors (although the sum of the powers must be even to be invariant under time reversal), as well as additional terms containing higher powers of the components of $\mathcal{E}$ and T and also derivatives. For the most part these additional terms are very small, and if they were included the number of terms would become so large that the utility of the general spin Hamiltonian would be considerably decreased.

Inclusion of $\mathcal{E}$ and $\mathbf{T}$ causes the spin Hamiltonian to differ for each symmetry considered. The actual forms of the several terms are not as easy to see in the present case as they were in Chapter 4. Let us list a few of the simpler ones.

For C_1 symmetry we have the maximum number of terms allowed. For example, there are three components of $\mathcal{E}$ and five of A^2, where $\mathbf{A}$ represents any angular momentum vector, so that we have 15 terms

Table 7-1

The Number of Independent Field-Dependent Terms of the Indicated Type Allowed by Symmetry in a Spin Hamiltonian

Symmetry	$\mathcal{E}A^2$	$\mathcal{E}AB$	TA^2	TAB
Spherical	0	0	1	2
O_h	0	0	2	3
O	0	1	2	3
T_d	1	1	2	3
T_h	0	0	3	5
T	1	2	3	5
$D_{6h}, D_{\infty h}$	0	0	4	7
D_6	1	3	4	7
$C_{6v}, C_{\infty v}$	2	4	4	7
D_{3h}	1	1	4	7
$C_{6h}, C_{\infty h}$	0	0	6	12
C_6	3	7	6	12
C_{3h}	2	2	6	12
D_{4h}	0	0	5	8
D_4	1	3	5	8
C_{4v}	2	4	5	8
D_{2d}	2	3	5	8
C_{4h}	0	0	8	14
S_4	4	6	8	14
C_4	3	7	8	14
D_{3d}	0	0	6	10
D_3	2	4	6	10
C_{3v}	3	5	6	10
S_6	0	0	12	20
C_3	5	9	12	20
D_{2h}	0	0	9	15
D_2	3	6	9	15
C_{2v}	4	7	9	15
C_{2h}	0	0	16	28
C_2	7	13	16	28
C_s	8	14	16	28
C_i	0	0	30	54
C_1	15	27	30	54

for $\mathcal{E}A^2$. If we write this for **S** we have [1]

$$\mathcal{K} = \sum_{\substack{i,j,k \\ j \leq k}} R_{ijk} \mathcal{E}_i (S_j S_k + S_k S_j),$$ (7-1)

where three relations between the R_{ijj} exist since $S_x^2 + S_y^2 + S_z^2$ is a constant $(\Sigma_j R_{ijj} = 0)$. All other symmetries are described by a particular form of Eq. (7-1). Similarly for C_1 symmetry we have $3 \times 3 \times 3 = 27$ $\mathcal{E}HS$ terms, which can be written [1] as

$$\mathcal{K} = \sum_{i,j,k} P_{ijk} \mathcal{E}_i H_j S_k.$$ (7-2)

Since stress is a symmetric second-rank tensor [2], it has six components: three shear, two uniaxial, and one hydrostatic. Thus there are $6 \times 5 = 30 T A^2$ terms in C_1 symmetry, and $6 \times 3 \times 3 = 54$ TAB terms. The spin Hamiltonian can then be written (for TS^2 and THS) as

$$\mathcal{K} = \sum_{\substack{i,j,k,l \\ i \leq j \\ k \leq l}} \mathcal{R}_{ijkl} T_{ij} (S_k S_l + S_l S_k) + \sum_{\substack{i,j,k,l \\ i \leq j}} \mathcal{S}_{ijkl} T_{ij} H_k S_l,$$ (7-3)

where six relationships exist among the $\mathcal{R}_{ijkk}$.

By contrast, in cubic symmetry there are many fewer terms in the spin Hamiltonian. For example, if the point group is O, only one electric field term is present and it is of the type $\mathcal{E}AB$. Writing it explicitly for $\mathcal{E}HS$, we have

$$\mathcal{K} = P[\mathcal{E}_x(H_y S_z - H_z S_y) + \mathcal{E}_y(H_z S_x - H_x S_z) + \mathcal{E}_z(H_x S_y - H_y S_x)].$$ (7-4)

For tetrahedral, T_d, symmetry there are two terms, one quadratic and one bilinear in the axial vectors. Thus in terms of $\mathcal{E}HS$ and $\mathcal{E}S^2$ we have

$$\mathcal{K} = P[\mathcal{E}_x(H_y S_z + H_z S_y) + \mathcal{E}_y(H_z S_x + H_x S_z) + \mathcal{E}_z(H_x S_y + H_y S_x)]$$
$$+ R[\mathcal{E}_x(S_y S_z + S_z S_y) + \mathcal{E}_y(S_z S_x + S_x S_z) + \mathcal{E}_z(S_x S_y + S_y S_x)].$$ (7-5)

The terms involving stress for O_h, O, and T_d symmetries written for THS are

$$\mathcal{K} = \mathcal{S}_1(T_{xx} + T_{yy} + T_{zz})\mathbf{H} \cdot \mathbf{S} + \mathcal{S}_2[\tfrac{1}{3}(2T_{zz} - T_{xx} - T_{yy})(2H_z S_z - H_x S_x - H_y S_y)$$
$$+ (T_{xx} - T_{yy})(H_x S_x - H_y S_y)] + \mathcal{S}_3[T_{yz}(H_y S_z + H_z S_y)$$
$$+ T_{zx}(H_z S_x + H_x S_z) + T_{xy}(H_x S_y + H_y S_x)].$$ (7-6)

The first term represents the g shift due to hydrostatic pressure. The second term represents the effect of uniaxial stress along the cubic axes; such a component of stress will lower the symmetry to tetragonal, and two principal values for the g factor will result. This may be somewhat easier to visualize if the second term in Eq. (7-6) is written as

$$\tfrac{2}{3}\mathcal{S}_2[T_{xx}(2H_x S_x - H_y S_y - H_z S_z) + T_{yy}(2H_y S_y - H_z S_z - H_x S_x)$$
$$+ T_{zz}(2H_z S_z - H_x S_x - H_y S_y)].$$ (7-7)

The TS^2 terms for O_h, O, and T_d symmetries are

$$\mathcal{H} = \mathcal{R}_1[\tfrac{1}{3}(2T_{zz} - T_{xx} - T_{yy})(2S_z^2 - S_x^2 - S_y^2) + (T_{xx} - T_{yy})(S_x^2 - S_y^2)]$$

$$+ \mathcal{R}_2[T_{yz}(S_yS_z + S_zS_y) + T_{zx}(S_zS_x + S_xS_z) + T_{xy}(S_xS_y + S_yS_x)]. \quad (7\text{-}8)$$

By contrast for spherical symmetry we would have

$$\mathcal{H} = \mathcal{S}_1(T_{xx} + T_{yy} + T_{zz})\mathbf{H} \cdot \mathbf{S} + \mathcal{S}_2[2T_{yz}(H_yS_z + H_zS_y)$$

$$+ 2T_{zx}(H_zS_x + H_xS_z) + 2T_{xy}(H_xS_y + H_yS_x) + (T_{xx} - T_{yy})(H_xS_x - H_yS_y)$$

$$+ \tfrac{1}{3}(2T_{zz} - T_{xx} - T_{yy})(2H_zS_z - H_xS_x - H_yS_y)]$$

$$+ \mathcal{R}[2T_{yz}(S_yS_z + S_zS_y) + 2T_{zx}(S_zS_x + S_xS_z) + 2T_{xy}(S_xS_y + S_yS_x)$$

$$+ (T_{xx} - T_{yy})(S_x^2 - S_y^2) + \tfrac{1}{3}(2T_{zz} - T_{xx} - T_{yy})(2S_z^2 - S_x^2 - S_y^2)]. \quad (7\text{-}9)$$

As a final example the four TS^2 terms for D_{6h}, D_6, C_{6v}, and D_{3h} symmetry are

$$\mathcal{H} = \mathcal{R}_1(T_{xx} + T_{yy} + T_{zz})(2S_z^2 - S_x^2 - S_y^2)$$

$$+ \mathcal{R}_2(2T_{zz} - T_{xx} - T_{yy})(2S_z^2 - S_x^2 - S_y^2)$$

$$+ \mathcal{R}_3[T_{zx}(S_zS_x + S_xS_z) + T_{yz}(S_yS_z + S_zS_y)]$$

$$+ \mathcal{R}_4[\tfrac{1}{2}(T_{xx} - T_{yy})(S_x^2 - S_y^2) + T_{xy}(S_xS_y + S_yS_x)]. \quad (7\text{-}10)$$

We should bear in mind that, although we have written only the terms of the types $\mathcal{E}S^2$, $\mathcal{E}HS$, TS^2, and THS, we could substitute any of the bilinear or quadratic axial vector terms of the types $\mathcal{E}I^2$, $\mathcal{E}SI$, $\mathcal{E}HI$, TI^2, TSI, and THI. These represent changes in the hyperfine terms produced by the fields.

We notice in Table 7-1 that all point symmetries which include the inversion operation possess no first-order effects of the electric field. There can be quadratic effects of electric fields, however, and the number of terms involved is the same as for the case of linear dependence on stress.

Although the approach we have described provides a quick and convenient way to obtain the most general form of the spin Hamiltonian, it affords little insight into the origin of these terms. One point of view that we might adopt is to say that the parameters in the spin Hamiltonian, such as g, **D**, and **A**, are field dependent. In nonzero field we can determine the parameters by a Taylor series expansion. Using g as an example, we obtain

$$\mathbf{g} = \mathbf{g}_0 + \sum_i \frac{\partial \mathbf{g}}{\partial \mathcal{E}_i}\bigg|_0 \mathcal{E}_i + \dots, \quad (7\text{-}11)$$

where g_0 is the g tensor for zero electric field, and $(\delta g/\delta \mathcal{E}_i)|_0$ is the value of the partial derivative of **g** with respect to the ith component of $\mathcal{E}$ as evaluated for zero field. Quadratic terms may be important, particularly when symmetry causes the linear terms to vanish. Similar expressions can be obtained for the effects of stress.

From this point of view we could attempt to explain the magnitude of the spin Hamiltonian parameters appearing in Eqs. (7-1) through (7-10) by use of the mechanisms which produced the field-free parameters. All that is necessary is to generalize the calculation to include the fields. For example, stress produces a strain around the paramagnetic entity that results in a crystal field, or its equivalent, which is modified in magnitude and symmetry.

7–2 The Influence of Fields on Electron Paramagnetic Resonance Spectra

From the point of view of symmetry, perhaps the simplest systems for which the effects on electron paramagnetic resonance of electric fields have been studied are transition-group impurity ions occupying interstitial sites in silicon [3-6]. The interstitial sites in the silicon crystal structure have tetrahedral symmetry about their centers (although the ordering of the d orbitals is the same as though it were six-coordinated with negative ions as shown in Fig. 3-8(a). There are two interstitial sites, each being carried

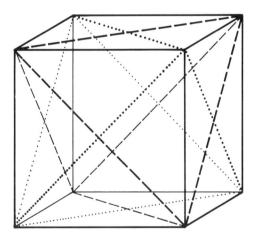

FIG. 7-1 Two inequivalent orientations of tetrahedra in a cube; one tetrahedron is dotted, and the other is dashed. The two tetrahedra are related by inversion through the center of the cube. These are the geometrical relationships of the two types of interstitial sites in silicon, a cubic crystal. They can be rendered inequivalent by any influence which destroys the inversion symmetry of the silicon crystal, such as an applied electric field.

into the other by the operation of inversion through the center of the interstice. Figure 7-1 shows two tetrahedra so related.

Of the many transition-group impurities for which the electric-field effects have been studied in silicon [3-6], two are simple because S is $\frac{1}{2}$. They are neutral manganese and positively charged iron, both with [Ar] $3d^7$ configurations. The spin Hamiltonian for Fe^+, if we ignore the 2.2% abundant ^{57}Fe, is

$$\mathcal{H} = g\beta \mathbf{H} \cdot \mathbf{S} + P[\mathcal{E}_x(H_y S_z + H_z S_y) + \mathcal{E}_y(H_z S_x + H_x S_z) + \mathcal{E}_z(H_x S_y + H_y S_x)],$$

$$(7\text{-}12)$$

where we have included the Zeeman interaction and the linear effect of the electric field on the g value [see Eq. (7-5)]. The difference between the two interstitial sites is that the sign of P is changed. This arises upon applying the inversion operator to Eq. (7-12) in order to generate the other site. Presumably the two interstitial sites will be occupied by impurities with equal probability, so that we expect to observe two lines of equal intensity, one for each type of site.

We may solve the eigenvalue problem arising from Eq. (7-12) in a manner similar to that employed in Section 5-1. By collecting together all of the coefficients of S_x, S_y, and S_z, we find that the Hamiltonian of Eq. (7-12) can be written as the scalar product of $\mathbf{S}$ with the vector

$$(g\beta H_x + P\mathcal{E}_y H_z + P\mathcal{E}_z H_y, \; g\beta H_y + P\mathcal{E}_z H_x + P\mathcal{E}_x H_z, \; g\beta H_z + P\mathcal{E}_x H_y + P\mathcal{E}_y H_x).$$

$$(7\text{-}13)$$

Thus

$$\mathcal{H} = [(g\beta H_x + P\mathcal{E}_y H_z + P\mathcal{E}_z H_y)^2 + (g\beta H_y + P\mathcal{E}_z H_x + P\mathcal{E}_x H_z)^2$$

$$+ (g\beta H_z + P\mathcal{E}_x H_y + P\mathcal{E}_y H_x)^2]^{1/2} S_\zeta. \qquad (7\text{-}14)$$

By equating the square root in Eq. (7-14) to $g\beta H$ we obtain the g factor in the presence of the electric field. The g factor is now anisotropic, that is, its principal values are not all equal. Also the principal axes of the g tensor are not the cubic axes in general. These two properties arise because the quadratic form within the square-root operation in Eq. (7-14) has unequal coefficients of H_x^2, H_y^2, and H_z^2 and also has cross terms of the form $H_x H_y$, and so on. Since we are usually dealing with terms arising from the electric field which are of the order of 1% or less of the Zeeman effect in zero electric field, we many expand Eq. (7-14) as a power series in P. Solving for the energy and obtaining an effective g value in the electric field, we have

$$g_{\text{eff}} = g + \frac{2P}{\beta H^2}(\mathcal{E}_x H_y H_z + \mathcal{E}_y H_z H_x + \mathcal{E}_z H_x H_y) = g + \frac{2P}{\beta}(\mathcal{E}_x mn + \mathcal{E}_y nl + \mathcal{E}_z lm),$$

$$(7\text{-}15)$$

where l, m, and n are the direction cosines of the magnetic field with respect to the cubic axes x, y, and z.

It is very useful in EPR studies of crystalline solids to take spectra as a function of the orientation of the magnetic field with respect to the crystal. The magnetic field (or the sample) is usually rotated so that the field may have any orientation in a particular crystallographic plane. The planes of greatest utility in studying cubic crystals are the {100} or {110} crystal planes because they are of high symmetry and because they contain more of the high-symmetry directions ($\langle 100 \rangle$, $\langle 111 \rangle$, and $\langle 110 \rangle$) than any other planes. Considering first a {100} plane, a plane normal to a cubic axis, we find that Eq. (7-15) now simplifies to

$$g_{\text{eff}} = g + \frac{2P}{\beta}\mathcal{E}_z lm, \qquad (7\text{-}16)$$

where the plane chosen is normal to z, that is, $H_z = n = 0$. We see immediately from this that only the component of the electric field normal to the (001) plane will cause g_{eff} to differ from g. For electric fields in the plane we get a single isotropic line at the same field as for $\mathcal{E} = 0$. For $\mathcal{E}$

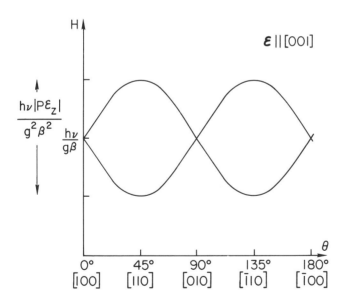

FIG. 7-2 Angular dependence of the EPR spectra of interstitial transition-group impurities with $S = \frac{1}{2}$ in silicon. The magnetic field is always normal to the electric field, which is along a cubic axis. The $\mathcal{E}HS$ term in the spin Hamiltonian of Eq. (7-12) produces the anisotropy and causes each of the two types of interstitial sites to contribute one of the two observed lines.

along [001] we obtain the angular variation of Fig. 7-2, where one curve results from each of the two inequivalent sites. Figure 2 in Ludwig and Woodbury [3] is similar to this figure.

By contrast, if we consider a {110} plane, we find that components of the electric field normal to the plane do not affect the g factor but that electric fields in the plane do. The angular dependence is somewhat more complicated, in part because the direction of $\mathcal{E}$ is now a parameter. Ham, Ludwig, and Woodbury [3-6] did not report measurements for this case.

If $S \geq 1$, then the largest electric-field effect usually arises through terms of the type $\mathcal{E}S^2$ [4-7]. Let us consider this circumstance for the high-symmetry case of transition-group impurities in silicon. If we also require $S \leq \frac{3}{2}$ so that quartic spin operators do not enter the problem, the dominant terms in the spin Hamiltonian are

$$\mathcal{H} = g\beta \mathbf{H} \cdot \mathbf{S} + R[(\mathcal{E}_x(S_yS_z + S_zS_y) + \mathcal{E}_y(S_zS_x + S_xS_z) + \mathcal{E}_z(S_xS_y + S_yS_x)].$$

$$(7\text{-}17)$$

To solve the resultant eigenvalue problem we follow the procedure of Section 5-2. We transform from the cubic axes as a coordinate system to one for which ζ is the direction of $\mathbf{H}$. Since, as was the case for Eq. (7-12), the electric-field contribution is always a small quantity compared to the Zeeman splitting, we need only retain terms which are diagonal. This first-order transformed version of Eq. (7-17) is

$$\mathcal{H} = g\beta H S_\zeta + R(\mathcal{E}_x mn + \mathcal{E}_y nl + \mathcal{E}_z lm)[3S_\zeta^2 - S(S+1)], \qquad (7\text{-}18)$$

where l, m, and n are the direction cosines of $\mathbf{H}$ with respect to the cubic axes x, y, and z.

A comparison of Eqs. (7-18) and (7-15) shows the same dependence on the angle of $\mathcal{E}$ and $\mathbf{H}$. Therefore we will discuss only the simple case found earlier for which $\mathbf{H}$ is in the xy or (001) plane. For this case the energy is

$$E = g\beta H M_S + R\mathcal{E}_z lm[3M_S^2 - S(S+1)], \qquad (7\text{-}19)$$

and the resonance ($M_S \rightleftharpoons M_S - 1$) occurs at

$$H = \frac{h\nu}{g\beta} - \frac{3R\mathcal{E}_z}{g\beta} lm(2M_S - 1). \qquad (7\text{-}20)$$

The dependence of H on angle for $S = 1$ is similar to that shown in Fig. 7-2, except that each site will produce both lines of the figure (the two sites lead to opposite signs for R). For $S = \frac{3}{2}$ there is an extra line which is isotropic. The figures in Ludwig and Woodbury [3] show the results for Fe^0, which has $S = 1$.

Many of the studies of the effects of electric fields on electron paramagnetic resonance have been carried out on Cr^{3+} in Al_2O_3 (ruby) [1], a crystal which has four inequivalent Al sites into which Cr^{3+} ions go. These sites have C_3 symmetry and thus require five $\mathcal{E}A^2$ terms and nine $\mathcal{E}AB$ terms according to Table 7-1. Hence a detailed description becomes lengthy and tedious and will not be attempted here.

Nonetheless many interesting experiments have been performed on $Al_2O_3:Cr^{3+}$. One of these is the observation of electron paramagnetic resonance by sweeping the electric field rather than the magnetic field [8].

By examination of Table 7-1 we see that the simplest problems concerning the effect of static applied stress on electron paramagnetic resonance are those for which the paramagnetic entity has O_h, O, or T_d point symmetry. Hence a large fraction of the work done in this field is carried out on cubic crystals such as MgO. The terms in the spin Hamiltonian describing the coupling of the spin to the stress are given in Eqs. (7-6) and (7-8).

Let us again consider the simplest case first: O_h symmetry, $S = \frac{1}{2}$, and no hyperfine structure. Tucker [9] has reported on Co^{2+} in MgO, which has all of these properties except for the hyperfine interaction with ^{59}Co which has $I = \frac{7}{2}$. Müller and Berlinger [10] have reported on Fe^+ in MgO, which also has these properties and does not have the hyperfine structure. The spin Hamiltonian for $MgO:Co^{2+}$, ignoring nuclear spin, and $MgO:Fe^+$ is [see Eqs. (7-6) and (7-7)]

$$\mathcal{H} = g\beta \mathbf{H} \cdot \mathbf{S} + \mathcal{I}_1 (T_{xx} + T_{yy} + T_{zz}) \mathbf{H} \cdot \mathbf{S}$$

$$+ \tfrac{2}{3}\mathcal{I}_2 [T_{xx}(2H_x S_x - H_y S_y - H_z S_z) + T_{yy}(2H_y S_y - H_z S_z - H_x S_x)$$

$$+ T_{zz}(2H_z S_z - H_x S_x - H_y S_y)]$$

$$+ \mathcal{I}_3 [T_{yz}(H_y S_z + H_z S_y) + T_{zx}(H_z S_x + H_x S_z) + T_{xy}(H_x S_y + H_y S_x)] . \quad (7\text{-}21)$$

Solving the eigenvalue problem just as was done for Eq. (7-15), we obtain the effective g value:

$$g_{\text{eff}} = g + \frac{\mathcal{I}_1}{\beta}(T_{xx} + T_{yy} + T_{zz})$$

$$+ \frac{2\mathcal{I}_2}{3\,\beta}[T_{xx}(3l^2 - 1) + T_{yy}(3m^2 - 1) + T_{zz}(3n^2 - 1)]$$

$$+ 2\frac{\mathcal{I}_3}{\beta}(T_{yz}mn + T_{zx}nl + T_{xy}lm). \quad (7\text{-}22)$$

Let us first consider what would happen if a uniaxial stress were applied along a cubic axis, say z. Then Eq. (7-22) becomes

$$g_{\text{eff}} = g + \frac{\mathcal{I}_1}{\beta} T_{zz} + \frac{2\mathcal{I}_2}{3\,\beta} T_{zz}(3n^2 - 1). \quad (7\text{-}23)$$

The effective g factor has axial symmetry with a small stress-induced anisotropy. Thus the angular dependence as **H** varies in angle relative to the z axis is the same as shown in Fig. 5-1 except that the anisotropy is much smaller. The anisotropy is directly proportional to T_{zz}. This result is very reasonable if we note that stress along z will produce in the crystal a strain which lowers the symmetry from cubic to tetragonal. Thus the spectrum is the same as if a tetragonal crystal field of any sort is present. This result can of course be generalized. By applying stress we produce a modified crystal structure for which the usual symmetry restrictions on the EPR spectra apply.

By measuring both the parallel and the perpendicular components of $g_{\rm eff}$ for Eq. (7-23) we have, together with the value of g from $T_{zz}=0$, the information required to determine $\mathfrak{I}_1$ and $\mathfrak{I}_2$. If in addition we apply uniaxial stress along a $\langle 110 \rangle$ direction and have the magnetic field parallel to the stress, we can then determine the third coefficient, $\mathfrak{I}_3$.

Analysis of Tucker's results [9] for MgO:Co^{2+} gives the results shown in Table 7-2. Also listed is the g value measured by Low [11]. However, the hyperfine parameters are not included, although they are given by Tucker [9].

Table 7-2

Parameters for Stress Coupling to MgO:Co^{2+}

$$g = 4.278$$
$$\mathfrak{I}_1/\beta = 5 \times 10^{-13} \text{ cm}^2/\text{dyn}$$
$$\mathfrak{I}_2/\beta = 240 \times 10^{-13} \text{ cm}^2/\text{dyn}$$
$$\mathfrak{I}_3/\beta = -66 \times 10^{-13} \text{ cm}^2/\text{dyn}$$

Normally the g value and other bilinear parameters are not very sensitive to stress, so that if any other coupling to stress exists it is likely to be stronger. In particular, for $S \geq 1$ there may be terms of the type TS^2, and these produce the dominant effects of stress in most cases. The spin Hamiltonian terms describing this coupling are given in Eq. (7-8). Let us consider a paramagnetic entity with $S \geq 1$ having O_h symmetry and described by the Hamiltonian

$$\mathcal{H} = g\beta \mathbf{H} \cdot \mathbf{S} + \tfrac{2}{3}\mathcal{R}_1 [T_{xx}(3S_x^2 - S^2) + T_{yy}(3S_y^2 - S^2) + T_{zz}(3S_z^2 - S^2)]$$

$$+ \mathcal{R}_2 [T_{yz}(S_yS_z + S_zS_y) + T_{zx}(S_zS_x + S_xS_z) + T_{xy}(S_xS_y + S_yS_x)].$$

$$(7\text{-}24)$$

The absence of quartic operators in the spin components which are independent of stress implies either that $S < \frac{3}{2}$ or that the quartic terms are negligible (the absence of quartic operators proportional to stress for the case $S > \frac{3}{2}$ is due to the fact that they would probably be much smaller than the quadratic ones). We now transform to a coordinate system with ζ parallel to **H**, as we did in going from Eq. (7-17) to Eq. (7-18). We obtain (keeping only the diagonal term since stress effects are usually small)

$$\mathcal{H} = g\beta H S_\zeta + \{\tfrac{1}{3}\mathcal{R}_1[T_{xx}(3l^2 - 1) + T_{yy}(3m^2 - 1) + T_{zz}(3n^2 - 1)]$$

$$+ \mathcal{R}_2(T_{yz}mn + T_{zx}nl + T_{xy}lm)\}[3S_\zeta^2 - S(S + 1)]. \qquad (7\text{-}25)$$

We can deduce a great deal from the form of Eq. (7-25). A shear stress produces an effect like an electric field for T_d symmetry, as we see by comparing Eq. (7-25) to Eq. (7-18). The behavior for all components of the stress equal to zero except T_{xy} would then be as expressed in Eq. (7-20) with $R\mathcal{E}_z$ replaced by $\mathcal{R}_2 T_{xy}$. The angular dependence in general will be similar to that obtained for *THS* terms in Eqs. (7-21) to (7-23) except that *THS* terms will only displace lines, making them anisotropic. By contrast TS^2 terms split lines, resulting in $2S$ anisotropic lines symmetrically situated about an isotropic centroid.

   Watkins and Feher [12] have measured the equivalent of the coupling constants $\mathcal{R}_1$ and $\mathcal{R}_2$ for Ni^{2+} $(S = 1)$ and Cr^{3+} $(S = \frac{3}{2})$ in MgO. Feher [13] has also studied Mn^{2+} and Fe^{3+} in MgO; these require the quartic operator of Eq. (4-8) as well as those in Eq. (7-24) (and hyperfine structure for Mn^{2+}).

   In addition to affecting the spectrum, stress or an electric field may change the number of paramagnetic entities having a specific orientation when several different orientations of the imperfection have the same energy. Usually this occurs when the temperature is high enough so that the paramagnetic entities can reorient by thermal activation over the energy barrier. The temperature must be low enough, however, to allow a different thermal equilibrium population for at least two orientations whose energies have been changed by the stress. The reader should not confuse this energy, which is proportional to the stress only and thus represents a shift of all spin states uniformly, with the stress-dependent terms in the spin Hamiltonian. The present case is sometimes represented as the interaction of the stress with an elastic dipole moment [14] of the paramagnetic entity.

   Several examples of this type of behavior have been studied by Watkins and Corbett [15] for imperfections in silicon, and similar studies in alkali halides have been carried out by Känzig [16]. Känzig made a thorough study of the O_2^- molecule ion which substitutes for a halide ion in several different alkali halide crystals. The O_2^- molecule ion is paramagnetic, and when occupying the halogen site (which would have O_h

symmetry if the halogen were present) it has D_{2h} symmetry (orthorhombic). Figure 7-3 shows the arrangement for a cut through a {100} plane containing the impurity molecule. There are six different orientations that the D_{2h} symmetry defect can assume in an O_h symmetry site. All of these are equivalent in the absence of stress. The application of stress, however, will render them inequivalent; and if the energy differences become comparable to kT, the molecules will reorient and the number having the orientation with lowest energy will increase. Since the EPR spectrum is very anisotropic, the intensities of the lines from differently oriented molecules can be monitored as a function of stress.

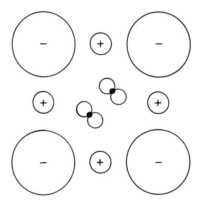

FIG. 7-3   An O_2^- molecule ion at a substitutional site in an alkali halide crystal such as KCl. The plane of atoms shown is a {100} plane through an impurity molecule. The two oxygen nuclei are on a $\langle 110 \rangle$ axis equidistant from the center of the negative-ion site. The ground state of the O_2^- ion is a molecular orbital consisting primarily of atomic p functions with lobes as shown.

Let us consider the effect of a uniaxial stress along a $\langle 100 \rangle$ direction. As we see from Fig. 7-4, the two orientations for which the oxygen-oxygen axis is at right angles to the stress differ from the four for which the angle is 45°. Thus we will have two energetically different cases with the energy levels (not showing any contributions arising from the spin Hamiltonian) as given in Fig. 7-5, where the 90° orientation is shown to have the lowest energy for compression, in agreement with Känzig's observations [16].

If the magnetic field were directed along the same cubic axis as the stress, then the defects at 45° and 90° would each produce one line, the two being well resolved. Hence we would expect the line corresponding to 90° to increase in intensity at the expense of the line corresponding to 45°.

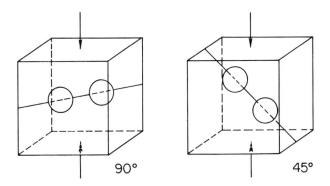

FIG. 7-4   The two possible geometrical arrangements of O_2^- molecule ions and the uniaxial stress for the case in which the stress is applied along a cubic axis. Because of the differences in geometry, we would expect that O_2^- molecule ions whose internuclear axis makes an angle of 90° with the force would differ in energy from those for which the angle is 45°. The resultant energies for compression are shown in Fig. 7-5.

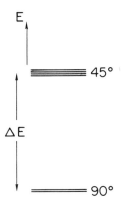

FIG. 7-5   The energies of the six distinct types of O_2^- molecule ions for a compressional stress applied along a cubic axis. The geometry is shown in Fig. 7-4. The two orientations corresponding to 90° are lower in energy, and thus more abundantly populated, than the four at 45°. No contributions arising from the spin Hamiltonian are shown.

7-3   Transitions Caused by Oscillating Electric Fields or Stresses

In Section 5-4 we took all of the terms in the spin Hamiltonian which involved **H** and argued that they (or the largest of them) would represent the Hamiltonian describing the interaction with an oscillating magnetic field. In this section we take the analogous step and describe the interaction with oscillating electric fields and stresses by the $\mathcal{E}$ or T-dependent terms in the spin Hamiltonian.

For transitions produced by an oscillating electric field there are few data [17]. We will discuss two examples. The first observation of transitions caused by an oscillating electric field was that of Ludwig and Ham [5] on Mn^+ in an interstitial site in silicon. The ground state has a spin of 1. The electromagnetic field in a microwave cavity has regions of large microwave electric field and other regions where the microwave magnetic field is large. Ludwig and Ham observed that the $\Delta M_S = \pm 2$ transition was much more intense when the sample was placed in a region of the cavity where the microwave magnetic field was at a minimum and the microwave electric field at a maximum than could be expected on the basis of magnetic dipole transitions alone (in this case magnetic dipole transitions can occur only because of effects of internal crystalline strains).

To see this we need only consider the second term in Eq. (7-5) since only quadratic spin operators can produce a $\Delta M_S = \pm 2$ transition if M_S is a good quantum number, which it is if strains are ignored and the static electric field is zero. Thus

$$\mathcal{H}_1 = \mathcal{H}_1' \cos \omega t,$$

$$\mathcal{H}_1' = R[\ _{1x}(S_y S_z + S_z S_y) + \mathcal{E}_{1y}(S_z S_x + S_x S_z) + \mathcal{E}_{1z}(S_x S_y + S_y S_x)], \tag{7-26}$$

where $\mathcal{E}_1 \cos \omega t$ is the oscillating electric field. If we consider the experimental geometry of Ludwig and Ham [5], then $\mathcal{E}_1$ is along y and $\mathbf{H}$ is along ζ in the xy plane. In that case

$$\mathcal{H}_1' = R\mathcal{E}_1(S_z S_x + S_x S_z). \tag{7-27}$$

Transforming to a coordinate system with ζ along $\mathbf{H}$ and $\mathbf{H}$ making an angle ϕ with x, we obtain the part of $\mathcal{H}_1'$ which contributes to the $\Delta M_S = \pm 2$ transitions as

$$\mathcal{H}_1' = -\frac{R}{2i}\mathcal{E}_1 \sin \phi \, (S_+^2 - S_-^2). \tag{7-28}$$

The intensity parameter I_{ij} defined by Eq. (5-103) becomes for this case of $\Delta M_S = \pm 2$ transitions (since $S = 1$)

$$I_{ij} = R^2 \mathcal{E}_1^2 \sin^2 \phi. \tag{7-29}$$

Ludwig and Ham [5] also observed the dependence on the angle ϕ.

Transitions caused by oscillating electric fields are probably of even greater importance in the non-Kramers doublets mentioned in Section 4–1. For the particular case of praseodymium in yttrium ethyl sulfate [18] and in lanthanum zinc double nitrate [19] we observe no magnetic dipole transitions for the ideal unstrained ionic complex. To see how this comes about, we will describe the non-Kramers doublet ground state in terms of a spin Hamiltonian, following Müller [20].

The simplest spin Hamiltonian description of a non-Kramers doublet regards the two states as the $M_S = \pm 1$ states resulting from $S = 1$. This is consistent with the transformation properties of the majority of non-Kramers doublets and is the only description we will employ. A spin-$\frac{1}{2}$ formalism is usually used [18-20] and is somewhat simpler to manipulate, although less transparent in its form and transformation properties. For Pr^{3+} in the two crystals mentioned above the symmetries are C_{3h} and C_{3v}, respectively. The term from an $S = 1$ spin Hamiltonian for these symmetries, which is required to describe the $M_S = \pm 1$ levels in a static magnetic field, is [20]

$$\mathcal{H} = \tfrac{1}{2} g_{\parallel} \beta H_z S_z, \tag{7-30}$$

where the factor of $\frac{1}{2}$ is used for consistency with parameters obtained from the spin-$\frac{1}{2}$ formalism. There can be no magnetic dipole transitions arising from this Hamiltonian [see the discussion following Eq. (5-46)]. However, an oscillating electric field will cause the required $\Delta M_S = \pm 2$ transitions as a result of the terms

$$\mathcal{H}_1' = \tfrac{1}{2} R \mathcal{E}_{1+} S_+^2 + \tfrac{1}{2} R^* \mathcal{E}_{1-} S_-^2 \qquad (C_{3h} \text{ symmetry}), \tag{7-31}$$

or

$$\mathcal{H}_1' = \tfrac{1}{2} R(\mathcal{E}_{1-} S_-^2 - \mathcal{E}_{1+} S_+^2) \qquad (C_{3v} \text{ symmetry}). \tag{7-32}$$

The intensity is thus proportional to

$$I_{ij} = |R|^2 \mathcal{E}_1^2, \tag{7-33}$$

where $\mathcal{E}_1$ is in the plane normal to z (the threefold axis).

In reality this description is too simple for non-Kramers doublets. Since the doublet can be split by stress, the random internal strain fields in the crystals will cause a distribution of zero-field splittings. If this effect is big, it usually produces a line with an asymmetric shape. It also can cause magnetic dipole transitions via the interaction of Eq. (7-30); these result because of the mixing of $M_S = \pm 1$ in the eigenstates by the terms producing the zero-field splitting. Then

$$\mathcal{H}_1' = \tfrac{1}{2} g_{\parallel} \beta H_{1z} S_z \tag{7-34}$$

will have matrix elements between the parts of the two eigenstates with $M_S = 1$ and also with $M_S = -1$. Nevertheless the transitions caused by oscillating electric fields are the dominant ones even in real (strained) samples.

The stimulation of transitions by electric fields has been referred to [18] as paraelectric resonance. We will not employ this terminology since the term fits another phenomenon somewhat better [21]. The stimulation of transitions by an applied oscillating stress is termed ultrasonic paramagnetic resonance or acoustic paramagnetic resonance. The literature on this subject is much more extensive than that on electrically stimulated transitions.

As we observed in Section 7–2, the TS^2 terms in the Hamiltonian are usually the largest of those linear in the components of $\mathbf{T}$. Thus, in seeking a system to produce strong ultrasonic paramagnetic resonance signals, it is logical to choose paramagnetic entities with $S \geq 1$. Again, for simplicity in understanding, O_h symmetry is employed. Let us consider specifically the cases of MgO containing either Ni^{2+} or Fe^{2+}, both with a spin (effective) of 1. The spin Hamiltonian for either ion in a perfect MgO crystal is simply

$$\mathcal{K} = g\beta \mathbf{H} \cdot \mathbf{S} \tag{7-35}$$

if no static electric fields or stresses are applied. The coupling to the oscillating stress is described by [see Eq. (7-8)]

$$\mathcal{K}_1' = \mathcal{R}_1[\tfrac{1}{3}(2T_{1zz} - T_{1xx} - T_{1yy})(2S_z^2 - S_x^2 - S_y^2) + (T_{1xx} - T_{1yy})(S_x^2 - S_y^2)]$$
$$+ \mathcal{R}_2[T_{1yz}(S_yS_z + S_zS_y) + T_{1zx}(S_zS_x + S_xS_z) + T_{1xy}(S_xS_y + S_yS_x)]. \tag{7-36}$$

Let us consider first an oscillating stress along one of the cubic axes, say the z axis. Then $\mathcal{K}_1'$ becomes

$$\mathcal{K}_1' = \tfrac{2}{3}\mathcal{R}_1 T_1[3S_z^2 - S(S+1)]. \tag{7-37}$$

If we write Eq. (7-37) in terms of ξ, η, ζ, where ζ is along $\mathbf{H}$ and ξ is in the z-ζ plane, we obtain

$$\mathcal{K}_1' = \tfrac{1}{3}\mathcal{R}_1(3n^2 - 1)T_1[3S_\zeta^2 - S(S+1)]$$
$$- \mathcal{R}_1 T_1 n\sqrt{1 - n^2}\,(S_\zeta S_+ + S_+ S_\zeta + S_\zeta S_- + S_- S_\zeta)$$
$$+ \tfrac{1}{2}\mathcal{R}_1 T_1(1 - n^2)(S_+^2 + S_-^2). \tag{7-38}$$

For this case, in which low-symmetry crystal fields or internal strains produce no zero-field splitting, the selection rules are simple. The first term produces no transitions, the second term causes $\Delta M_S = \pm 1$ transitions, and the last term results in $\Delta M_S = \pm 2$ transitions. Calculating the relative intensities of the two types of transitions involved, we obtain

$$I_{ij} = \tfrac{1}{2}\mathcal{R}_1^2 T_1^2 \sin^2 2\theta \qquad (\Delta M_S = \pm 1), \tag{7-39}$$

and

$$I_{ij} = \mathcal{R}_1^2 T_1^2 \sin^4 \theta \qquad (\Delta M_S = \pm 2), \tag{7-40}$$

where θ is the angle between the magnetic field and the z axis, the cubic axis along which the oscillating uniaxial stress is applied. Plotting the intensities as a function of θ, we obtain the curves in Fig. 7-6. We note that for $\theta = 0$ or π the field is parallel to the stress and no transitions occur. When the field is normal to the stress only transitions with $\Delta M_S = \pm 2$ are allowed. For other directions both types of transitions occur.

If transitions are caused by a pure shear component of oscillating stress in the cubic axis system, the angular dependence is more complicated, although, in general, transitions for which both $\Delta M_S = \pm 1$ and $\Delta M_S = \pm 2$ occur. A general discussion of this topic has been given by Dobrov [22].

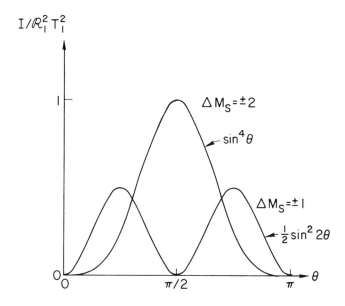

FIG. 7-6 Relative intensities of ultrasonic paramagnetic resonance transitions for a system with $S \geq 1$ and O_h symmetry. The oscillating stress is a uniaxial component along a cubic axis, and the angle θ is measured from that cubic axis. The TS^2 terms are assumed to provide the largest coupling to the oscillating stress and are the only ones considered.

7–4 Supplemental Bibliography

1. K. W. H. Stevens, *Rept. Progr. Phys.* **30** (Part 1), 189 (1967). Section 5 calculates the Hamiltonian coupling the effective spin to the phonons, a problem closely related to the one handled in this chapter, as we will see in Chapter 8.

References Cited in Chapter 7

[1] E. B. Boyce and N. Bloembergen, *Phys. Rev.* **131**, 1912 (1963).
[2] C. Kittel, *Introduction to Solid State Physics*, 3rd ed., Wiley, New York, 1966, p. 115.
[3] G. W. Ludwig and H. H. Woodbury, *Phys. Rev. Letters* **7**, 240 (1961).
[4] F. S. Ham, *Phys. Rev. Letters* **7**, 242 (1961).
[5] G. W. Ludwig and F. S. Ham, *Phys. Rev. Letters* **8**, 210 (1962).
[6] G. W. Ludwig and F. S. Ham, *Paramagnetic Resonance* (W. Low, ed.), Academic, New York, 1963, Vol. II, p. 620.
[7] J. J. Krebs, *Phys. Rev.* **155**, 246 (1967).
[8] A. A. Bugai and A. B. Roitsin, *JETP Letters* **5**, 67 (1967).
[9] E. B. Tucker, *Phys. Rev.* **143**, 264 (1966).
[10] K. A. Müller and W. Berlinger, *Bull. Am. Phys. Soc.* **12**, 40 (1967).
[11] W. Low, *Phys. Rev.* **109**, 256 (1958).
[12] G. D. Watkins and E. Feher, *Bull. Am. Phys. Soc.* **7**, 29 (1962).
[13] E. R. Feher, *Phys. Rev.* **136**, A145 (1964).
[14] A. S. Nowick and W. R. Heller, *Advan. Phys.* **12**, 251 (1963); *Advan. Phys.* **14**, 101 (1965).
[15] G. D. Watkins and J. W. Corbett, *Phys. Rev.* **121**, 1001 (1961); G. D. Watkins, *J. Phys. Soc. Japan* **18**, Suppl. II, 22 (1963); G. D. Watkins and J. W. Corbett, *Phys. Rev.* **134**, A1359 (1964).
[16] W. Känzig, *J. Phys. Chem. Solids* **23**, 479 (1962).
[17] For a recent example see S. H. Christensen, *Phys. Rev.* **180**, 498 (1969).
[18] F. I. B. Williams, *Proc. Phys. Soc.* **91**, 111 (1967).
[19] J. N. Culvahouse, D. P. Shinke, and D. L. Foster, *Phys. Rev. Letters* **18**, 117 (1967).
[20] K. A. Müller, *Phys. Rev.* **171**, 350 (1968).
[21] T. L. Estle, *Phys. Rev.* **176**, 1056 (1968).
[22] W. I. Dobrov, *Phys. Rev.* **134**, A734 (1964).

CHAPTER 8

Spin-Lattice Relaxation

In Section 7–3 we studied transitions between spin states caused by an oscillating stress. Implicit in our discussion was the monochromaticity of the stress. Spin-lattice relaxation is the same kind of process, that is, transitions caused by oscillating elastic fields, but all lattice modes are excited and may participate in causing the transitions. The excitation of the lattice modes occurs because we assume a thermal equilibrium distribution of all excitations (some exceptions occur). If lattice vibrations are in thermal equilibrium, then spin-lattice relaxation will cause the spin system to be in thermal equilibrium if transitions caused by applied fields are not significant. Our main task in this chapter, then, is to re-examine transitions stimulated by stress when a thermal distribution of lattice vibrations causes the stress (strain). After doing this, we will elaborate on some of the many ways in which spin-lattice relaxation is actually more complicated than this simple description implies.

8–1 Spin-Phonon Hamiltonian

Aside from some more or less obvious modifications, the Hamiltonian describing the coupling of the spin system to the quantized lattice vibrations (phonons) is essentially the same as the Hamiltonian coupling stress to the spin system, which is discussed in Section 7–1. The main difference is that in all previous calculations of transition probabilities the fields were dealt with classically. It would have been more elegant to employ photons or phonons instead of oscillating fields, with the same results. However, now that we must deal with a statistical distribution of lattice vibrations, it is useful to write the Hamiltonian in terms of phonon creation and annihilation operators instead of stress or strain. To do this we must write the stress in terms of phonon creation and annihilation operators and insert the result in the appropriate spin Hamiltonian as given in Section 7–1. We could have employed the strain rather than the stress as the basic variable in our spin Hamiltonian, and this is frequently done in the literature.

According to Maradudin, Montroll, and Weiss [1], or Weinreich [2], the displacement, $\mathbf{q}_{\mathbf{R}i}$, of the ith atom in the unit cell located at the lattice point **R** is related to the amplitude of the normal modes with wave vectors **k** and polarization indices μ by

$$\mathbf{q}_{\mathbf{R}i} = \frac{1}{\sqrt{NM_i}} \sum_{\mathbf{k},\mu} e^{i\mathbf{k}\cdot\mathbf{R}} Q_{\mathbf{k}\mu} \varepsilon_{\mathbf{k}\mu i}, \tag{8-1}$$

where N is the number of unit cells in the crystal, M_i is the mass of the ith atom in a unit cell, and $Q_{\mathbf{k}\mu}$ is the amplitude of a normal mode. The amplitudes of the normal modes may be expressed in terms of phonon creation and annihilation operators

$$Q_{\mathbf{k},\mu} = \left(\frac{\hbar}{2\omega_{\mathbf{k}\mu}}\right)^{1/2} [a^*_{-\mathbf{k}\mu} + a_{\mathbf{k}\mu}], \tag{8-2}$$

where $a^*_{\mathbf{k}\mu}$ is the creation operator, $a_{\mathbf{k}\mu}$ the annihilation operator, and $\omega_{\mathbf{k}\mu}$ the characteristic frequency for phonons with wave vector **k** and polarization index μ. Combining Eqs. (8-1) and (8-2), we obtain

$$\mathbf{q}_{\mathbf{R}i} = \frac{1}{\sqrt{NM_i}} \sum_{\mathbf{k},\mu} \left(\frac{\hbar}{2\omega_{\mathbf{k}\mu}}\right)^{1/2} e^{i\mathbf{k}\cdot\mathbf{R}} [a^*_{-\mathbf{k}\mu} + a_{\mathbf{k}\mu}] \varepsilon_{\mathbf{k}\mu i}. \tag{8-3}$$

There is a considerable similarity between applied static stress and lattice vibrations in crystals if long-wavelength acoustic phonons are considered. For such phonons all atoms in a unit cell are displaced approximately equally, and the differences in their displacements are nearly constant over several atomic spacings, the region which is usually of primary interest for the interaction of a spin with its environment. Thus no difference occurs locally between a static stress and low-energy acoustic vibrations. Although the discussion of lattice vibrations has been given in terms of a perfect crystal, the crystal is obviously not perfect near a paramagnetic imperfection. However, the difference in the displacements near the imperfection from those in a perfect crystal will be the same for both the static and the low-energy acoustic case. Therefore, if we know the response of the system to a static stress, we also know the response to low-energy acoustic vibrations. The displacements for low-energy acoustic phonons are given by

$$\mathbf{q}_{\mathbf{R}i} = \frac{1}{\sqrt{NM}} \sum_{\mathbf{k},\mu} \left(\frac{\hbar}{2\omega_{\mathbf{k}\mu}}\right)^{1/2} e^{i\mathbf{k}\cdot\mathbf{R}} [a^*_{-\mathbf{k}\mu} + a_{\mathbf{k}\mu}] \hat{\varepsilon}_{\mathbf{k}\mu}, \tag{8-4}$$

where $\hat{\varepsilon}_{\mathbf{k}\mu}$ is a unit vector in the direction of the polarization vector, $\varepsilon_{\mathbf{k}\mu i}$, and $M = \Sigma_i M_i$. Equation (8-4) has no dependence on the index i (note that the i in $e^{i\mathbf{k}\cdot\mathbf{R}}$ is $\sqrt{-1}$), just as required for long-wavelength acoustic modes. From this it is very easy to calculate the components of the strain tensor given by

$$e_{\alpha\beta} = \frac{1}{2}\left(\frac{\partial q_\alpha}{\partial R_\beta} + \frac{\partial q_\beta}{\partial R_\alpha}\right). \tag{8-5}$$

Dropping the subscripts **R**, i, μ, and **k** (except for a minus sign for a^* to indicate $-\mathbf{k}$), we obtain

$$e_{\alpha\beta} = \frac{i}{2\sqrt{NM}} \sum_{\mathbf{k},\mu} \left(\frac{\hbar}{2\omega}\right)^{1/2} e^{i\mathbf{k}\cdot\mathbf{R}}[a_-^* + a](\hat{\varepsilon}_\alpha k_\beta + \hat{\varepsilon}_\beta k_\alpha). \tag{8-6}$$

The strain can be related to the stress by means of the elastic stiffness constants [3],

$$T_{\alpha\beta} = \sum_{\gamma,\delta} C_{\alpha\beta\gamma\delta} e_{\gamma\delta}. \tag{8-7}$$

The stress, which is now an operator, can then be inserted into the spin Hamiltonian terms which contain the stress, yielding the terms in the spin-phonon Hamiltonian. These terms have coefficients that can be obtained from static stress measurements or from ultrasonic paramagnetic resonance. As an example consider the two terms in Eq. (7-8) which represent the dominant coupling between stress and a paramagnetic entity with $S > \frac{1}{2}$. The Hamiltonian could have been written in terms of the strain rather than the stress, although with modified coefficients. If we do this, for simplicity, we obtain

$$\begin{aligned}
\mathcal{H} = {}& \tilde{\mathcal{R}}_1[\tfrac{1}{3}(2e_{zz}-e_{xx}-e_{yy})(2S_z^2-S_x^2-S_y^2)+(e_{xx}-e_{yy})(S_x^2-S_y^2)] \\
& + \tilde{\mathcal{R}}_2[e_{yz}(S_yS_z+S_zS_y)+e_{zx}(S_zS_x+S_xS_z)+e_{xy}(S_xS_y+S_yS_x)] \\
= {}& \frac{i}{\sqrt{NM}} \sum_{\mathbf{k},\mu} \left(\frac{\hbar}{2\omega}\right)^{1/2} e^{i\mathbf{k}\cdot\mathbf{R}}[a_-^* + a]\{\tilde{\mathcal{R}}_1[(2\hat{\varepsilon}_z k_z-\hat{\varepsilon}_x k_x-\hat{\varepsilon}_y k_y)(2S_z^2-S_x^2-S_y^2) \\
& + (\hat{\varepsilon}_x k_x-\hat{\varepsilon}_y k_y)(S_x^2-S_y^2)]+\tilde{\mathcal{R}}_2[\tfrac{1}{2}(\hat{\varepsilon}_y k_z+\hat{\varepsilon}_z k_y)(S_yS_z+S_zS_y) \\
& + \tfrac{1}{2}(\hat{\varepsilon}_z k_x+\hat{\varepsilon}_x k_z)(S_zS_x+S_xS_z)+\tfrac{1}{2}(\hat{\varepsilon}_x k_y+\hat{\varepsilon}_y k_x)(S_xS_y+S_yS_x)]\} \\
= {}& \sum_{\mathbf{k},\mu} \mathcal{H}(\mathbf{k},\mu). \tag{8-8}
\end{aligned}$$

This spin-phonon Hamiltonian, which applies to O_h, O, and T_d point symmetry, will have matrix elements between states which differ by one phonon and with $\Delta M_S = \pm 1, \pm 2$. The phonon will have an energy equal to the difference in energy of the two states of the paramagnet between which transitions occur. Such a process is termed a direct process because only one phonon is involved in the transition. This point will be discussed in more detail in Section 8–2.

If we write down all possible terms, in analogy to Eq. (8-8), which arise from spin Hamiltonian terms linear in the components of **T**, we will have no first-order effects involving more than one phonon. The phonons in resonance with typical energy differences are near the peak in the phonon distribution if the temperature is near 1 °K. At higher temperatures there are many phonons with energies greater than the resonance energy. Multiphonon processes, especially those involving two phonons, then become much more probable. Of these processes the most common is called the Raman process; it can occur as a result of terms quadratic in the components of **T**, thus allowing operators of the form $a^*_{\mathbf{k}'\mu'}\, a_{\mathbf{k}\mu}$, etc. Hence our simple picture must be modified by including all spin Hamiltonian terms proportional to T^2. The process for accomplishing this is straightforward but usually quite tedious.

A substantial part of the subject of spin-lattice relaxation can be understood with terms of the type just introduced. It may be desirable to include higher powers of T, or the derivative with respect to time. However, whenever phonons of a wavelength of several atomic spacings or less or phonons from nonacoustic modes are involved, the formulation is much more complicated. We will say little about this; rather, we will concentrate on the low-temperature results.

Discussions are often encountered in the literature of relaxation via spin-orbit coupling or some other basic interaction. These interactions are not distinct from the ones which we describe above, because, for example, the spin-orbit interaction may contribute substantially to the TS^2 term in the spin Hamiltonian. Rather, the distinction is semantic, one description being couched in terms of the spin Hamiltonian and the other in terms of the actual Hamiltonian.

8-2 Elementary Relaxation Rates

By using time-dependent perturbation theory, usually to first order, it is possible to calculate the transition rates between the energy levels of a spin system resulting from absorbing, emitting, or scattering phonons. The result is given by Fermi's "Golden Rule" [4] as

$$\frac{dW_{fi}}{d\Omega} = \frac{2\pi}{\hbar}|\mathcal{H}_{fi}(\mathbf{k}, \mu)|^2 \rho(\hbar\omega_{fi}),\qquad(8\text{-}9)$$

where $\rho(\hbar\omega_{fi})$ is the density of phonon states with a given direction for **k** and value for μ at the energy $\hbar\omega_{fi}$, and $\mathcal{H}_{fi}(\mathbf{k}, \mu)$ is the matrix element of $\mathcal{H}(\mathbf{k}, \mu)$. This expression must be integrated over all orientations of **k** and summed over all polarization indices μ to obtain the desired elementary relaxation rate between states i and f (the result will depend on whether the transition is i to f or f to i). The value of $\rho(\hbar\omega_{fi})$ to be used may be obtained from the Debye model of lattice vibrations because it is an accurate description for long-wavelength acoustic phonons while also being very simple. In particular we take $\omega = kv$ but allow v to vary with the angle of $\mathbf{k}$ and the polarization μ, but not with the magnitude of $\mathbf{k}$. Note that v is not the magnitude of the group velocity but is the proportionality constant in $\omega = kv$. The result is

$$\rho(\hbar\omega_{fi}) = \frac{V\omega_{fi}^2}{(2\pi)^3 \hbar v_\mu^3(\theta, \phi)}, \tag{8-10}$$

where V is the volume of the crystal, and $v_\mu(\theta, \phi)$ is the velocity for a $\mathbf{k}$ with angular coordinates θ and ϕ and for a polarization μ. If we also include the average value of the phonon occupation number whenever it appears in the matrix element,

$$\bar{n}_{\mathbf{k},\mu} = \frac{1}{e^{\hbar\omega/kT} - 1}, \tag{8-11}$$

we obtain explicit and usually convenient expressions for the elementary relaxation rates (do not confuse k and T in this context, as Boltzmann's constant and temperature, with their more frequent use as wave vector and stress) of the form

$$W_{fi} = \frac{V}{(2\pi)^2 \hbar^2} \omega_{fi}^2 \int d\Omega \sum_\mu \frac{|\mathcal{H}_{fi}(\mathbf{k}, \mu)|^2}{v_\mu^3(\theta, \phi)}. \tag{8-12}$$

Using the Hamiltonian of Eq. (8-8), we obtain

$$|\mathcal{H}_{fi}(\mathbf{k}, \mu)| = \frac{k}{\sqrt{NM}}\left(\frac{\hbar}{2\omega_{fi}}\right)^{1/2} \sqrt{\bar{n}_{\mathbf{k},\mu} + \tfrac{1}{2} \pm \tfrac{1}{2}} \left| \tilde{\mathcal{R}}_1[(2\hat{e}_z\hat{k}_z - \hat{e}_x\hat{k}_x - \hat{e}_y\hat{k}_y) \right.$$

$$\times \langle f|2S_z^2 - S_x^2 - S_y^2|i\rangle + (\hat{e}_x\hat{k}_x - \hat{e}_y\hat{k}_y)$$

$$\times \langle f|S_x^2 - S_y^2|i\rangle] + \tilde{\mathcal{R}}_2[\tfrac{1}{2}(\hat{e}_y\hat{k}_z + \hat{e}_z\hat{k}_y)\langle f|S_yS_z + S_zS_y|i\rangle$$

$$+ \tfrac{1}{2}(\hat{e}_z\hat{k}_x + \hat{e}_x\hat{k}_z)\langle f|S_zS_x + S_xS_z|i\rangle$$

$$\left. + \tfrac{1}{2}(\hat{e}_x\hat{k}_y + \hat{e}_y\hat{k}_x)\langle f|S_xS_y + S_yS_x|i\rangle] \right|, \tag{8-13}$$

where the upper sign is for emission of a phonon and the lower one is for absorption. The quantity $\hat{\mathbf{k}}$ is a unit vector parallel to $\mathbf{k}$. The quantity within the absolute value signs will be denoted as $\mathbb{M}$ (note that $\mathbb{M}$ depends on θ, ϕ, and μ). Hence

$$W_{fi} = \frac{\omega_{fi}^3}{8\pi^2 \hbar \rho} \, \bar{n}_{\mathbf{k},\mu} \int d\Omega \sum_{\mu} \frac{1}{v_{\mu}^5(\theta, \phi)} |\mathbb{M}|^2$$

$$= \frac{\omega_{fi}^3}{8\pi^2 \hbar \rho} \frac{1}{e^{\hbar \omega_{fi}/kT} - 1} \int d\Omega \sum_{\mu} \frac{1}{v_{\mu}^5(\theta, \phi)} |\mathbb{M}|^2, \qquad (8\text{-}14)$$

where only the expression for phonon absorption is given, and ρ is the density. To obtain the result for emission we merely multiply by $e^{\hbar \omega_{fi}/kT}$. Unless the zero-field splittings due to fine or hyperfine structure are comparable to $\hbar \omega_{fi}$, $\mathbb{M}$ will be independent of ω_{fi}. The only dependence on ω_{fi} that can occur for $\mathbb{M}$ is for the wave function corresponding to i and f to depend on ω_{fi}. This does not occur for a system dominated by the Zeeman interaction since in that case the wave functions are independent of H and thus of ω_{fi}. A case in which the Zeeman interaction does not dominate has been analyzed by Donoho [5].

The quantity $\mathbb{M}$ is always independent of T. Hence we may examine the energy and temperature dependence of this direct process by studying the behavior of the coefficient of the integral in Eq. (8-14). Of particular interest is the high-temperature limit, for which $kT \gg \hbar \omega_{fi}$. This condition is at least approximately satisfied at all temperatures obtained by standard liquid-helium cryogenics if the experimental frequency is 10 GHz or less. For temperatures greater than 4.2 °K (the temperature of liquid helium at STP) it is good for almost all frequencies obtainable by microwave techniques. Thus in the high-temperature limit we have

$$W_{fi} \propto \omega_{fi}^2 T. \qquad (8\text{-}15)$$

This expression is the same for emission and absorption of phonons because the stimulated processes occur much more frequently than spontaneous emission. This argument can be generalized to give the result that all direct relaxation processes occur at a rate directly proportional to the temperature in the high-temperature limit. Another consequence is that, if the relaxation occurs via the Hamiltonian of Eq. (8-8), the relaxation rate is proportional to H^2. This assumes $\omega_{fi} \propto H$, an assumption identical to that yielding no dependence of $\mathbb{M}$ on ω_{fi}.

The spin-phonon Hamiltonian of Eq. (8-8) used for the above calculations will have no matrix elements between the states for a spin of $\frac{1}{2}$. In that case it becomes more likely that an operator such as that of Eq. (7-6) will produce the relaxation (still considering cubic symmetry for simplicity). The resultant analysis then gives

$$W_{fi} \propto \omega_{fi}^2 H^2 T \propto H^4 T \qquad (8\text{-}16)$$

in the high-temperature limit. This dependence occurs for Kramers doublets, and it may be a term in the relaxation rate for higher spins. If the effect of stress on the hyperfine interaction (a term of the form TSI) is dominant, then the field and temperature dependence for an isolated Kramers doublet is H^2T, as deduced for TS^2 above.

We have considered here only the simplest of the elementary relaxation processes, the direct process. At higher temperatures one or more additional relaxation processes may occur. One of the most important of these is the Raman process, mentioned in Section 8–1, which usually arises from terms quadratic in stress in the spin Hamiltonian or from linear terms carried to second order in perturbation theory. The important parts of such terms are those consisting of a creation operator for one phonon mode and an annihilation operator for another ($a^*_{\mathbf{k}'\mu'}a_{\mathbf{k}\mu}$, for example). These will result in a process in which a phonon is scattered inelastically with the difference in its energy being $\hbar\omega_{fi}$, the energy difference of the two states involved. This is the vibrational analog of the optical Raman effect. The reason that the Raman process is so important is that the density of states for phonons is proportional to the square of their energy. Thus there are more phonons with energy near kT than at any other energy. If kT is much greater than $\hbar\omega_{fi}$, there are many more pairs of phonons with their energy difference equal to $\hbar\omega_{fi}$ than there are phonons whose energy equals $\hbar\omega_{fi}$. This overcomes the reduced coupling associated with terms quadratic in the stress.

The detailed calculation of Raman relaxation rates is a lengthy and tedious process. It is easier to obtain the temperature and field dependences in much the same way as for direct processes. If $S > \frac{1}{2}$, the T^2S^2 terms in the spin-phonon Hamiltonian will give a relaxation rate proportional to T^7 but independent of H. For $S = \frac{1}{2}$ a similar calculation, but using T^2HS instead, gives the relaxation rate as proportional to T^7H^2. This term is usually dominated by another process whose rate varies as T^9. This field-independent relaxation for Kramers doublets arises from a $T(\partial T/\partial t)S$ term in the spin-phonon Hamiltonian, a term missing for the static spin Hamiltonian. This term represents a magnetic coupling to the spin that results from the motion of the charged ions in the crystal (which motion produces an oscillating magnetic field). Finally, for paramagnetic entities which have several low-lying levels, the Raman relaxation rate may vary as T^5, as has been shown both theoretically [6] and experimentally [7].

8–3 Observed Relaxation Times

If we ignore all of the possible complications which can modify the results of an experimental determination of spin-lattice relaxation times or rates, many of which are discussed in Sections 8–4 and 8–5, we still have the problem of relating the elementary relaxation rates to the experimentally determined properties of the system. We encountered this problem briefly in Section 2–4, where the behavior was obtained from the solution of rate equations. The basic ideas can be understood by considering the four-level system of Fig. 8-1.

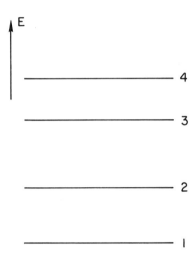

FIG. 8-1 Energy level diagram employed to distinguish between elementary relaxation rates associated with transitions between a pair of levels, say $1 \rightarrow 2$, and multistep contributions with one or more intermediate levels involved, such as $1 \rightarrow 3$ followed by $3 \rightarrow 2$.

Let us assume that we are observing the return to thermal equilibrium of the population difference for levels 1 and 2. We can do this by observing the intensity of an EPR signal for the transition between levels 1 and 2 as a function of time and as a function of the way in which nonthermal populations are produced. The elementary relaxation rates for all processes causing transitions between levels 1 and 2 will of course make contributions. However, we will also get contributions from relaxation proceeding from level 1 to 3 via an elementary process and then from level 3 to level 2. Similarly $1 \rightarrow 4$ followed by $4 \rightarrow 2$ will contribute, as will processes involving three or more elementary steps (such as $1 \rightarrow 4$, $4 \rightarrow 3$, $3 \rightarrow 2$). The exact way in which these will combine to yield the observed rate will depend on the way in which the populations were disturbed from equilibrium. For example, if at a given instant the population difference between levels 1 and 2 has its equilibrium value, then the elementary processes connecting these levels do not influence the rate of change of this population difference, but other processes may do so if levels 3 and 4 do not have their equilibrium populations. From this we see that the rate at which the population difference between levels 1 and 2 returns to thermal equilibrium will depend on time in a fairly complicated way. In fact the only simple solution for a general set of rate equations occurs for two levels (see Section 2–4).

One composite relaxation process stands out because of its special properties. Called the Orbach process, it consists of two successive transitions [8] and is illustrated in Fig. 8-2. The direct transition from

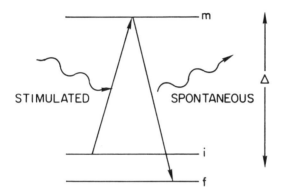

FIG. 8-2   An illustration of some of the essential features of relaxation via the Orbach process. We are usually interested in cases in which levels i and f are part of the ground manifold of spin states and relatively close in energy. The intermediate level, m, is higher in energy by an amount, Δ, which is much greater than the splitting between i and f and also much greater than kT. Under these conditions the stimulated excitation will be followed by a spontaneous de-excitation leading to a composite relaxation rate proportional to $\exp(-\Delta/kT)$.

level i to level m is stimulated, leading to an $e^{-\Delta/kT}$ temperature dependence in the transition rate if $\Delta \gg kT$ [see Eq. (8-14) and the discussion following it]. The direct transition from level m to level f is accompanied by the spontaneous emission of a phonon and thus proceeds at a rate independent of temperature. For the spontaneous process to dominate we must also have $\Delta \gg kT$. Normally level m refers to a level not described by the effective spin describing the ground manifold. Such low-lying excited states are common for many rare-earth impurities in crystals. Since the composite rate is approximately equal to the much slower stimulated rate, it follows that the transition rate for the Orbach process is proportional to $e^{-\Delta/kT}$. It is in fact this characteristic exponential temperature dependence which is usually used to identify Orbach relaxation. From the point of view of the ground manifold of levels (the effective-spin states) the Orbach process is elementary and is usually used in this way.

8–4 Other Relaxation Mechanisms

For a collection of noninteracting paramagnetic entities spin-lattice relaxation is as we have described it above, except that occasional simplifications and approximations were made. One approximation was that the lattice vibrations were in internal thermal equilibrium and in equilibrium with the dominant thermal reservoir (the "bath"). We will consider deviations from this simple behavior in Section 8–5.

For isolated spins we have hitherto assumed that only long-wavelength acoustic phonons are involved in the relaxation processes. At higher temperatures this is not necessarily a good approximation. Huang [9] has calculated the effect of the most drastic breakdown of this assumption. He shows that optical phonons, if such modes exist, may be effective in relaxing spins via the Raman process and that the rate for such a process should depend on temperature in a way similar to that characterizing the Orbach process, namely, as $e^{-\hbar\omega_0/kT}$, where $\hbar\omega_0$ is the optical phonon energy at $\mathbf{k} = 0$.

When the concentration of spins is high enough so that they interact, several other more complicated processes may occur. One of these, discussed in Section 6–2, is frequently described by introducing a relaxation time, T_2. Physically this means that interactions cause a line width greater than that caused by the finite life time of the state, T_1, using the uncertainty principle. A related property is the possibility of transferring energy from one region of the sample to another by diffusion of the polarization of the dipoles.

The ability to transfer energy because of interactions suggests an important spin-lattice relaxation mechanism. Consider a crystal with two paramagnetic species present. One paramagnet has a long spin-lattice relaxation time when isolated, and its relaxation is being studied by an EPR experiment. The second has a very short spin-lattice relaxation time and is not being directly observed in the experiment. Under these circumstances the observed paramagnetic species can relax by transferring energy to the lattice or by having it diffuse to where it can couple to the other spin, which then rapidly transfers it to the lattice. The latter mechanism is the dominant one in many substances. The rapidly relaxing species can be an impurity ion or other imperfection. It can also be a pair or triple of strongly interacting spins of the same species. In this case we frequently find that terms in the spin Hamiltonian of the type TS_1S_2 are the strongest coupling to stress, and hence they lead to very rapid spin-lattice relaxation. The description of this process is similar to the descriptions given earlier in this chapter, although it is more complicated. An essential ingredient in this process is the transfer of energy between the slowly relaxing species and the rapidly relaxing one. This process is known as cross relaxation.

The diffusion of energy through a weakly interacting spin system can be thought of as consisting of a number of energy-conserving mutual spin flips. Consider diagram (a) of Fig. 8-3. A downward transition occurs for dipole A, accompanied by an upward transition for dipole A'. Since A and A' are the same species, the process conserves energy and no phonons are involved. This may be regarded as causing a finite lifetime and hence a width of the transition. This T_2 process is only the simplest of such energy-conserving processes. They can occur for more than two spins and for like or unlike species, and may involve more than one transition for a given species. In some cases conservation of energy would not occur save for the breadth produced by the interactions.

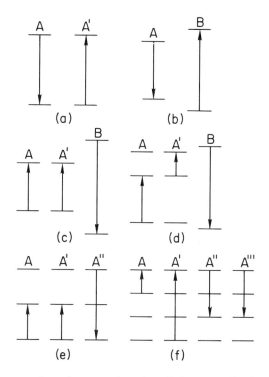

FIG. 8-3 Six examples of cross relaxation. Primes on the letter A indicate other paramagnets of the same kind; the letter B denotes an entirely different kind of paramagnet. Diagram (a) illustrates the type of process which can lead to a value of T_2 less than T_1. Diagrams (a) and (b) depict processes involving two interacting spins; (c) through (e) depict processes involving three interacting spins; and (f) depicts a process in which four interacting spins are involved.

In Fig. 8-3, parts (b) through (d), we illustrate a few cross-relaxation processes which are more complicated than the one in (a). These processes occur because the transitions have widths sufficient for the lines to overlap. In parts (e) and (f) we show processes which conserve energy because of the exact or approximate equality in the spacings. Some insight into the effect of cross relaxation can be obtained by including this process in the rate equations [10] presented in Section 2–4. For example, using the process shown diagramatically in Fig. 8-3(b) and presented in more detail in Fig. 8-4, we may write the rate equations including cross relaxation, but neglecting transitions caused by the electromagnetic field, as

$$\frac{dN_1}{dt} = -W_{12}N_1 + W_{21}N_2 + \frac{W_x}{N_B}(N_2N_3 - N_1N_4) \qquad (8\text{-}17)$$

with analogous equations for the other three levels. The quantities N_1, N_2, N_3, and N_4 are the populations of the four levels, N_B is the total number of the B species, W_x is the cross-relaxation rate, and W_{12} and W_{21} are the probabilities for thermally stimulated transitions (W_{21} also has a spontaneous contribution—see Section 2–4).

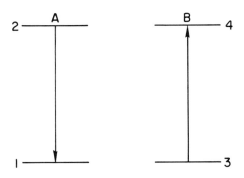

FIG. 8-4   Diagram (b) of Fig. 8-3 in more detail. The two interacting paramagnets are of different types and may have quite different properties except for the accidental near equality of their energy differences. These energy differences are unequal by an amount comparable to or less than the interaction energy so that energy can be conserved without phonon involvement.

These and similar equations can be analyzed and used to interpret the various observations attributed to cross relaxation. We will consider here only the simple case in which the spin-lattice relaxation is much more rapid for B spins than the cross relaxation. In this case the B-spin populations will have their thermal equilibrium values, N_3^0 and N_4^0. Thus

$$\frac{dN_1}{dt} = -\left(W_{12} + W_x \frac{N_4^0}{N_B}\right)N_1 + \left(W_{21} + W_x \frac{N_3^0}{N_B}\right)N_2. \qquad (8\text{-}18)$$

This equation is the same as would result for no cross relaxation except that the relaxation rate is now the sum of two contributions, the relaxation to the lattice and to the B spins. If cross relaxation is the faster of the two, we have the case mentioned above of relaxation via a more rapidly relaxing species.

8–5 Phonon Bottleneck

We have considered explicitly only relaxation in which all the vibrational modes of the lattice are in thermal equilibrium with a large thermal reservoir (the bath) but not necessarily in equilibrium with the spin system. Such thermal equilibrium requires time to establish; and if energy is absorbed by certain modes at a rate faster than they can transfer it to the remaining modes or the bath, the so-called phonon bottleneck [11] is encountered.

Actually there may be several thermal reservoirs somewhat in cascade between the spin system and the bath (the dominant thermal reservoir). Such a situation is illustrated in Fig. 8-5, which shows direct relaxation coupling only to modes resonant with the transition but Raman processes coupling to all modes. If we associate with each thermal reservoir a heat capacity, and if we associate a thermal conductance with each coupling process, then a simple thermodynamic description [12] can be given which indicates the main features of the phonon bottleneck. For example, consider the simpler case shown in Fig. 8-6 with an infinite heat capacity associated with the nonresonant lattice modes plus the bath. If we assume that C_i, the heat capacities, and α_i, the thermal conductances, are indepen-

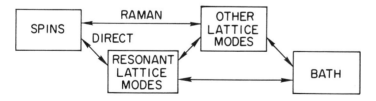

FIG. 8-5 Diagrammatic representation of relaxation as coupled thermal reservoirs. The spin system couples directly to resonant lattice modes, but via the Raman process it can also couple to the other lattice modes. The lattice may in turn be coupled to a still larger thermal reservoir, the bath.

dent of T_i and t (temperatures and time), that is, if we assume that all reservoirs are at nearly the same temperature, we may write

$$C_S \frac{dT_S}{dt} = \alpha_{SL}(T_L - T_S),$$

(8-19)

$$C_L \frac{dT_L}{dt} = \alpha_{SL}(T_S - T_L) + \alpha_{LB}(T_B - T_L).$$

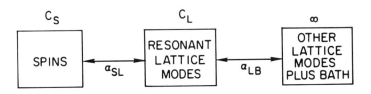

FIG. 8-6 A simplified version of Fig. 8-5. This thermal problem is analyzed in the text and leads to a description of the phonon bottleneck. In simple terms, this occurs when energy can be coupled from the spin system into the resonant lattice modes faster than it can be coupled on out into the other lattice modes and the bath.

Of course T_B is constant since C_B is infinite. The solution of Eq. (8-19) is relatively easy, both T_S and T_L consisting of two exponentially decaying components and a constant term, T_B.

The simplest behavior occurs when the resonant lattice modes and the lattice plus bath form one thermal reservoir. Then the spin temperature decays with a rate α_{SL}/C_S, which we will regard as the reciprocal of the spin-lattice relaxation time since it corresponds to our previous use of the term. More generally two time constants are associated with the decay of T_S from some initial value to T_B. One is longer and one is shorter than the spin-lattice relaxation time. Hence the decay of a system with a phonon bottleneck is qualitatively like that shown in Fig. 8-7 (which is strictly valid only for small variations in signal).

Probably the simplest case to analyze for a phonon bottleneck is one in which the heat capacity, C_L, for the resonant modes is very small. Then Eq. (8-19) can be solved to give a decay rate of $\alpha_{SL}\alpha_{LB}/C_S(\alpha_{SL} + \alpha_{LB})$, which is slower than the spin-lattice relaxation rate. A more complete analysis yields a second and more rapid rate with a value of $(\alpha_{SL} + \alpha_{LB})/C_L$. This rate is much faster than the spin-lattice relaxation rate, although in this case there is a very small change in the spin temperature resulting from this fast decay.

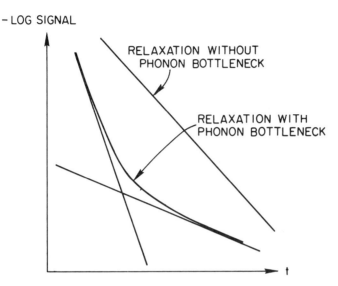

−LOG SIGNAL

RELAXATION WITHOUT
PHONON BOTTLENECK

RELAXATION WITH
PHONON BOTTLENECK

t

FIG. 8-7   Schematic representation of relaxation with and without a phonon
bottleneck. With a phonon bottleneck there are two characteristic relaxation
rates, one faster and one slower than the rate in the absence of a phonon bottleneck. We have assumed recovery from partial saturation in this figure.

Although the simple analysis used here and embodied in Eq. (8-19)
cannot be generalized to large temperature differences without some
modification, the basic physical ideas can be applied more widely. By doing
this we can explain one of the most dramatic aspects of the phonon
bottleneck, a process descriptively labeled as the phonon avalanche. To
understand the phonon avalanche consider a two-level paramagnetic
species in a crystal in which the lattice modes resonant with the paramagnetic species couple energy only very slowly into other modes or the
bath. Now invert the population of the spins, using, for example, fast
passage (see Section 2–2). Since a two-level system can always be
described by a temperature, we can describe the condition of inverted
population by saying that the system has a negative absolute temperature.
More to the point, the spins have a much higher internal energy than when
in thermal equilibrium. The first process that occurs is that the spins
transfer some of this energy to the resonant vibrational modes. The rate
at which this transfer occurs increases with the resonant mode temperature
(presumably linearly). The temperature of the resonant modes cannot
become negative because any number of phonons are allowed, thus
making it possible for any amount of energy to be absorbed. But as the

resonant mode temperature increases toward infinity, the relaxation rate increases. This avalanche effect causes the spin temperature to approach infinity very rapidly, although after a delay. Thereafter the spins and the resonant vibrational modes approach equilibrium at a much slower rate typical of the second stage of a phonon bottleneck. Figure 8-8 shows roughly the behavior for a phonon avalanche.

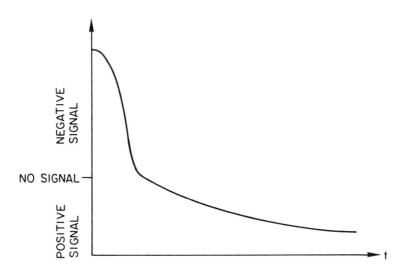

FIG. 8-8 Schematic representation of an EPR signal in the case of a phonon avalanche following population inversion. Three stages are evident. Initially the relaxation is to cool resonant lattice modes and is relatively slow. As the resonant lattice modes heat up, the relaxation rate increases and the "avalanche" occurs. This stops when the spin system is at a very high, but not negative, temperature and the signal is small. Subsequent changes are again slow as the coupled system of spins and resonant lattice modes approaches equilibrium with the other modes and the bath.

Possibly the most convincing demonstration of the phonon bottleneck was its observation by Brillouin scattering of light [13]. When the electron paramagnetic resonance of Ni^{2+} impurities in MgO single crystals was saturated, the effective temperature of phonons in a narrow band near 25.6 GHz (the microwave frequency) was observed to rise to about 60°K while the other phonons remained at the 2°K bath temperature.

It should be kept in mind that the phonon bottleneck is a manifestation of the difficulty which can arise in heat transport across an interface between two thermal reservoirs. A more obvious interface of this sort is the one between the crystal and the bath. The effects of the crystal-bath interface may be particularly apparent at liquid-helium temperatures, where the lattice heat capacity is low and the spin heat capacity is large. Larson and Jeffries [14] observed a decrease of approximately three orders of magnitude in the relaxation rate as the temperature was varied from just below the λ point of liquid helium to just above. The thermal conductivity of helium changes drastically at the λ point, the temperature at which all superfluid properties disappear.

8–6 Supplemental Bibliography

1. K. W. H. Stevens, Rep. Prog. Phys. **30** (part 1), 189 (1967).

2. K. J. Standley and R. A. Vaughan, *Electron Spin Relaxation Phenomena in Solids*, Plenum, New York, 1969.

3. A. A. Manenkov and R. Orbach, eds., *Spin-Lattice Relaxation in Ionic Solids*, Harper and Row, New York, 1966.

References Cited in Chapter 8

[1] A. A. Maradudin, E. W. Montroll, and G. H. Weiss, *Theory of Lattice Dynamics in the Harmonic Approximation*, Academic, New York, 1963, Suppl. 3 of *Solid State Physics*.
[2] G. Weinreich, *Solids: Elementary Theory for Advanced Students*, Wiley, New York, 1965, p. 56.
[3] C. Kittel, *Introduction to Solid State Physics*, 3rd ed., Wiley, New York, 1966, p. 115.
[4] E. Merzbacher, *Quantum Mechanics*, 2nd ed., Wiley, New York, 1970, p. 470.
[5] P. L. Donoho, *Phys. Rev.* **133**, A1080 (1964).
[6] R. Orbach and M. Blume, *Phys. Rev. Letters* **8**, 478 (1962).
[7] R. W. Bierig, M. J. Weber, and S. I. Warshaw, *Phys. Rev.* **134**, A1504 (1964); Chao-Yuan Huang, *Phys. Rev.* **139**, A241 (1965); J. B. Horak and A. W. Nolle, *Phys. Rev.* **153**, 372 (1967).
[8] C. B. P. Finn, R. Orbach, and W. P. Wolf, *Proc. Phys. Soc.* **77**, 261 (1961).
[9] Chao-Yuan Huang, *Phys. Rev.* **154**, 215 (1967); *Phys. Rev.* **161**, 272 (1967); *J. Phys. Chem. Solids* **28**, 1339 (1967).
[10] W. J. C. Grant, *J. Phys. Chem. Solids* **25**, 751 (1964).
[11] A recent discussion of the status of research on the phonon bottleneck is given in A. Abragam, *Comments Solid State Phys.* **2**, 1 (1969).
[12] A. M. Stoneham, *Proc. Phys. Soc.* **86**, 1163 (1965).
[13] W. J. Brya, S. Geschwind, and G. E. Devlin, *Phys. Rev. Letters* **21**, 1800 (1968). References are given therein to several other experimental studies of the phonon bottleneck.
[14] G. H. Larson and C. D. Jeffries, *Phys. Rev.* **141**, 461 (1966).

CHAPTER 9

The Effects of Motion; Liquids

Most considerations of Chapters 1 through 8 imply that the paramagnetic species in question is in a well-defined environment whose orientation is fixed in the laboratory. This is usually the case for paramagnets in solids but is certainly not true of liquids. In this chapter we will examine a few of the consequences of motion of the paramagnet, particularly the Brownian or random motion in liquids. We will develop these ideas in a way which follows naturally from our treatment of fixed paramagnets.

9–1 The Tumbling Paramagnetic Complex

As a basis for our analysis, we will assume that the paramagnetic complexes in question have well-defined short-range order when in liquid solution. Such is the case for many solvated ions and also for many other paramagnets of interest. These complexes, which are similar to those associated with imperfections in single crystals, may have symmetries as high as cubic but are more frequently axial or even lower in symmetry. By contrast to the situation in solids, the complexes within the liquid tumble in a random way as they are jostled by the molecular motion of the solvent liquid.

The paramagnets may therefore be described by a spin Hamiltonian which can have the same complexity as for single crystals. Hence we may represent it by the appropriate terms drawn from those in Chapter 4. To be specific let us consider the Hamiltonian for axial symmetry of Eq. (4-5):

$$\mathcal{H} = g_{\parallel}\beta H_z S_z + g_{\perp}\beta(H_x S_x + H_y S_y) + D[S_z^2 - \tfrac{1}{3}S(S+1)]$$

$$+ AS_z I_z + B(S_x I_x + S_y I_y). \tag{9-1}$$

Since the complex tumbles, we would expect the symmetry axis z to have equal probability of being in any element of solid angle and to vary randomly in orientation. If we assume only a small anisotropy in the Zeeman and hyperfine interactions and further assume $D \ll g\beta H$, then the spins are quantized very close to the direction of **H**. Thus the Hamiltonian can be written in the 123-coordinate system, where the 3 axis is parallel to **H** [this has already been done for the Zeeman interaction in Eq. (5-14)].

If we keep only the 3 components of the spin operators because they give the lowest-order contribution, we can use the methods of Chapter 5 to write the Hamiltonian in a more convenient form:

$$\mathcal{H} = \beta \frac{\mathbf{H} \cdot \mathbf{g} \cdot \mathbf{H}}{H} S_3 + \frac{\mathbf{H} \cdot \mathbf{A} \cdot \mathbf{H}}{H^2} S_3 I_3 + \frac{\mathbf{H} \cdot \mathbf{D} \cdot \mathbf{H}}{H^2} \tfrac{1}{2}(3S_3^2 - S^2), \quad (9\text{-}2)$$

where only the operators with diagonal matrix elements are given.

Equation (9-2) is valid for any symmetry. For the axial symmetry of Eq. (9-1), and using the *xyz* coordinate system for obtaining the components of the vector and tensor quantities, we have

$$\mathbf{H} = H(\sin \theta \cos \phi, \sin \theta \sin \phi, \cos \theta),$$

$$\mathbf{g} = \begin{pmatrix} g_\perp & 0 & 0 \\ 0 & g_\perp & 0 \\ 0 & 0 & g_\parallel \end{pmatrix},$$

$$\mathbf{A} = \begin{pmatrix} B & 0 & 0 \\ 0 & B & 0 \\ 0 & 0 & A \end{pmatrix},$$

$$\mathbf{D} = \begin{pmatrix} -\tfrac{1}{3}D & 0 & 0 \\ 0 & -\tfrac{1}{3}D & 0 \\ 0 & 0 & \tfrac{2}{3}D \end{pmatrix}, \quad (9\text{-}3)$$

$$\frac{\mathbf{H} \cdot \mathbf{g} \cdot \mathbf{H}}{H^2} = g_\perp \sin^2 \theta + g_\parallel \cos^2 \theta,$$

$$\frac{\mathbf{H} \cdot \mathbf{A} \cdot \mathbf{H}}{H^2} = B \sin^2 \theta + A \cos^2 \theta,$$

$$\frac{\mathbf{H} \cdot \mathbf{D} \cdot \mathbf{H}}{H^2} = -\tfrac{1}{3}D \sin^2 \theta + \tfrac{2}{3}D \cos^2 \theta.$$

If we substitute

$$\cos^2 \theta = \tfrac{1}{3}(3 \cos^2 \theta - 1) + \tfrac{1}{3}$$

$$\sin^2 \theta = -\tfrac{1}{3}(3 \cos^2 \theta - 1) + \tfrac{2}{3} \quad (9\text{-}4)$$

into Eq. (9-3), we obtain

$$\frac{\mathbf{H} \cdot \mathbf{g} \cdot \mathbf{H}}{H^2} = \frac{2g_\perp + g_\parallel}{3} + \tfrac{1}{3}(g_\parallel - g_\perp)(3\cos^2\theta - 1),$$

$$\frac{\mathbf{H} \cdot \mathbf{A} \cdot \mathbf{H}}{H^2} = \frac{2B + A}{3} + \tfrac{1}{3}(A - B)(3\cos^2\theta - 1), \tag{9-5}$$

$$\frac{\mathbf{H} \cdot \mathbf{D} \cdot \mathbf{H}}{H^2} = \tfrac{1}{3}D(3\cos^2\theta - 1).$$

The Hamiltonian of Eq. (9-2) then becomes

$$\mathcal{H} = g_a\beta HS_3 + aI_3S_3 + g_b\beta HS_3(3\cos^2\theta - 1) + bI_3S_3(3\cos^2\theta - 1)$$

$$+ \tfrac{1}{2}D[S_3^2 - \tfrac{1}{3}S(S+1)](3\cos^2\theta - 1), \tag{9-6}$$

where

$$g_a \equiv \tfrac{1}{3}g_\parallel + \tfrac{2}{3}g_\perp, \qquad g_b \equiv \tfrac{1}{3}(g_\parallel - g_\perp),$$

$$a \equiv \tfrac{1}{3}A + \tfrac{2}{3}B, \qquad b \equiv \tfrac{1}{3}(A - B). \tag{9-7}$$

The resultant expression for the energy will contain terms independent of orientation and terms which vary with angle as $3\cos^2\theta - 1$, that is,

$$E = g_a\beta HM_S + aM_SM_I + \{g_b\beta HM_S + bM_SM_I$$

$$+ \tfrac{1}{2}D[M_S^2 - \tfrac{1}{3}S(S+1)]\}(3\cos^2\theta - 1). \tag{9-8}$$

The terms which depend on the orientation of the magnetic field with the complex average to zero when integrated over all solid angles (it was for this reason that we expressed the angular dependence in terms of $3\cos^2\theta - 1$, a spherical harmonic apart from a multiplicative constant, instead of $\sin^2\theta$ and $\cos^2\theta$).

Several relatively simple limiting cases for the application of Eq. (9-8) exist and provide some insight into the general situation. In addition to the possibility that this formulation might be useful for a single crystal, there are two extremes for randomly oriented complexes. The first consists of the stationary but randomly oriented complexes in amorphous solids, polycrystalline solids, and powders, as well as the slowly tumbling complexes in viscous liquids. At the other extreme are the rapidly tumbling complexes in low-viscosity liquids or gases.

If a complex tumbles slowly enough, or not at all, the EPR spectrum observed will be that associated with its instantaneous orientation at the moment of observation. The result for a bulk sample of randomly oriented complexes is observation of the superposed spectra corresponding to all

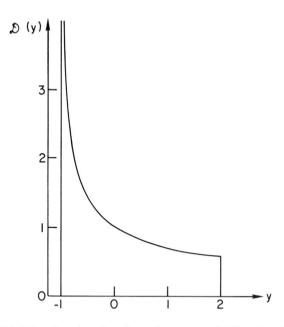

FIG. 9-1 Weighting function for "powder spectra." The function $\mathfrak{D}(y)$ is $(y+1)^{-\frac{1}{2}}$, where $y = 3\cos^2\theta - 1$. This weighting function applies to each component of the fine or hyperfine structure described by Eq. (9-8), that is, if the anisotropy and fine structure are sufficiently small. If the resonance lines had infinitesimal widths, the absorption would have the form shown. For finite line widths one obtains a more rounded absorption which is just the superposition of lines distributed between the two extremes of the graph and having intensities proportional to the values of $\mathfrak{D}(y)$ corresponding to their positions.

possible orientations, each increment of solid angle being weighted equally. Expressed in terms of $y = 3\cos^2\theta - 1$, the weighting then becomes $(y+1)^{-1/2}$, which is shown in Fig. 9-1. The resulting "powder spectra" have been the subject of several papers [1]. It is more difficult to extract information from "powder spectra" than from single-crystal spectra because of the poor resolution usually produced by the distribution shown in Fig. 9-1 and because of inability to correlate the spectra with a particular orientation of crystal and field.

If the complex tumbles rapidly, however, it will simply produce a spectrum in which all orientation-dependent terms have their average value, that is, zero. The result is a simple spectrum described by the first two terms in Eq. (9-8). The process by which the powder spectrum narrows to produce the averaged spectrum is termed motional averaging or motional narrowing [2]. Figure 9-2 shows spectra for a solution of $CuSO_4 \cdot xH_2O$

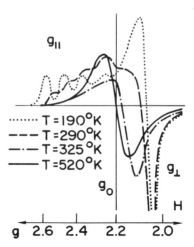

FIG. 9-2   First derivative of the absorption of a solution of $CuSO_4 \cdot xH_2O$ ($x = 0$–5) in glycerol at several temperatures [1]. Despite the complication of the hyperfine structure, one can see a continuous transition from a "powder spectrum" at low temperatures to a motionally averaged spectrum at high temperatures. This is a consequence of the decreased viscosity of glycerol and the resultant increased tumbling rate of the Cu^{2+} complexes as the temperature is raised.

in glycerol at several temperatures as observed by Kneubühl [1]. Spectra corresponding to both limits, as well as two intermediate cases, can be seen.

The answer as to whether a given complex tumbles slowly or rapidly depends on whether the characteristic time for tumbling is longer or shorter than the reciprocal of the frequency associated with the terms which depend on orientation. This characteristic time or correlation time, τ_c, is roughly the time required to alter the orientation significantly, that is, to change $3 \cos^2 \theta - 1$ by about 1. Thus, if h/τ_c were much greater than $g_b \beta H + b M_I + \frac{1}{2} D(2M_S - 1)$, that particular line ($M_S, M_I \rightleftharpoons M_S - 1, M_I$) would be averaged. By contrast, if h/τ_c were much smaller than $g_b \beta H + b M_I + \frac{1}{2} D(2M_S - 1)$, no averaging would occur. We will discuss the problem of randomly time-varying functions in the next section.

9-2   Random Functions and Correlations [3]

To illustrate the problem now before us, a problem similar to that treated by Bloembergen, Purcell, and Pound [4] for nuclear resonance in liquids, we consider as an example the function $3 \cos^2 \theta - 1$, which appears as a coefficient in Eq. (9-8). If θ is the angle between a fixed direction in space and an axis within a randomly tumbling molecule, over sufficiently long times the axis will point with equal likelihood through all equal surface elements of the unit sphere, and the mean value of $3 \cos^2 \theta - 1$ will be

$$\overline{3 \cos^2 \theta - 1} = \frac{\displaystyle\int_0^\pi (3 \cos^2 \theta - 1) 2\pi \sin \theta \, d\theta}{\displaystyle\int_0^\pi 2\pi \sin \theta \, d\theta} = 0. \qquad (9\text{-}9)$$

The question arises as to how long a time one must wait to have the tumbling axis sample all orientations, or at least enough of them for the average to tend closely to zero. For concreteness, suppose that Fig. 9-3 represents the variation of $[3 \cos^2 \theta(t) - 1] \sin \theta(t)$ with time, as θ in turn varies with time. Over the time interval, t_0, shown, $[3 \cos^2 \theta(t) - 1] \sin \theta(t)$ surely does not appear to average very close to zero, and it seems likely that one would have to observe the motion for perhaps several t_0 before the average would be zero, within 5% of the amplitude from -1 to $+2$. It is also apparent that there is a length of interval—choose, for example, $t_0/10$ or smaller—such that the value of the function at the end of the

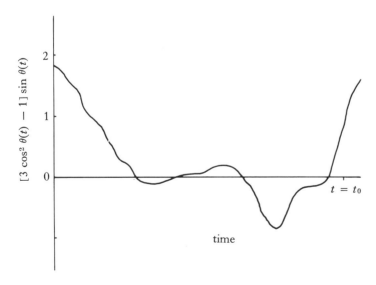

FIG. 9-3 An imagined random variation with time of $3 \cos^2 \theta(t) - 1$, with proper spherical weighting, $\sin \theta(t)$, as a molecular complex tumbles in a liquid.

interval is quite probably of the same sign, and perhaps even of similar magnitude, as at the beginning of the interval. This latter statement is true in a statistical sense for any choice of starting point for the small interval. We say that over such an interval the values of the function are correlated. Clearly the correlation is better the shorter the interval.

We can try to be more quantitative by defining a correlation function, $K(t_1, t_2)$, for a random function, $f(x(t))$. We now have in mind that f is a prescribed function of x, which, however, varies randomly with t, where $f(x(t))$ has an average value, $(1/T) \int_{t_1}^{t_1+T} f(x(t))\,dt$, of zero over a long time interval, T. The correlation function is defined as

$$K(t_1, t_2) = \overline{f(x(t_1))f^*(x(t_2))}, \qquad (9\text{-}10)$$

where the asterisk indicates a complex conjugate, since $f(x(t))$ may in general be complex, and the bar denotes an ensemble average; that is, we suppose that there are many identical systems (here our molecular complex) and we average the product for the two instants, t_1 and t_2, over all the molecules.

In terms of the conditional probability, $p(x_1, t_1; x_2, t_2)\,dx_1\,dx_2$, that a molecule has x_1 in dx_1 at t_1 and x_2 in dx_2 at time t_2,

$$K(t_1, t_2) = \iint p(x_1, t_1; x_2, t_2)f(x_1)f^*(x_2)\,dx_1\,dx_2. \qquad (9\text{-}11)$$

We shall suppose that we deal with a stationary random process, one which depends not at all on the origin in time but only on $\tau = |t_1 - t_2|$. Then

$$p(x_1, x_2, \tau) = p(x_1, x_2, -\tau) = p(x_2, x_1, \tau), \qquad (9\text{-}12)$$

and from

$$K(\tau) = \iint p(x_1, x_2, \tau)f(x_1)f^*(x_2)\,dx_1\,dx_2 \qquad (9\text{-}13)$$

it follows that

$$K(-\tau) = K^*(\tau) = K(\tau). \qquad (9\text{-}14)$$

Then Eq. (9-10) becomes for stationary random processes

$$K(\tau) = \overline{f(x(t))f^*(x(t+\tau))}. \qquad (9\text{-}15)$$

We define now $k(\tau)$ such that $k(0) = 1$ as follows:

$$K(\tau) = K(0)k(\tau) = \overline{|f(x(t))|^2}\,k(\tau). \qquad (9\text{-}16)$$

Since the process is stationary, the ensemble average of $|f(x(t))|^2$ can be performed for any instant of time. In our ensemble all orientations of the molecular axis are equally likely, and the ensemble average of $|3\cos^2\theta(t) - 1|^2$ is simply the average of $(3\cos\theta - 1)^2$ over a sphere.

Abragam [2] illustrates the calculation of the correlation function for a model in which the complex is considered to be a sphere of radius a immersed in a fluid of viscosity η, with the viscous resisting torque on the sphere given by Stokes's law [5]. The r axis is taken to be a particular direction fixed in the tumbling sphere. If $f(\cos \theta(t))$ is any second-order spherical harmonic, Abragam finds, by using the diffusion equations to examine the flow of $p(x_1, x_2, \tau)$ with time, that

$$K(\tau) = \overline{|f(\cos \theta(t))|^2} \exp\left(\frac{-|\tau|}{\tau_c}\right) \qquad (9\text{-}17)$$

where

$$\tau_c = \frac{4\pi\eta a^3}{3kT}. \qquad (9\text{-}18)$$

For our example of $3 \cos^2 \theta - 1 = f(\cos \theta(t))$ we suppose that there is an isotropic distribution of the axis directions within the ensemble of molecular systems, giving $\overline{(3 \cos^2 \theta - 1)^2} = \frac{4}{5}$.

The function $k(\tau)$ certainly need not have the simple exponential form of Eq. (9-17). Sometimes a Gaussian is used, and in more general cases $k(\tau)$ oscillates. In any case, it depends in detail on the model that is used, and it is common practice to assume a form for $k(\tau)$ that is mathematically convenient and has the properties $k(0) = 1$, $k(\tau \to \infty) \to 0$, and $k(\tau_c) \approx k(0)/2$. Although the mathematical definition of τ_c is thus not precise, it is clear that τ_c is a measure of the length of time over which some correlation persists. Therefore τ_c is the correlation time mentioned in Section 9–1 and it is evidently much longer for a sugar molecule in molasses in January than for the same molecule dissolved in water at room temperature. The value for a typical molecule in water is $\sim 10^{-11}$ sec.

The correlation function lends mathematical precision to some of our qualitative ideas about the loss of correlation within an assembly of tumbling molecules. Moreover, it is directly useful in a quantitative description of relaxation processes within the liquid. We wish next to demonstrate this fact by calculating the transition probability for electron spins under the influence of a random perturbation.

Let us consider $\mathcal{H} = \mathcal{H}_0 + \mathcal{H}_1(t)$, where $\mathcal{H}_1(t)$ arises from a perturbing interaction between the spins and the lattice. The spins are, in effect, a subsystem of the entire system, which includes in addition the many degrees of freedom of atomic and molecular motions. The interaction $\mathcal{H}_1$ in our problem will contain the angle-dependent terms of Eq. (9-6), which are those having diagonal matrix elements for our choice of the 3 axis, and will also contain the angle-dependent terms omitted from Eq. (9-6) because they have off-diagonal matrix elements (these terms can be obtained in a manner similar to that developed in Appendix B). An example of such an omitted term is shown in Eq. (5-14). The perturbation $\mathcal{K}_1$ becomes a time-dependent operator in the Heisenberg sense, with the time dependence introduced by the Hamiltonian for the lattice motions. Because the liquid "lattice" has very many degrees of freedom, we suppose that $\mathcal{K}_1(t)$, incorporating this time dependence, can be treated as a random function of time instead of performing the more rigorous but impossibly difficult quantum-mechanical calculation for the entire system consisting of spin subsystem and lattice.

To demonstrate how we handle $\mathcal{K}_1(t)$ as a random function, we begin by using standard time-dependent perturbation theory as discussed in Section 2–3. We expand the perturbed spin functions in terms of the eigenfunctions of $\mathcal{K}_0$ [thereby obtaining Eq. (2-70)]:

$$\psi = \sum_{M''} a_{M''}(t)\Phi_{M''} \exp\left(-\frac{i}{\hbar}E_{M''}t\right). \tag{9-19}$$

Substituting into the Schrödinger equation, we obtain the equivalent of Eq. (2-71):

$$i\hbar\frac{da_{M'}}{dt} = \sum_{M''} \langle M'|\mathcal{K}_1(t)|M''\rangle a_{M''}(t) \exp i\omega_{M'M''}t, \tag{9-20}$$

where

$$\omega_{M'M''} = \frac{1}{\hbar}(E_{M'} - E_{M''}). \tag{9-21}$$

If the system is initially in the stationary state M, that is, $a_{M''}(0) = \delta_{M''M}$, the $a_{M'}(t)$ for $M' \neq M$ initially unfold in time as

$$a_{M'}(t) = \frac{1}{i\hbar} \int_0^t \langle M'|\mathcal{K}_1(t')|M\rangle \exp\left(i\omega_{M'M}t'\right) dt'. \tag{9-22}$$

The probability that, after t seconds, a system initially in state M will be found in M' is

$$P_{MM'} = a_{M'}a_{M'}^*, \tag{9-23}$$

and we seek a transition rate, $w_{MM'} = dP_{MM'}/dt$:

$$w_{MM'} = a_{M'}\frac{da_{M'}^*}{dt} + \text{c.c.} \tag{9-24}$$

Placing Eq. (9-22) into Eq. (9-24) and using the Hermitian property of $\mathcal{H}_1$ gives

$$w_{MM'} = \hbar^{-2}\langle M|\mathcal{H}_1(t)|M'\rangle \exp(-i\omega_{M'M}t)$$

$$\times \int_0^t \langle M'|\mathcal{H}_1(t')|M\rangle \exp(i\omega_{M'M}t')\, dt' + \text{c.c.}$$

$$= \hbar^{-2}\int_0^t \langle M'|\mathcal{H}_1(t')|M\rangle$$

$$\times \langle M|\mathcal{H}_1(t)|M'\rangle \exp[-i\omega_{M'M}(t-t')]\, dt' + \text{c.c.} \quad (9\text{-}25)$$

Up to this point we have simply reproduced a very familiar calculation of time-dependent perturbation theory, using steps differing little from those employed in Section 2–3. Now we want to consider that the $\mathcal{H}_1(t)$ in Eq. (9-25) is a random function, and so therefore is its matrix element. The measurable quantity in our assembly of molecular complexes is the ensemble average, $\overline{w_{MM'}}$. Taking such an average of Eq. (9-25), while at the same time transforming to the variable $\tau = t - t'$, yields

$$\overline{w_{MM'}} = \hbar^{-2}\int_0^t \overline{f^*(t-\tau)f(t)}\exp(-i\omega_{M'M}\tau)\, d\tau + \text{c.c.} \quad (9\text{-}26)$$

In Eq. (9-26) we have written $f(t)$ for $\langle M|\mathcal{H}_1(t)|M'\rangle$ in order to emphasize that the integrand contains in fact the correlation function $K(\tau)$ as defined in Eq. (9-15). Making use of $K(\tau) = K(-\tau)$, Eq. (9-14), one can cast Eq. (9-26) into the form

$$\overline{w_{MM'}} = \hbar^{-2}\int_{-t}^t K(\tau)\exp(-i\omega_{M'M}\tau)\, d\tau. \quad (9\text{-}27)$$

If we suppose that the correlation time, τ_c, is short compared to the times, t, of interest (which means for this calculation $\tau_c \ll t$), loss of correlation will carry the integrand to zero before τ reaches t, and the limits can be called $\pm\infty$. Equation (2-102) relates the spin-lattice relaxation time, T_1, to the transition probabilities. For high temperatures we have therefore

$$\left(\frac{1}{2T_1}\right)_{MM'} = \overline{w_{MM'}} = \hbar^{-2}\int_{-\infty}^{\infty} K(\tau)\exp(-i\omega_{M'M}\tau)\, d\tau. \quad (9\text{-}28)$$

The contribution of $M \to M'$ transitions to the relaxation rate, $1/T_1$, is thus proportional to the Fourier transform of the correlation function.

As an example we will select as our $\mathcal{H}_1(t)$ one of the off-diagonal terms omitted in Eq. (9-6) but present in Eq. (9-1):

$$\mathcal{H}_1(t) = \tfrac{3}{2}(g_b\beta H + bI_3)\sin\theta\cos\theta(S_+e^{-i\phi} + S_-e^{i\phi}), \quad (9\text{-}29)$$

letting $S = \frac{1}{2}$ for simplicity. The operator in Eq. (9-29) will produce transitions for which $\Delta M_S = \pm 1$ and $\Delta M_I = 0$. For such a transition we obtain

$$K(\tau) = \overline{\langle -\tfrac{1}{2}, M_I | \mathcal{K}_1(t) | \tfrac{1}{2}, M_I \rangle \langle \tfrac{1}{2}, M_I | \mathcal{K}_1(t+\tau) | -\tfrac{1}{2}, M_I \rangle}. \quad (9\text{-}30)$$

Using Eqs. (9-29) and (9-17), we find

$$K(\tau) = \tfrac{4}{9}(g_b\beta H + bM_I)^2 |\langle -\tfrac{1}{2}|S_-|\tfrac{1}{2}\rangle|^2 \, \overline{|\sin\theta \cos\theta \, e^{i\phi}|^2} \exp\left(\frac{-|\tau|}{\tau_c}\right)$$

$$= \tfrac{3}{10}(g_b\beta H + bM_I)^2 \exp\left(\frac{-|\tau|}{\tau_c}\right). \quad (9\text{-}31)$$

Finally, the contribution to the relaxation rate is found by placing Eq. (9-31) into Eq. (9-28):

$$\frac{1}{2T_1} = \frac{3}{10\hbar^2}(g_b\beta H + bM_I)^2 \frac{2\tau_c}{1+\omega^2\tau_c^2}. \quad (9\text{-}32)$$

Figure 9-4 shows plots of the correlation spectrum,

$$j(\omega) = \frac{2\tau_c}{1+\omega^2\tau_c^2}, \quad (9\text{-}33)$$

for three different values of τ_c.

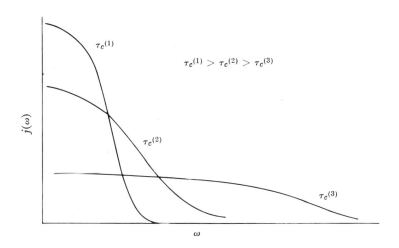

FIG. 9-4 Graphs of the correlation function of Eq. (9-33) for three values of τ_c.

This correlation-function treatment of liquids has been extremely successful in nuclear magnetic resonance [2], giving, in fact, far more precise quantitative agreement than the crudeness of the Stokes model would suggest. In addition, a number of features of electronic paramagnetic resonance are explained by the model. We shall describe some of these in Section 9–3.

9–3 Influence of Molecular Tumbling on Hyperfine Structure

Consider the effect of a term such as $b(3 \cos^2 \theta - 1)I_3 S_3$ in Eq. (9-6). If the molecular complex is fixed in space and if the coupling $b \ll g_a \beta H$ so that simple first-order perturbation theory applies, this term for a state M_S, M_I corresponds to a local hyperfine magnetic field displacing the electron resonance frequency by an amount $\delta v = \delta \omega / 2\pi$:

$$\hbar \, \delta \omega = b(3 \cos^2 \theta - 1)M_I. \tag{9-34}$$

If rapid tumbling occurs, the angular factor averages to zero and the resonance is undisplaced by this term. The critical question is: How rapidly must the molecule tumble, or, more precisely, how small must τ_c of Eq. (9-17) be to average away $(3 \cos^2 \theta - 1)$?

This factor occurs in dipole-dipole coupling, and the question was answered correctly for nuclear magnetic resonance in a qualitative way by Bloembergen *et al.* [4] in 1948. Recent general theories, summarized in Abragam's book [2], make the argument more precise. Our purpose here is not to provide such precision but rather to try to establish a plausible physical argument for the qualitative answer.

Both in the present example and in the picture of exchange narrowing by Anderson and Weiss [6], narrowing is brought on by a fluctuating magnetic environment of the paramagnetic ion. Let us idealize the situation to one in which each ion, instead of resonating at ω_0, has available to it only two possible magnetic locales, which shift the resonance from ω_0 by $+\delta$ and $-\delta$ radians per second, respectively. Let us suppose that the ion jumps randomly between these two locales (or equivalently that the magnetic nature of a given locale alternates randomly) with a mean time τ_c for the existence of the ion in either kind of environment. It is now possible to deduce the effect upon the splitting or broadening of the resonance by recalling the basic definition of T_2 as the lifetime for the decay of transverse components of magnetization [see Eqs. (2-24) and (2-29)].

Consider an assembly of these ions which may have precession frequencies $\omega_0 + \delta$ or $\omega_0 - \delta$, and suppose that somehow they have been prepared in an initial state having **M** (or total **S**) along the x' axis of a frame rotating at ω_0. Of course some spins precess at $+\delta$ and some at $-\delta$ with respect to the primed frame, and it is clear that, if the environment did not fluctuate, the vector sum of the precessing components would decay in a time $T_2^0 \approx 1/\delta$.

On the other hand, if the environment of a given spin fluctuates between $+\delta$ and $-\delta$ with a mean time τ_c, each precessing spin executes a random walk in phase angle with respect to the rotating frame. By the simple properties of the random walk [7], the mean-square phase difference, $\overline{\Delta\phi^2}$, accumulated by the spins after n changes of environment is

$$\overline{\Delta\phi^2} \approx n(\tau_c\delta)^2, \tag{9-35}$$

where $\tau_c\delta$ is the magnitude of the mean phase accumulation, in radians, per step. Now the definition of the relaxation time, T_2, is the time in which the spins, initially precessing in phase, get out of phase to the extent that their vector sum is decreased in magnitude by $1/e$. This requires $\overline{(\Delta\phi^2)}^{1/2}$ to be of the order of 1 radian. If the elapsed time is T_2, we can write $n = T_2/\tau_c$, which converts Eq. (9-35) to

$$1^2 \approx \frac{T_2}{\tau_c}(\tau_c\delta)^2. \tag{9-36}$$

Thus we have, for the measure of line width or splitting,

$$\frac{1}{T_2} \approx \tau_c\delta^2 \qquad \left(\tau_c < \frac{1}{\delta}\right). \tag{9-37}$$

This result is valid providing the environment has fluctuated before the transverse spin component decayed in consequence of the $T_2^0 \approx 1/\delta$ decay. In other words, when $\tau_c < 1/\delta$, $1/T_2 = 1/T_2^0 \approx \delta$. When $\tau_c < 1/\delta$, Eq. (9-37) applies. Evidently, $\tau_c < 1/\delta$ is the criterion for averaging away broadening effects, and the averaging toward zero is more complete the shorter τ_c, in accordance with Eq. (9-37).

If we return to the correlation spectrum of Fig. 9-4 and Eq. (9-33), which applies to the spherical harmonic $3\cos^2\theta - 1$ for random molecular tumbling, we can interpret Eq. (9-37) as telling us that

$$\frac{1}{T_2} \approx \delta^2 j(0) \qquad \left(\tau_c < \frac{1}{\delta}\right) \tag{9-38}$$

since $j(0) = 2\tau_c$. This is not surprising because the line width (that is, $1/T_2$) arises from static local fields which distribute the precession angular frequencies over an interval near ω_0. Equation (9-38) simply says that $j(0)$ is a measure of the static portion of the correlation spectrum of local fields—this is of course a truism.

The exchange-narrowing expression (Eq. 6-51) is clearly a special case of Eq. (9-37) with $\omega_e = 1/\tau_c$, as is entirely consistent with the Anderson-Weiss model [6], in which the magnetic environment fluctuates at a rate ω_e. In this case, δ is the frequency measure of dipolar coupling.

General theories [8] have verified Eq. (9-37) as a quite general result, showing that δ can be taken to be the amplitude of any randomly fluctuating perturbation diagonal in M_S, which averages to zero over long times and has a correlation time τ_c. The expression does not apply, however, to a rigid lattice (τ_c very long), for which the line width (in angular frequency units) is δ. The criterion for narrowing is that $\tau_c < 1/\delta$, where δ is the angular frequency magnitude of a diagonal term in the spin Hamiltonian.

Off-diagonal random perturbations contribute to spin-lattice relaxation, as we illustrated in Section 9–2. Under conditions of extreme narrowing, $\tau_c \ll 1/\delta$, $1/T_1$ can contribute a term comparable to $1/T_2$ of Eq. (9-37) to the total line width because the finite spin state lifetime, T_1, broadens energy levels in accordance with $T_1 \Delta E \approx \hbar$. When this effect is included, Eq. (9-37) still has order-of-magnitude validity as an expression for the narrow width.

If the molecular tumbling is very rapid, corresponding to a τ_c value much less than $1/\delta$, the averaging of the anisotropic terms in the Hamiltonian Eq. (9-6) will be nearly complete. Rapid tumbling of the complex in effect renders the symmetry spherical by averaging away anisotropic g-factor and anisotropic hyperfine effects. The resonance lines are then located by the very simple Hamiltonian

$$\mathcal{H} = g_a \beta \mathbf{H} \cdot \mathbf{S} + a\mathbf{I} \cdot \mathbf{S}. \qquad (9\text{-}39)$$

This situation is frequently encountered in the paramagnetic resonances of organic free radicals, molecules such as those mentioned at the end of Section 6–2, which are stable even though they have unsatisfied chemical valences. These molecules are paramagnetic because they possess an odd number of electrons (except for certain ones, biradicals, having two unpaired electrons that may be located in different parts of the same molecule, and except for molecules that are readily excited into triplet states). The study of these free-radical molecules has been exceptionally fruitful for theoretical chemistry, especially when the technique of dissolving the molecule in a liquid solvent is used to "tumble away" the anisotropic hyperfine couplings. Anisotropic g values are also tumbled away, but because these organic molecules normally possess very small spin-orbit coupling, all principal values of the g tensor are very near $g_e = 2.0023$ and so, therefore, are the isotropic averages. A typical value is $g = 2.0037$. In this sense, the electrons of the organic radicals have spins that are among the "most free in captivity". Figure 9-5 shows the first of these well-resolved hyperfine splittings observed for such a molecule in a liquid [9]. Studies of the same molecule ion in solid solutions have shown an anisotropic hyperfine coupling comparable to the isotropic coupling responsible for the liquid spectrum in Fig. 9-5.

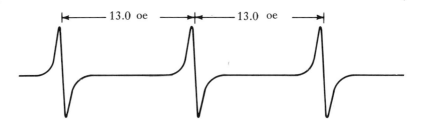

FIG. 9-5 The EPR spectrum of $ON(SO_3)_2^{2-}$ ions in $0.01M$ aqueous solution, observed at 10 GHz and 300°K [9]. The 13 G splitting between adjacent lines arises from hyperfine interaction with the ^{14}N nucleus $(2I+1=3)$.

As an example, we can check to see whether the criterion $\tau_c \ll 1/\delta$ is met. The anisotropic splitting is comparable [10] to the isotropic splitting of 13 G and corresponds, for a g near 2, to 36 MHz, or to $\delta = 2.3 \times 10^8$ sec^{-1}; then $1/\delta = 4 \times 10^{-9}$ sec. If the equivalent spherical radius of the $ON(SO_3)_3^{2-}$ ion is guessed to be 3Å, and if water at 300°K having $\eta \approx 10^{-2}$ poise is the solvent, Eq. (9-18) gives

$$\tau_c = \frac{4\pi\eta a^3}{3kT} \approx 3 \times 10^{-11} \text{ sec}, \qquad (9\text{-}40)$$

which is certainly less than 4×10^{-9} sec, as required.

Such tumbling molecules in liquid solution can indeed have a very rich hyperfine structure if they contain a number of nuclear moments.

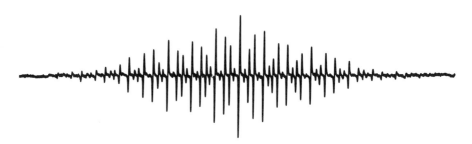

FIG. 9-6 The EPR spectrum of a $3 \times 10^{-4}M$ solution of tetracene in concentrated sulfuric acid at 65°C [11]. The structure results from hyperfine interaction with three different groups of four protons, each group having a different hyperfine splitting. An analogous but simpler spectrum is shown in Fig. 5-12 and discussed in Section 5-3. For tetracene some of the 125 possible lines are accidentally coincident, a consequence of the particular values of the hyperfine splittings.

Figure 9-6 shows the hyperfine structure for the cation of tetracene [11]. The spectrum results from three distinct groups of four equivalent protons. It was taken at $65\,°C$ in a $3 \times 10^{-4}\ M$ solution of tetracene in concentrated H_2SO_4.

Another illustration of correlation spectrum effects is provided by VO^{2+} ion in aqueous solution. Figure 9-7 shows the resonance observed at about 10 GHz. The presence of eight lines is in accordance with the nuclear spin of ^{51}V, $I = \frac{7}{2}$. However, there is a puzzling feature, namely, the variation of line width from line to line of the spectrum. It is also remarkable that the width variation lacks symmetry with respect to the center of the pattern. Why should a line off the center of the spectrum be the sharpest?

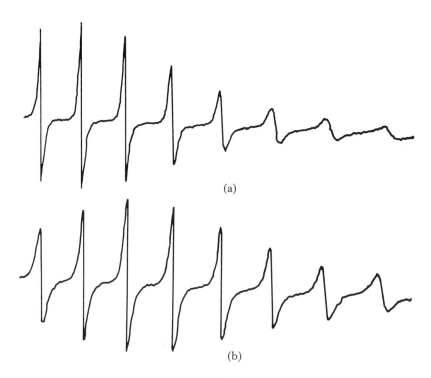

(a)

(b)

FIG. 9-7 The EPR spectrum of the VO^{2+} ion in aqueous solution [13] at (a) 24.3 GHz and (b) 9.25 GHz. The hyperfine splitting is approximately 120 G.

The answer was suggested by McConnell [12] and was verified experimentally by Rogers and Pake [13]. The VO^{2+} ion is doubtless surrounded by a complex of H_2O molecules, and there are strong grounds for believing that the oxygen atom and the H_2O complex place the ion in a site of axial symmetry. Thus the Hamiltonian of Eq. (9-6) should apply. For tetravalent vanadium, $3d^1$, $S = \frac{1}{2}$, and the fine-structure terms may be dropped.

Consider the terms in Eq. (9-6) that have the form

$$(g_b\beta H + bI_3)(3\cos^2\theta - 1)S_3. \tag{9-41}$$

Such terms will, for sufficiently rapid tumbling, be averaged away except for a residual contribution given by Eq. (9-37) with $\delta = (g_b\beta H + bM_I)/\hbar$:

$$\frac{1}{T_2} \approx \frac{\tau_c(g_b\beta H + bM_I)^2}{\hbar^2}. \tag{9-42}$$

In large fields the isotropic hyperfine coupling splits the resonance into $2I + 1$ lines, and Eq. (9-42) predicts a different width contribution, in general, for each hyperfine line. The minimum width should occur for the M_I that most nearly makes the bracket zero. Of course $g_b = \frac{1}{3}(g_\parallel - g_\perp)$ and $b = \frac{1}{3}(A - B)$ are fixed by the nature of the VO^{2+} complex. However, the external field can be varied; and, if Eq. (9-42) describes the situation, it should be possible to shift the point of narrowest width from one line to another within the pattern by observing the resonance in higher or lower fields. This is exactly what is demonstrated by Fig. 9-7.

Again we must keep the record straight by reiterating that T_1 processes arising from off-diagonal terms may also contribute to the total observed line width if τ_c has the proper magnitude. One of these terms has the same dependence on $(g_b\beta H + bI_3)$ as does Eq. (9-41). The effect of all terms was taken into account in the work of reference 12. A general theoretical discussion of the many interactions that may influence the magnetic resonance in liquids and the ways in which they are to be taken into account is given by Kivelson [14]. Carrington and McLachlan [15] describe the results rather generally.

References Cited in Chapter 9

[1] F. K. Kneubühl, *J. Chem. Phys.* **33**, 1074 (1960) and references therein.

[2] A. Abragam, *The Principles of Nuclear Magnetism*, Oxford, New York, 1961.

[3] In this section the authors parallel to some extent a discussion by A. Abragam, *The Principles of Nuclear Magnetism*, Oxford, New York, 1961. A more systematic and detailed development is given in *Selected Papers on Noise and Stochastic Processes* (N. Wax, ed.), Dover, New York, 1954. The papers by S. Chandrasekhar [*Rev. Mod. Phys.* **15**, 1 (1943) and M. C. Wang and G. E. Uhlenbeck [*Rev. Mod. Phys.* **17**, 323 (1945)] in the Wax volume are especially recommended.

[4] N. Bloembergen, E. M. Purcell, and R. V. Pound, *Phys. Rev.* **73**, 679 (1948).

[5] A. Sommerfeld, *Mechanics of Deformable Bodies*, Academic, New York, 1950, p. 251.

[6] P. W. Anderson and P. R. Weiss, *Rev. Mod. Phys.* **25**, 269 (1953).

[7] See, for example, the Chandrasekhar paper of reference 3.

[8] See, for example, Chapter 7 of the earlier version of this volume.

[9] G. E. Pake, J. Townsend, and S. I. Weissman, *Phys. Rev.* **85**, 682 (1952).

[10] S. I. Weissman and D. Banfill, *J. Am. Chem. Soc.* **75**, 2534 (1953).

[11] J. S. Hyde and H. W. Brown, *J. Chem. Phys.* **37**, 368 (1962).

[12] H. M. McConnell, *J. Chem. Phys.* **25**, 709 (1956).

[13] R. N. Rogers and G. E. Pake, *J. Chem. Phys.* **33**, 1107 (1960).

[14] D. Kivelson, *J. Chem. Phys.* **27**, 1087 (1957); **33**, 1094 (1960).

[15] A. Carrington and A. D. McLachlan, *Introduction to Magnetic Resonance*, Harper and Row, New York, 1967.

CHAPTER 10

Examples of Electron Paramagnetic Resonance Spectra

The experimentalist studying the electron paramagnetic resonance of some sample ordinarily obtains his information in the form of spectra. From these he attempts to determine the nature of the paramagnetic entity or entities producing the spectra. In this chapter (and, in fact, in most of the book) we employ the reverse of this "natural" order. We start from a knowledge of the system under study and deduce the spectra, because in this way it is relatively simple and easy to compress a large amount of information into a small space. The "natural" order is much more complicated, and its implementation varies among individual investigators. It is safe to say, however, that part of the process consists of comparing the observed spectra with the investigator's catalog of information (mental and otherwise). For this reason we will give some examples of paramagnetic entities and their EPR spectra. The examples are intended to be sufficiently varied so as to indicate some of the scope of the subject. It is hoped that some useful new ideas will also be presented.

10–1 Atomic Hydrogen

To anyone who has studied the physics or chemistry of atoms it is obvious how much physical insight comes from understanding atomic hydrogen. In order to start with a subject which may provide a somewhat similar basis for electron paramagnetic resonance, we will discuss atomic hydrogen as our first example [1].

Free atomic hydrogen, essentially unperturbed, has been observed in gaseous discharges and in atomic beams. In addition atomic hydrogen is a stable paramagnetic species in a wide variety of substances if the temperature is sufficiently low. Under these conditions the paramagnetism is very similar to that of the free atom.

Atomic hydrogen has a single $1s$ electron, the simplest possible paramagnet. The paramagnetism of hydrogen is complicated somewhat by the fact that the three isotopes of this element all have nonzero nuclear spins, together with rather sizable hyperfine couplings with the $1s$ electron. This coupling arises from the Fermi contact interaction discussed in Section 4–4 [see Eq. (4-47)]. Table 10-1 gives various pertinent parameters for the three isotopes of hydrogen.

Table 10-1
Hyperfine Parameters for the Isotopes of Hydrogen

Isotope	Nuclear Spin	Nuclear Magnetic Dipole Moment in Units of Nuclear Magnetons [2]	Nuclear Electric Quadrupole Moment in Units of $e \times 10^{-24}$ cm^2 [2]	A, Free-Atom Hyperfine Constant
Hydrogen, ^{1}H	$\frac{1}{2}$	2.79268	...	1420.40573(5) MHz [3], 506.83 G
Deuterium, ^{2}H	1	0.857386	2.77×10^{-3}	218.25620(2) MHz [3], 77.880 G
Tritium, ^{3}H	$\frac{1}{2}$	2.9788	...	1516.70(1) MHz [4], 541.19 G

The Hamiltonian describing the lowest four states of free hydrogen in a magnetic field is

$$\mathcal{K} = g\beta\mathbf{H}\cdot\mathbf{S} + A\mathbf{S}\cdot\mathbf{I} - g_n\beta_n\mathbf{H}\cdot\mathbf{I}, \tag{10-1}$$

the same form as the spin Hamiltonian of Eq. (5-93). Atomic hydrogen which is not free may be described by the Hamiltonian of Eq. (10-1) also, but now this is a spin Hamiltonian and therefore the quantities g and A are parameters that differ from the free-hydrogen values (in principle g_n could differ as well). The solution of the eigenvalue equation resulting from Eq. (10-1) for $S = \frac{1}{2}$ is carried out in Section 5–3 immediately after Eq. (5-93). The solutions, referred to as Breit-Rabi levels, are exact for free atoms or atoms in cubic hosts (the spin Hamiltonian may be somewhat different in lower symmetry). For hydrogen with $A = 1.42$ GHz it is not necessary to use the exact form if the measuring frequency is about 8 GHz or above, the frequency range in which almost all experimental data are obtained. A power series expansion in $A/g\beta H$ and $g_n\beta_n/g\beta$ is then useful [see Eqs. (5-97) and (5-98)]. In the limit of very high field we find that the separation in field of the two allowed $\Delta M_S = \pm 1$ lines in $A/g\beta = 506.83$ G for the free ion. All known cases of atomic hydrogen paramagnetism, no matter what the host, result in lines split by roughly 500 G (variations of A from the free-atom value of as much as 5% have been reported).

Hydrogen is not usually atomic in nature. Most hydrogen is bonded in molecules, or, when present as an impurity in a crystal, it is an ion. Atomic hydrogen is formed in one of two ways. The hydrogen-ion impurities present in some crystals become atoms under the influence of ionizing radiation. Another mechanism is the creation of atomic hydrogen by dissociation of a molecule or a molecular impurity by radiation.

In the first category are hydrogen impurities in single crystals of the following:

1. Alkali halides.
2. Alkaline-earth fluorides.
3. Quartz.

The various kinds of hydrogen-containing imperfections in alkali halides are termed U centers and constitute an important class of color centers. The category containing the hydrogen produced by dissociation includes the following:

1. OH⁻ decomposition in alkali halides (again forming U centers).
2. Condensation of hydrogen discharge products in an amorphous Van der Waals solid.
3. Decomposition of condensed molecules (by light or other radiation).
4. Amorphous solids of bulk H_2O, H_2O-acid solutions, and adsorbed H_2O.
5. Water of hydration in crystals.
6. Organic substances.

Atomic hydrogen which is not free will have its wave function modified somewhat from the atomic $1s$ wave function by the crystalline field, that is, by its environment. These changes may include admixture of other free-hydrogen wave functions, of ligand or nearest-neighbor wave functions, and of polyelectronic configurations. These changes may result in a departure from the simple spin-only behavior of free hydrogen. Yet we continue to describe the ground state by a spin of $\frac{1}{2}$. We must now use an effective Hamiltonian, the spin Hamiltonian. For cubic symmetry the spin Hamiltonian is identical with Eq. (10-1) except that frequently additional terms representing hyperfine structure from host crystal nuclei are included to explain more fully all of the observed details.

In Table 10-2 we list spin Hamiltonian parameters for atomic hydrogen in several solid-state environments. All data except those for crystalline quartz [5] are analyzed using Eq. (10-1), even though in many cases the symmetry is unlikely to be cubic. However, the anisotropy is small, and the orientation of the local symmetry axes and the magnitude of the anisotropy are both distributed. Thus only an isotropic average value is observed. It is readily seen from Table 10-2 that there is only a small varia-

Table 10-2

Spin Hamiltonian Parameters for Atomic Hydrogen in Solids

Species	Host	Temperature (°K)	g	A (MHz)	$\frac{A - A_{free}}{A_{free}}$ (%)	Reference
H	Free			1420.40573(5)		3
D	Free			218.25620(2)		"
T	Free			1516.70(1)		4
H	CaF$_2$ (subst.)	77	2.00235(6)	1439.4(3)	1.34	6
D	"	77	2.0825(1)	221.4(2)	1.4	"
H	CaF$_2$ (inter.)	77	2.0029(1)	1465.0(1)	3.14	7
D	"	300	2.0025(1)	224.9(3)	3.0	8
H	SrF$_2$ (subst.)	77	2.003(1)	1437.8(5)	1.22	6
D	"	77	2.0028(1)	221.3(2)	1.4	"
H	SrF$_2$ (inter.)	77	2.0029(1)	1444.2(2)	1.68	9
D	"	300	2.002(2)	221.5(5)	1.5	7
H	BaF$_2$ (inter.)	77	2.0023(1)	1426.1(1)	0.40	9
D	"	300	2.002(2)	219.0(5)	0.3	9
H	NaCl (subst.)	66	2.0032(3)	1398.2(2)	−1.57	10
H	NaCl (inter.)	20	2.002(2)	1362(2)	−4.1	11
H	KCl (subst.)	20	2.0024(1)	1408.53(8)	−0.835	10
H	KCl (inter.)	20	2.002(1)	1387(2)	−2.3	11
H	KBr (inter.)	20	2.008(2)	1347(3)	−5.1	"
H	RbCl (inter.)	20		1389(3)	−2.2	12
H	SiO$_2$ (cryst.)	77	2.0021(5)	1453.1(1)	2.30	5
H	SiO$_2$ (fused)	77	2.003(1)	1409.1(2)	−0.80	"
H	Beryl	77	2.00265(5)	1408.0(3)	−0.87	13

Table 10-2 (cont'd.)

Species	Host	Temperature (°K)	g	A (MHz)	$\dfrac{A - A_{free}}{A_{free}}$ (%)	Reference
H	Pyrex glass	77	2.002	1411(15)		14
H	Sodium tetraborate glass	77	2.002	1400(15)		"
H	Solid Ne	4.2	2.00207(8)	1426.6(2)	0.44	15
H	Solid Ar	4.2	2.00220(8)	1413.8(4)	−0.47	"
H	"	4.2	2.0022(1)	1416.3(8)	−0.29	"
H	"	4.2	2.00161(8)	1436.2(4)	1.11	"
H	Solid Kr	4.2	2.00179(8)	1411.8(3)	−0.61	"
H	"	4.2	1.9997(3)	1427(3)	0.5	"
H	Solid Xe	4.2	2.00178(8)	1405.0(3)	−1.09	"
H	"	4.2	2.000578(8)	1405.6(3)	−1.04	"
H	Solid H$_2$	4.2	2.00230(8)	1417.1(2)	−0.23	16
H	Solid D$_2$	4.2	2.0021(2)	1418.6(4)	−0.13	17
D	"	4.2	2.0019(2)	218.1(2)	−0.1	"
D	"	4.2	2.0022(2)	218.9(2)	0.3	"
T	Solid T$_2$	4.2	2.0019(2)	1515.3(4)	−0.09	"
T	"	4.2	2.002(2)	1515(2)	−0.1	18
H	Frozen H$_2$SO$_4$-H$_2$O sol'n	77	2.00217(2)	1415.16(3)	−0.370	19
D	"	77	2.00219(2)	217.37(3)	−0.41	"
H	Frozen H$_3$PO$_4$-H$_2$O sol'n	77	2.00213(3)	1411.74(5)	−0.611	"
D	"	77	2.00215(3)	216.80(3)	−0.67	"
H	Frozen HClO$_4$-H$_2$O sol'n	77	2.00210(2)	1406.98(6)	−0.947	"
D	"	77	2.00208(2)	216.30(3)	−0.90	"

tion of the parameters from the free-atom values. This small variation suggests a very small departure in the wave function from the free-atom 1s orbital, thereby implying a tightly bound electron confined largely to the immediate vicinity of the proton. Such an electron would have only a small hyperfine interaction with the nearer neighbors in the solid. This behavior can be seen very clearly by examining the data obtained for hydrogen in single crystals and discussed below.

The two most extensively studied crystalline hosts for hydrogen are the alkali halides (NaCl, KCl, etc.) and the alkaline-earth fluorides (CaF_2, SrF_2, etc.). In both types of crystal the hydrogen has been observed to occupy an interstitial site (a site "in between" normal lattice sites) and a site in which it is substitutional for the halogen (see Fig. 10-1). The superhyperfine interaction with the nearer neighbors is summarized in Table 10-3. The data were obtained by a technique called ENDOR, described in Section 5–4 and discussed more fully in Section 11–4. All we need to know now is that it allows one to observe transitions with $\Delta M_S = 0$, $\Delta M_I = \pm 1$. In this way hyperfine interactions can be measured directly with great precision. The data of Table 10-3 show clearly the rapid decrease in the superhyperfine interaction as the nuclei get farther from the hydrogen. In fact, beyond about the next-nearest neighbors the hyperfine interaction is almost entirely the value expected for the dipole-dipole interaction [see Eq. (4-45)] of point dipoles separated by a distance equal to the corresponding perfect crystal distances. The variation of the nearest-neighbor hyperfine interaction is roughly consistent with the proportionality of $a = \frac{1}{3}A + \frac{2}{3}B$ to g_n and $|\psi(0)|^2$ and similarly the proportionality of $b = \frac{1}{3}(A - B)$ to g_n and $\langle r^{-3} \rangle$. These arise from Eq. (4-48).

The superhyperfine structure resolved in the EPR spectra gives a clear picture of the surroundings of the hydrogen. It was this information which allowed the sites to be identified as either substitutional or interstitial. In CaF_2 the largest superhyperfine interaction had a $\langle 100 \rangle$ axis of symmetry for the substitutional site and a $\langle 111 \rangle$ axis of symmetry for the interstitial site, as expected from the location of the nearest neighbors shown in Fig. 10-1. In the alkali halides the interstitial site had a $\langle 111 \rangle$ axis of symmetry for the largest superhyperfine interaction, and no resolved superhyperfine structure was observed for the substitutional site. The lack of structure in the latter case occurred because the hydrogen was much farther from the halogen ions than in any of the other three sites.

Some of the hosts for atomic hydrogen listed in Table 10-2 contain large amounts of hydrogen in other forms (bonded in molecules). In some of these cases the hydrogen EPR lines are flanked by satellites spaced from the main line by an amount $\Delta H = (g_n \beta_n / g\beta)H$. This occurs because a small anisotropic (probably dipolar) hyperfine interaction with these distant protons causes the nuclear spin selection rules for the distant protons to break down [22] [see Eq. (5-78) and the following discussion]. The spin

Hamiltonian for atomic hydrogen interacting with one distant proton can be written as

$$\mathcal{H} = g\beta\mathbf{H}\cdot\mathbf{S} + A\mathbf{S}\cdot\mathbf{I} - g_n\beta_n\mathbf{H}\cdot\mathbf{I} - g_n'\beta_n\mathbf{H}\cdot\mathbf{I}', \qquad (10\text{-}2)$$

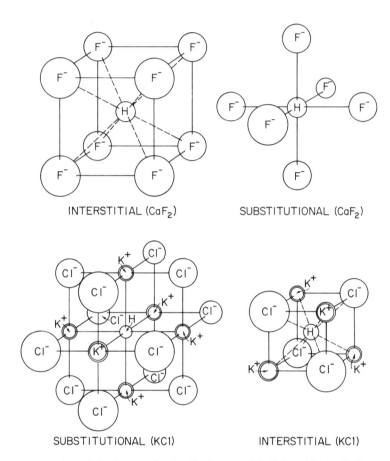

INTERSTITIAL (CaF$_2$)   SUBSTITUTIONAL (CaF$_2$)

SUBSTITUTIONAL (KCl)   INTERSTITIAL (KCl)

FIG. 10-1 Atomic hydrogen sites in alkaline-earth halides with the CaF$_2$ crystal structure and in alkali halides with the KCl crystal structure. In CaF$_2$ the F$^-$ ions form a simple cubic lattice. The Ca^{2+} ions occupy every other body center. Interstitial hydrogen occupies one of the empty body centers and has eight F$^-$ ions as nearest neighbors. Substitutional atomic hydrogen occupies a F$^-$ site and has four nearest-neighbor Ca^{2+} ions and six next-nearest-neighbor F$^-$ ions, which are almost as close and are shown in the figure. Hydrogen, which substitutes for Cl$^-$ in KCl, has six K$^+$ nearest neighbors and twelve Cl$^-$ ions as next-nearest neighbors. Interstitial atomic hydrogen in KCl is surrounded by four Cl$^-$ ions and four K$^+$ ions. Displacements from the perfect crystal sites determines which of these groups of ions is nearest the hydrogen. These displacements must maintain the cubic symmetry, but they can be different for the K$^+$ and Cl$^-$.

Table 10-3

Superhyperfine Parameters for Atomic Hydrogen in Selected Host Crystals

Host Crystal	Site	Temperature (°K)	Nucleus	Shell	Orientation	a (MHz)	b (MHz)	b' (MHz)	Reference
CaF_2	Subst.	77	^{19}F	1	$\langle 100 \rangle$	91.2(3)	38.4(3)	—	20
				2	$\langle 110 \rangle$	−0.02(1)	1.22(2)	—	
				3	$\langle 111 \rangle$	1.37(1)	1.34(1)	—	
				4	$\langle 100 \rangle$	0.81(2)	0.82(2)	—	
CaF_2	Inter.	77	^{19}F	1	$\langle 111 \rangle$	104.0(2)	34.9(2)	—	8
				2	$\sim\langle 311 \rangle$	0.42(2)	0.87(2)	—	
				3	$\sim\langle 331 \rangle$	0.02(2)	0.36(2)	—	
KCl	Inter.	77	^{35}Cl	1	$\langle 111 \rangle$	23.74	6.71	—	21
			^{39}K	1	$\langle 111 \rangle$	0.983	0.457	—	
			^{35}Cl	2	$\sim\langle 311 \rangle$	$\sim$0.01	$\sim$0.05	—	
			^{39}K	2	$\sim\langle 311 \rangle$	0.123(2)	0.032(2)	0.010(1)	
			^{35}Cl	3	$\sim\langle 331 \rangle$	0.00(1)	0.06(1)	—	
RbCl	Inter.	20	^{35}Cl	1	$\langle 111 \rangle$	17.34	5.47	—	12
			^{87}Rb	1	$\langle 111 \rangle$	18.25	6.76	—	
			^{35}Cl	2	$\sim\langle 311 \rangle$	<0.07	$\sim$0.05	—	
			^{87}Rb	2	$\sim\langle 311 \rangle$	1.428(3)	0.271(6)	0.088(3)	
			^{35}Cl	3	$\sim\langle 331 \rangle$	<0.06	$\sim$0.02	—	
			^{87}Rb	3	$\sim\langle 331 \rangle$	<0.17	$\sim$0.1	—	

where g'_n and $\mathbf{I}'$ refer to the distant proton, and the hyperfine interaction with this distant proton is neglected as making an unobservably small contribution to the energy. Thus the equation for the energy in lowest order,

$$E = g\beta H M_S + A M_S M_I - g_n \beta_n H M_I - g'_n \beta_n H M'_I, \qquad (10\text{-}3)$$

shows that $\Delta M_S = \pm 1$, $\Delta M_I = 0$, $\Delta M'_I = 0$, ± 1 transitions occur at

$$h\nu = \Delta E = \begin{cases} g\beta H + A M_I \\ g\beta H + A M_I \pm g'_n \beta_n H \end{cases} \qquad (10\text{-}4)$$

or

$$H = \begin{cases} \dfrac{h\nu}{g\beta} - \dfrac{A}{g\beta} M_I \\[2ex] \dfrac{h\nu}{g\beta} - \dfrac{A}{g\beta} M_I \mp \dfrac{g'_n \beta_n H}{g\beta}, \end{cases} \qquad (10\text{-}5)$$

and

$$\Delta H = \frac{g'_n \beta_n H}{g\beta}, \qquad (10\text{-}6)$$

the observed splitting.

Because of the inherent simplicity of atomic hydrogen, many types of experiments have been performed on these paramagnetic centers. Relaxation times have been measured [23], nuclear polarization resulting from saturating EPR lines has been observed [9, 24], and the effects of pressure have been studied [25].

10-2 Other $^2S_{1/2}$-State Atoms and Ions

Atomic hydrogen is only one of many atoms and ions whose paramagnetism arises from a single s electron. Many of these have been observed by electron paramagnetic resonance, including the alkali- and noble-metal atoms and the monopositive alkaline-earth ions. Like hydrogen, they are described by the spin Hamiltonian of Eq. (10-1) or a generalization for lower symmetry.

In Table 10-4 we give some of the observed data for $^2S_{1/2}$-state atoms and ions. In addition to reinforcing some of the characteristics observed for hydrogen, new features appear. By combining the observations of Table 10-4 with those for hydrogen (neither are exhaustive lists) we see that $^2S_{1/2}$-state paramagnetism is relatively common.

Table 10-4

Spin Hamiltonian Parameters for $^2S_{1/2}$-State Atoms or Ions

Species	Host	g	A (MHz)	Reference
^{7}Li	Free	2.00231	401.77	26
^{7}Li	Solid Ar	1.9992	264	27
^{23}Na	Free	2.00231	885.88	26
^{23}Na	Solid Ar	2.0000	928	27
^{23}Na	"	2.0005	892	"
^{23}Na	"	2.0013	878	"
^{23}Na	"	1.9992	735	"
^{23}Na	"	1.9997	696	"
^{23}Na	Solid C_6H_6	2.0029(6)	719(3)	28
^{23}Na	"	2.0036(6)	808(3)	"
^{39}K	Free	2.00231	230.88	26
^{39}K	Solid Ar	1.9993	252	27
^{39}K	"	1.9998	244	"
^{39}K	"	1.9998	241	"
^{39}K	"	1.9984	199	"
^{39}K	"	1.9977	154	"
^{39}K	Solid Kr	1.9870	272(15)	"
^{39}K	"	1.9920	201(51)	"
^{39}K	Solid Xe	1.980	225(15)	"
^{39}K	Solid C_6H_6	2.0024(8)	181.7(5)	28
^{85}Rb	Free	2.00241	1,011.90	26
^{85}Rb	Solid Ar	1.9981	1,087	27
^{85}Rb	"	1.9990	1,072	"
^{85}Rb	"	1.9974	916	"
^{85}Rb	Solid C_6H_6	2.0046(12)	816(4)	28
^{133}Cs	Free	2.00258	2,297.8	26
^{63}Cu	"	2.002	5,866.915(5)	
^{63}Cu	LiCl	1.998(2)	5,876(5)	29
^{63}Cu	NaCl	1.997(2)	5,561(5)	"
^{63}Cu	KCl	2.000(2)	4,844(4)	"
^{63}Cu	Solid H_2O	2.018(4)	3,043(9)	30
^{63}Cu	Solid C_2H_5OH	2.018(4)	3,752(8)	"
^{63}Cu	Solid C_6H_6	2.0050(5)	4,158(4)	"
^{63}Cu	"	2.004	4,346	"
^{109}Ag	Free	2.00224	1,976.94(4)	
^{109}Ag	LiCl	2.001(3)	1,927(7)	31
^{909}Ag	NaCl	1.999(3)	1,870(7)	"
^{109}Ag	KCl	2.000(3)	1,890(7)	32
^{109}Ag	RbCl	2.001(3)	1,878(12)	31
^{109}Ag	Solid H_2O	1.999(2)	1,512(17)	33
^{109}Ag	"	1.999(1)	1,655(9)	"
^{109}Ag	"	2.0020(6)	2,005(3)	34
^{109}Ag	Solid C_2H_5OH	2.0004(9)	1,733(2)	"
^{109}Ag	Solid C_6H_6	2.001(2)	1,827(5)	35
^{109}Ag	"	2.000(2)	1,772(5)	"
^{109}Ag	Pyrex glass	1.999(5)	1,925(15)	14

Table 10-4 (cont'd.)

Species	Host	g	A (MHz)	Reference
^{109}Au	Pyrex glass	2.003(5)	2,000(15)	14
^{109}Ag	Tetraborate glass	2.006(5)	1,582(15)	"
^{109}Ag	"	2.003(5)	1,635(15)	"
^{197}Au	Free	2.00412	3,053.6(5)	
^{197}Au	Solid C_6H_6	2.000(2)	2,692(5)	35
^{197}Au	Solid H_2O	2.0031(15)	3,053(2)	36
^{197}Au	Solid C_2H_5OH	2.0715(10)	2,073(7)	"
$^{113}Cd^+$	Solid Ar	2.0006(2)	15,048	37
$^{27}Al^{2+}$	Si (inter.)	2.0019	1,320(2)	38
$^{27}Al^{2+}$	Si (inter. assoc. with subs. Al^-)	2.0006($\parallel$), 2.0009($\perp$)	1,187(2) ($\parallel$), 1,178(2) ($\perp$)	"
$^{27}Al^{2+}$	"	2.0014($\parallel$), 2.0025($\perp$)	1,168(2) ($\parallel$), 1,159(2) ($\perp$)	"
$^{71}Ga^{2+}$	ZnS (cubic)	1.9974(5)	7,716(3)	39, 40
$^{71}Ga^{2+}$	ZnS (hexagonal)		7,870 (avg.)	39
$^{71}Ga^{2+}$	Si (inter. assoc. with subs. Ga^-)	2.0014($\parallel$), 1.9973($\perp$)	4,181(3) ($\parallel$), 4,131(3) ($\perp$)	38
$^{115}In^{2+}$	ZnS (cubic)	1.9930(5)	9,362(5)	39
$^{115}In^{2+}$	ZnS (hexagonal)		9,720 (avg.)	"
$^{205}Tl^{2+}$	KCl	2.010(2)	105,400(100)	41
$^{205}Tl^{2+}$	ZnS (cubic)	2.0095(5)	71,530	39
$^{205}Tl^{2+}$	ZnS (hexagonal)	2.0093(5) ($\parallel$), 2.0103(5) ($\perp$)	71,980(30) $B-A = 16(2)$	"
$^{29}Si^{3+}$	ZnS (cubic)	2.0047(3)	1,961	42
Si^{3+}	ZnS (hexagonal)	2.0045(5) ($\parallel$), 2.0062(2) ($\perp$)		"
$^{73}Ge^{3+}$	CdS	2.0021(5) ($\parallel$), 2.0059(5) ($\perp$)	~990	43
$^{73}Ge^{3+}$	ZnS (cubic)	2.0086(3)	914	42
Ge^{3+}	ZnS (hexagonal)	2.0087(3) ($\parallel$), 2.0096(3) ($\perp$)		"
$^{73}Ge^{3+}$	ZnSe	2.403(5)	782(2)	40
$^{73}Ge^{3+}$	ZnTe	2.1375	657	44
$^{73}Ge^{3+}$	SiO_2	1.9941, 2.0012, 2.0023	776 (avg.)	45
$^{73}Ge^{3+}$	"	1.9936, 2.0010, 2.0015	782 (avg.)	"
$^{73}Ge^{3+}$	"	1.9907, 2.003, 2.0019	785 (avg.)	"
$^{73}Ge^{3+}$	"	1.9918, 2.0002, 2.0015	758 (avg.)	"

Table 10-4 (cont'd.)

Species	Host	g	A (MHz)	Reference
$^{73}Ge^{3+}$	SiO_2	1.9947, 1.9983, 2.0014	887, 806, 818	45
$^{117}Sn^{3+}$	CdS	2.0024(5) ($\parallel$), 2.0031(5) ($\perp$)	15,125(15) ($\parallel$), 14,540(15) ($\perp$)	43
$^{117}Sn^{3+}$	CdSe	2.0059(5) ($\parallel$), 2.0160(5) ($\perp$)	13,059(15) ($\parallel$), 13,008(15) ($\perp$)	"
$^{117}Sn^{3+}$	ZnS	2.0075(5)	15,610(15)	46
$^{117}Sn^{3+}$	ZnSe	2.0251(4)	13,659(15)	40
Sn^{3+}	ZnTe	2.094		44
Pb^{3+}	CdS	2.0020(5) ($\parallel$), 2.0049(5) ($\perp$)		43
$^{207}Pb^{3+}$	ThO_2	1.967	36,810	47
$^{207}Pb^{3+}$	"	1.9703(3) ($\parallel$), 1.9637(3) ($\perp$)	35,645 ($\parallel$), 35,424($\perp$)	"
$^{207}Pb^{3+}$	ZnSe	2.0729(5)	18,734(15)	40
$^{207}Pb^{3+}$	ZnTe	2.167(1)	15,680(30)	48

Another point which is quickly obvious on inspection of Table 10-4 is that in many cases the hyperfine parameter is much larger than for hydrogen. This is particularly true for Tl^{2+}. In addition, the isotopes of Pb^{3+}, Sn^{3+}, and Cd^{+} with nonzero nuclear spin have hyperfine constants greater than the frequency of about 10 GHz commonly employed in electron paramagnetic resonance. In such cases use of the Breit-Rabi formula [see Eq. (5-96)] is required to explain the spectra. In Fig. 10-2 we reproduce the Breit-Rabi energy levels for $I = \frac{1}{2}$, shown originally in Fig. 5-17. For any value of the frequency exactly two lines will always be observable. The three possible cases are presented in Fig. 10-2. In Fig. 10-3 we show the field at which these lines would occur as a function of the the frequency. We note that the dotted line signifying $H = h\nu/g\beta$ is the location of the resonance for any $I = 0$ isotopes of the same paramagnetic species (normally $g = 2$, giving about 3300 G for 9.3 GHz). Only in the limit of large $h\nu/A$ do we have a doublet almost equally spaced about the $I = 0$ line position. For small values of $h\nu/A$ lines at field values higher than those for $g = 2$ (assuming that the g values are close to 2) would be anticipated. If they were to be assigned a g value as if they arose from an $I = 0$ Kramers doublet (after all, they are isotropic and would be easily confused with the spectrum for a Kramers doublet), one g value would lie between 1 and 2 and the other could take on any value.

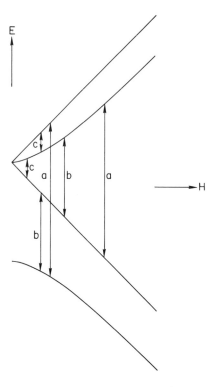

FIG. 10-2   The energy of a paramagnet with $S = \frac{1}{2}$ and $I = \frac{1}{2}$ as a function of the magnetic field. This diagram is equivalent to the one on the left of Fig. 5-17. It assumes an isotropic electronic Zeeman and hyperfine interaction and neglects the nuclear Zeeman interaction. If the frequency is fixed and the magnetic field is varied to obtain magnetic resonance, two lines will be observed. For different values of the frequency these lines can correspond to different transitions. The three possibilities are shown. The transitions labeled a occur for $h\nu > A$, those labeled b occur for $A > h\nu > \frac{1}{2}A$, and those labeled c occur for $\frac{1}{2}A > h\nu$. The position in the field of these lines is plotted in Fig. 10-3.

There is only a very small anisotropy in g and A for spectra in noncubic sites, even such noncubic sites as those with a neighbor having an extra positive charge, as for $Ge^{3+}-Li^+$ associates in SiO_2 [45]. The anisotropy in A is usually less than 1% (although it is easily measured because of the fact that A and $h\nu$ are comparable). Not only are the spectra for Ge^{3+} in SiO_2 anisotropic but also there is considerable variation (A varies by about 10% for ^{73}Ge) for different types of sites (different charge-compensating alkali ions) [45]. A similar variation occurs for interstitial Al^{2+} in silicon [38].

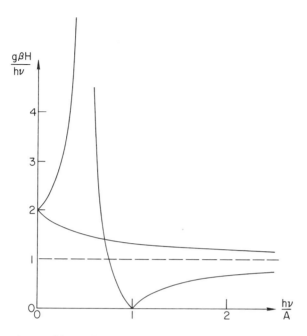

FIG. 10-3 The position of the fixed-frequency EPR lines for an isotropic paramagnet with $S = I = \frac{1}{2}$. The energy levels for this system are shown in Fig. 10-2. The dotted line locates the transition expected if I were zero.

In Fig. 10-4 we show the spectrum for Cd^+ in an argon matrix at $4°K$ (the strong lines at the left go off scale) [37]. The identification of the spectrum (ignoring the part due to H) is unambiguous. Cadmium consists of several isotopes, two of which (^{111}Cd and ^{113}Cd) have $I = \frac{1}{2}$ with approximately $12\frac{1}{2}\%$ abundance each. The remaining isotopes ($\sim 75\%$) have $I = 0$. The magnetic moments of the two $I = \frac{1}{2}$ isotopes differ by about 4%; hence presumably so would the A values. The three lines attributed to Cd^+ in Fig. 10-4 arise from the three types of isotopes and agree in both position and intensity if $h\nu/A \simeq 0.65$. By consulting Fig. 10-3 we see that the other two hyperfine lines would be near 8000 G and were not observed [37].

Not all cases are as unambiguous as Cd^+. Occasionally indirect information is required to make an identification, such as the similarity of the observed values of A and I to known atomic or ionic values. In the majority of cases studied, A differs by only a few per cent from the corresponding atomic values (recall the corresponding characteristic for atomic hydrogen). This is so because s orbitals are relatively unaffected in

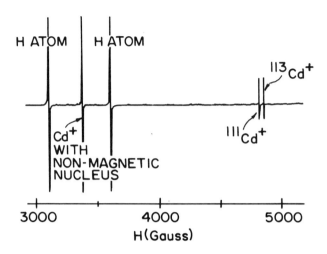

FIG. 10-4   The EPR spectrum of Cd^+ ions in an argon matrix at about 4°K [37]. In addition to the three lines arising from ^{111}Cd, ^{113}Cd, and the Cd isotopes with $I = 0$, a doublet arising from atomic hydrogen is seen. The hydrogen was present to trap the electrons photoexcited from the Cd atoms.

the environments in which they are seen and identified. Although most cases lie somewhere between a few per cent above to 30% below the free-ion value, very large reductions occur for Pb^{3+} in ZnSe and ZnTe: roughly one fifth of the free-ion value and one half of the value observed for Pb^{3+} in ThO_2. Accompanying this large reduction in A for ^{207}Pb is a fairly large superhyperfine interaction observed with the four nearest tellurium nuclei in ZnTe. Iida and Watanabe [49] have attributed this to a large admixture of a state in which a hole is shared by the four closest Te neighbors.

In addition to the many paramagnets similar to atomic hydrogen, cases have been observed which are analogous to molecular hydrogen. For neutral silver in glasses [50] and frozen solutions [51] spectra have been observed consisting of three lines (or groups of lines) with a splitting about one half of the atomic Ag hyperfine splitting (^{107}Ag and ^{109}Ag both have $I = \frac{1}{2}$ and magnetic moments which differ by about 15%). Two explanations are possible, Ag_2 and Ag_2^+. The latter, by analogy with H_2^+, would be an $S = \frac{1}{2}$ species and would probably have about one half the hyperfine interaction of Ag. The Ag_2 would be an analog of H_2 (although the Ag–Ag interaction would be weak) and could possibly be described as in Eqs. (6-13) to (6-15). The triplet state would give the observed spectrum. Further study would be necessary to distinguish the two.

Other types of paramagnetic species are related to $^2S_{1/2}$-state atoms and ions. For example, hydrogen, gallium, and indium, which can be localized $^2S_{1/2}$-state species in some crystals, can occur as shallow donors in others. In the latter case their wave functions, although s-like, are highly delocalized. For example, Ga and In in ZnS are localized $^2S_{1/2}$-state ions, but Ga in CdS and In in ZnO are shallow donors. Another variation occurs for boron in BeO [52]. Instead of B^{2+} the electron occurs in an antibonding orbital shared between the boron and one of three equivalent nearest-neighbor oxygens. A more extreme case of this variation occurs for nitrogen in diamond [53].

10–3 **Associates**

The simplicity of the paramagnets discussed in Sections 10–1 and 10–2 cannot be generalized to most paramagnetic species. To illustrate one way in which more complicated paramagnets and hence spectra can arise we consider ZnS crystals in which Ga^{2+} has been observed [39, 40]. The Ga^{3+} ion consists of closed electron shells, but it has one more positive charge than the Zn^{2+} ion for which it substitutes. This charge excess may be uncompensated locally (although of course the crystal as a whole must be nearly electrically neutral), or an electron may be attracted and the Ga^{2+} ion discussed in Section 10–2 is formed. Another possibility is that some other negatively charged entity may be attracted. A zinc vacancy (a missing Zn^{2+} ion) has a double negative charge, as can be seen from the fact that, if the Zn^{2+} were returned, the region of the crystal near the former vacancy would be neutral. If the Ga^{3+} ion attracts the zinc vacancy, the associate then has one unit of negative charge. Again this may go uncompensated locally, or it may attract a hole (that is, lose an electron). If it attracts a hole, it will be neutral and also paramagnetic. This associate is one of a class of defects in II-VI semiconducting compounds which produces a luminescence commonly called "self-activated" luminescence [54].

These associated centers have been seen in crystals of two different structures. Both have tetrahedral coordination about any site, the cubic zinc blende structure being the simpler and hence the one that we will describe. (The wurtzite structure results in a distortion of the tetrahedron along with more significant differences in the arrangement of neighbors farther than the nearest ones.) The two associating defects, the impurity and the vacancy, are observed to occupy the closest possible sites to each other (this seemingly reasonable behavior is not always found for defects attracted by their opposite net charges). We illustrate this in Fig. 10-5(a) (for the case of cubic ZnS).

The hole is attracted by the negative charge arising from the vacancy. It resides where the electrons are most loosely bound, that is, on the sulfurs. In this way it occurs on the sulfur nearest the vacancy but farthest from the positively charged aluminum, as shown in Fig. 10-5(a). An analogous center can occur if the positive charge attracting the vacancy arises from a halogen impurity substituting for sulfur [see Fig. 10-5(b)]. In this case the other three sulfur sites are all equivalent, so that the hole can occupy any of the three or all of them.

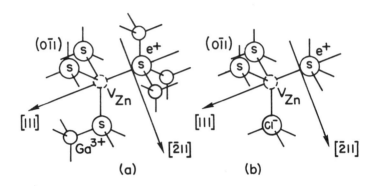

FIG. 10-5 Associated centers in cubic zinc sulfide [57]. In (a) the association occurs between a Ga^{3+} ion substituting for Zn^{2+} and a Zn vacancy. This negatively charged associate can bind a hole, which is located on the S^{2-} ion closest to the vacancy but farthest from the Ga^{3+}. This sulfur site is the one which minimizes the electrostatic energy of the positively charged hole interacting with the doubly negatively charged Zn vacancy and the positively charged Ga^{3+} ion. In (b) is shown an analogous center which results from the association of a Zn vacancy and a halogen ion substituting for a sulfur. Any of the three sulfurs adjacent to the Zn vacancy could be occupied by the hole. At low temperatures the hole will be on one of the three, the choices being random throughout the crystal.

At temperatures low enough to minimize the effects of any thermal processes involving activation energies, the two types of paramagnetic centers are very similar [55]. For the halogen centers the hole is on only one sulfur. The vacancy which is close and has a large net charge produces a nearly axial environment for the hole. The actual symmetry is rather low, C_s, and small features of the spectra reflect this deviation from the approximate axial symmetry. A small hyperfine interaction has been observed with the group III or VII impurity establishing its presence [56]. Also the hyperfine interaction with the nucleus of the atom containing the hole is occasionally observed, giving further confirmation to the structure [57]. The spin Hamiltonian describing such a system (neglecting hyperfine structure) is

$$\mathcal{H} = \beta \mathbf{H} \cdot \mathbf{g} \cdot \mathbf{S}, \qquad (10\text{-}7)$$

where the x principal axis of **g** is very close to the axis from the vacancy to the hole, except in the two selenium centers in alloys of ZnS and ZnSe, and the y axis is perpendicular to the {110} plane of reflection symmetry. The principal values of **g** are listed in Table 10-5.

Table 10-5

Principal Values of **g** for Associates of Group III or VII Impurities and Zinc Vacancies

Species	Host	g_x	g_y	g_z	Reference
VS_3Cl	ZnS	2.0027	2.0502	2.0565	56
VS_3Br	"	2.0029	2.0537	2.0569	"
$VS_4Zn_{11}Al$	"	2.0030	2.0513	2.0560	"
$VS_4Zn_{11}Ga$	"	2.0025	2.0509	2.0557	"
VS_2SeCl	$ZnS_{1-x}Se_x$	1.9708	2.1742	2.1941	58
VS_2SeBr	"	1.9708	2.1825	2.1922	"
$VS\,Se_2Cl$	"	2.1786	2.0125	2.0976	"
$VS\,Se_2Br$	"	2.1840	2.0060	2.1039	"
VSe_3Cl	ZnSe	1.9597	2.1612	2.2449	57
$VTe_4Zn_{11}Al$	ZnTe	2.045	2.088	2.091	59
$VS_4Zn_{11}Ga$	ZnS (hexagonal)	2.004	2.0534	2.0587	60

At temperatures near $100\,°K$ thermal excitation causes the hole to move so rapidly between the three sulfur sites adjacent to the vacancy in the halogen-doped ZnS crystals that the spectrum becomes axial as if the hole is shared equally by the equivalent sulfurs [61]. The changes in the ZnS:Cl spectrum for **H** parallel to a $\langle 111 \rangle$ axis are illustrated in Fig. 10-6. This motional averaging occurs when the hole "hopping" rate exceeds the difference in the resonant frequencies (at fixed field) of the particular localized hole magnetic resonance transitions contributing to the average under consideration.

If one examines alloys of ZnS and ZnSe in which ZnSe is the minority constituent and which are doped with group III or VII impurities, centers similar to those discussed above are observed. In particular, centers occur corresponding to one chlorine, two sulfurs, and one selenium surrounding a Zn vacancy. The hole shows a preference for the Se site because the Se^{2-} electrons are the most loosely bound. The resultant center has a spectrum similar to the Cl center in a ZnSe crystal (see Table 10-5). However, if two Se ions and only one sulfur surround the vacancy, the hole is located equally on the two Se ions even at temperatures near $1\,°K$.

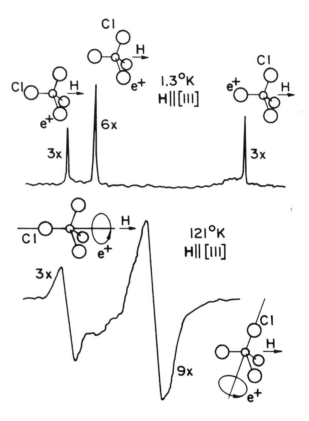

FIG. 10-6   The EPR spectrum [61] for the Zn-vacancy chlorine associate shown in Fig. 10-5(b). The upper spectrum arises from holes occupying single sulfur sites at low temperatures. The lower spectrum arises because at temperatures of the order of 100°K the hole hops between the three S sites nearest the vacancy, and the resonance lines occur at the average positions of the lines for the single S sites.

A center very similar to the associates described above occurs in silicon. This center, originally designated the Si–E center but more recently termed the Si–G8 center [38], arises from electron irradiation of phosphorus-doped silicon single crystals. Structurally it consists of a Si vacancy adjacent to a substitutional phosphorus. It is neutral and has a hole which is localized primarily on one of the other three equivalent silicons. Hence the structure is the same as for the associate in chlorine-doped ZnS. Most properties are similar for the two. Both are nearly axial, and both display a similar motional averaging at temperatures near 100°K. The influence of applied uniaxial stress on the intensity of the EPR lines of the Si–G8 center has been studied in the manner discussed at the end of Section 7–2.

Many other kinds of defect associates have been observed by electron paramagnetic resonance. A rather different kind, which also occurs in silicon, is the divacancy, two vacancies at the nearest possible sites. Such a defect is shown in Fig. 10-7. Two charge states of the divacancy have been observed by EPR. The positive charge state has one electron in the bonding orbital involving the starred atoms of Fig. 10-7, whereas the negative charge state has two electrons in the bonding orbital and one in the

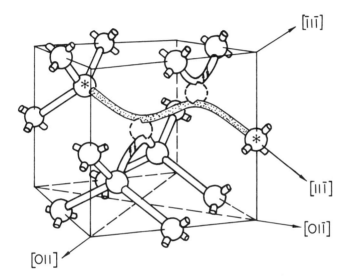

FIG. 10-7   An associated center in silicon formed by two vacancies. Two charge states of the divacancy have been observed by electron paramagnetic resonance. The paramagnetism results from an electron in a bonding orbital or in an antibonding orbital linking the two starred atoms as shown [38]. This figure was taken from J. W. Corbett and G. D. Watkins, *Phys. Rev. Letters* **7**, 314 (1961).

antibonding orbital involving the starred atoms. These have been called Si–G6 and Si–G7, respectively [38]. As is usual for associates the symmetry is low. The g values are near 2, and there are hyperfine interactions with the two starred Si nuclei. Since the two are identical, the presence of two could be determined only by the intensity of the hyperfine structure in relation to the lines without such structure (see Fig. 5-15). Silicon has three isotopes, two with $I = 0$. The third, ^{29}Si, has $I = \frac{1}{2}$ and a 4.7% natural abundance. If only one Si nucleus produces the hyperfine structure, then each intense line will be surrounded by two hyperfine lines with an intensity approximately $2\frac{1}{2}\%$ of the main line. If two Si nuclei are involved, these lines will be approximately twice as big in comparison to the intense line. In the latter case there should be two other lines about three times as far from the intense line. However, their intensity will be only 0.06% of that of the main line, and they may be unobservable.

10–4 The Dynamic Jahn-Teller Effect

The effective Hamiltonians which we have formulated and used so far have literally been spin Hamiltonians, that is, the operator parts of the Hamiltonians have been angular momentum operators of various kinds. It is possible, although not necessarily convenient, to describe any manifold of states in any point symmetry by a spin Hamiltonian. When there is insufficient similarity to the usual behavior of angular momenta, it may be useful to adopt a new finite set of operators to give a general description of the manifold of states under consideration. The dynamic Jahn-Teller effect for an orbital doublet in cubic symmetry is a case in point.

We alluded to the basic feature of the Jahn-Teller effect in Section 3–9: energetic arguments favor a distortion of an orbitally degenerate state of a nonlinear molecule or imperfection. If the imperfection produces an EPR spectrum, then one may observe several superimposed spectra from the several distorted paramagnets (see, for example, Fig. 5-2). This is referred to as the static Jahn-Teller effect. If the distinctiveness of the distortions is blurred because of zero-point motion, one has the dynamic Jahn-Teller effect.

As we can see by examining Table 3-3 or Fig. 3-8(b), a single d electron on an ion occupying an eight-coordinated cubic site in a crystal will have a doublet ground state (there are two degenerate e orbitals). Such a ^2E state (the superscript 2 is just the value of $2S+1$) is unstable against distortion (the Jahn-Teller theorem). The ground state remains a ^2E state even after the distortion (for a discussion of this point and others in more detail see reference 62). The ^2E state that results is vibronic, that is, partially electronic and partially vibrational in character, rather than purely electronic as was the original state considered. Thus an effective Hamiltonian for such a system must describe the manifold of four states arising from a twofold spin degeneracy and a twofold vibronic degeneracy. The spin part is handled as discussed in Chapter 4 and subsequent chapters with $S = \frac{1}{2}$. To describe the vibronic part we need operators which operate within the two-dimensional Hilbert space of the vibronic states. There are four such operators, analogous to the three independent spin operators plus the identity, and they can be written in matrix form in terms of the four possible matrix elements of the 2×2 matrix. Each operator term must be linear in these vibronic operators, which we will symbolize generically by U. Using symmetry arguments (group theory), it can be shown that the numbers of invariant terms allowed for cubic symmetry are those shown in Table 10-6. To ensure invariance under time reversal it is necessary to recognize that one of the four U operators is time-reversal odd.

Table 10-6

Number of Independent Terms of a Given Type in the Effective Hamiltonian for a ^2E State in O_h, O, and T_d Symmetry

Symbolic Operator Type	Number	Specific Examples
U	0	...
UA	0	...
UT	1	UT
UA^2	1	UI^2
UAB	2	UHS, USI
UTA	1	UTH, UTS
$UTAB$	8	$UTHS$
UAB^2	1	USI^2

The dominant terms are UT, UHS, and USI. These take the form

$$\mathcal{H} = g_1\beta\mathbf{H}\cdot\mathbf{SJ}+\tfrac{1}{2}qg_2\beta[(3H_zS_z-\mathbf{H}\cdot\mathbf{S})\mathcal{E}_\theta+\sqrt{3}(H_xS_x-H_yS_y)\mathcal{E}_\varepsilon]$$

$$+ A_1\mathbf{S}\cdot\mathbf{IJ}+\tfrac{1}{2}qA_2[(3S_zI_z-\mathbf{S}\cdot\mathbf{I})\mathcal{E}_\theta+\sqrt{3}(S_xI_x-S_yI_y)\mathcal{E}_\varepsilon]$$

$$+ qV_2(e_\theta\mathcal{E}_\theta+e_\varepsilon\mathcal{E}_\varepsilon), \tag{10-8}$$

where $\mathfrak{J}$, $\mathcal{E}_\theta$, and $\mathcal{E}_\varepsilon$ are the required vibronic operators, and e_θ and e_ε are components of the strain. The operator $\mathfrak{J}$ is the identity operator, $\mathcal{E}_\theta$ and e_θ transform like $3z^2-r^2$, and $\mathcal{E}_\varepsilon$ and e_ε transform like $\sqrt{3}(x^2-y^2)$. To illustrate the observed behavior [63] we ignore the hyperfine structure and assume that the vibronic states in the presence of strain are determined by the last term in Eq. (10-8). Then each of the strain-split vibronic levels (which are still spin doublets) can be described by the Hamiltonian

$$\mathcal{H} = g_1\beta\mathbf{H}\cdot\mathbf{S}+\tfrac{1}{2}qg_2\beta[\langle\mathcal{E}_\theta\rangle(3H_zS_z-\mathbf{H}\cdot\mathbf{S})+\sqrt{3}\langle\mathcal{E}_\varepsilon\rangle(H_xS_x-H_yS_y)], \tag{10-9}$$

where $\langle\mathcal{E}_\theta\rangle$ and $\langle\mathcal{E}_\varepsilon\rangle$ are the expectation values of the two vibronic operators. This can be written in the standard form used in Chapters 4 and 5:

$$\mathcal{H} = \beta\mathbf{H}\cdot\mathbf{g}\cdot\mathbf{S}. \tag{10-10}$$

If **g** is expressed in terms of the cubic axes, we have

$$\mathbf{g} = \begin{vmatrix} g_1 - \tfrac{1}{2}qg_2\langle \mathcal{E}_\theta \rangle + \dfrac{\sqrt{3}}{2}qg_2\langle \mathcal{E}_\varepsilon \rangle & 0 & 0 \\ 0 & g_1 - \tfrac{1}{2}qg_2\langle \mathcal{E}_\theta \rangle - \dfrac{\sqrt{3}}{2}qg_2\langle \mathcal{E}_\varepsilon \rangle & 0 \\ 0 & 0 & g_1 + qg_2\langle \mathcal{E}_\theta \rangle \end{vmatrix}.$$

(10-11)

If we assume $qg_2 \ll g_1$, we can calculate the energy, keeping only the first two terms in a power series expansion:

$$E = \left\{ g_1 + qg_2 \left[\tfrac{1}{2}(3n^2 - 1)\langle \mathcal{E}_\theta \rangle + \dfrac{\sqrt{3}}{2}(l^2 - m^2)\langle \mathcal{E}_\varepsilon \rangle \right] \right\} \beta H M_S. \quad (10\text{-}12)$$

The resultant spectrum [62, 63] consists of absorption lines, as shown in Fig. 10-8. The distribution of absorption intensity between the extremes occurs because of the distribution in $\langle \mathcal{E}_\theta \rangle$ and $\langle \mathcal{E}_\varepsilon \rangle$, which in

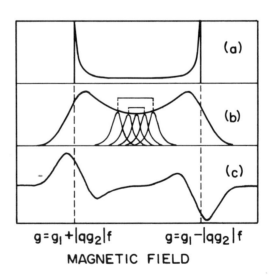

$$g = g_1 + |qg_2|f \qquad g = g_1 - |qg_2|f$$

MAGNETIC FIELD

FIG. 10-8   Electron paramagnetic resonance absorption for a vibronic doublet in cubic symmetry [63]. This inhomogeneous line shape results from large random strains. In (a) the absorption is shown for the case of no inherent line width. In (b) the effect of a nonzero line width is included, and in (c) the first derivative of the absorption is shown. The quantity f stands for $\sqrt{1 - 3(m^2 n^2 + n^2 l^2 + l^2 m^2)}$.

turn arises from a distribution of e_θ/e_ε. The angular dependence of the two peaks in the absorption is shown in Fig. 10-9. In first order the displacement of the peaks from the center of the pattern is proportional to $\sqrt{1-3(m^2n^2+n^2l^2+l^2m^2)}$.

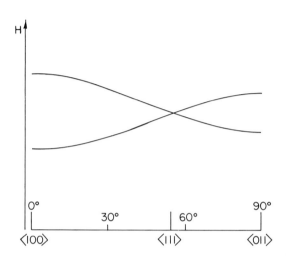

FIG. 10-9   The angular dependence of the two peaks of Fig. 10-8. The magnetic field is rotated in a $\{110\}$ plane.

10–5 Transition-Group Impurities in Ferroelectric Crystals

In Sections 10–1 and 10–2 we discussed crystalline impurities whose free-ion ground state was $^2S_{1/2}$. These paramagnets were rather insensitive to details of their environments, partly because $S=\frac{1}{2}$ and partly because there is very little orbital contribution to the magnetic moments.

In Section 5–2 we mentioned briefly (during a discussion of quartic terms in the fine structure) impurity ions with an [Ar] $3d^5$ configuration. Free ions with an [Ar] $3d^5$ configuration have a $^6S_{5/2}$ ground state. These ions, such as Cr^+, Mn^{2+}, or Fe^{3+}, and their rare-earth counterparts, Eu^{2+} and Gd^{3+} with a $^8S_{7/2}$ ground state, are quite sensitive to their crystalline environment because $S>\frac{1}{2}$, resulting in fine structure. For the $^6S_{5/2}$-state ions it is possible to have fine structure terms in the spin Hamiltonian which are quadratic in the spin and terms quartic in the spin. Usually the quadratic terms dominate the spectra for noncubic symmetry. For cubic symmetry, however, there are no quadratic terms, leaving only the quartic terms to produce the fine structure.

The point here is that ferroelectric crystals [64] have phase transitions resulting from changes in crystal structure. In the case of $BaTiO_3$, an extensively studied ferroelectric, the high-temperature crystal structure is the cubic perovskite structure. At about 120 °C there is a phase transition, and just below this temperature the crystal structure is tetragonal. Usually there are three types of tetragonal regions, corresponding to the three cubic axes of the perovskite lattice. If Fe^{3+} or Gd^{3+} is substituted into $BaTiO_3$, it is possible to see the changes in crystal structure at the transition and the change in the crystalline environment with temperature below 120°C.

Above 120 °C Fe^{3+} in $BaTiO_3$ is described [65] by Eq. (5-50) with $g = 2.003$ and $|a| = 0.0102(12)$ cm^{-1}. No detectable change occurs in g and a up to 170°C. Below 120°C the Fe^{3+} impurity ions can be described [65] approximately by Eq. (5-33) with $g = g_{\parallel} = 2.003$. However, the tetragonal crystal field and thus D vary rapidly with temperature, abruptly dropping to zero at the transition temperature.

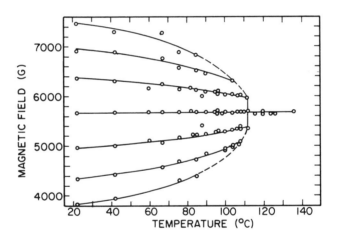

FIG. 10-10 The temperature dependence of the Gd^{3+} EPR spectrum in $BaTiO_3$ [66]. The fine structure resulting from the tetragonal crystal field disappears near 110°C, the temperature of the tetragonal to cubic phase transition in $BaTiO_3$. The magnetic field was parallel to the tetragonal axis, and the microwave frequency was 16 GHz.

A qualitatively similar behavior occurs with $BaTiO_3$ doped with Gd [66]. Figure 10-10 shows the temperature dependence of the EPR spectrum of Gd^{3+} in a single tetragonally distorted region of the crystal for the case in which the magnetic field is along the tetragonal axis. Other impurities and crystals have also been studied. Low and Offenbacher [67] have reviewed the work on perovskite-type crystals as of about 1964.

10–6 Rare-Earth Impurities in Alkaline-Earth Halide Crystals

A given impurity can produce many different point imperfections in a particular crystal. One of the best examples is the case of rare-earth-doped alkaline-earth halides with the fluorite crystal structure. The crystals studied by electron paramagnetic resonance have been CaF_2, SrF_2, BaF_2, CdF_2, and $SrCl_2$. Of these more is known about CaF_2, and therefore most of our discussion will concern this crystal.

In Section 10–1 we discussed hydrogen in CaF_2, and Fig. 10-1 shows a part of the structure of this crystal. In the fluorite crystal structure the F^- ions form a simple cubic structure with every alternate cube body center occupied by a Ca^{2+} ion. It appears that the rare-earth impurities always occupy calcium-ion sites.

The common charges for rare-earth ions are tripositive and dipositive with the trivalent form much more common. Thus a rare-earth ion will normally have one more unit of positive charge than the calcium ion it replaces. Since the crystal as a whole must be neutral (or nearly so), this means that an equal number of negative charges must exist somewhere in the crystal. This process is termed charge compensation. Although the charge-compensating negative charge can be many lattice constants from the rare-earth ion (and thus not influence the cubic symmetry of the rare earth's environment), it can also be attracted to the positively charged rare-earth ion, forming an associate. We speak of remote or local charge compensation in these two cases. The various possible imperfections correspond to the many ways in which local charge compensation can occur.

Let us start by considering an ion with the configuration $[Xe] 4f^{13}$, that is, a single hole in the $4f$ shell (which is filled with 14 electrons). The ions Yb^{3+} and Tm^{2+} have this ground configuration. Since the spin-orbit coupling constant is negative for a shell more than half full, we expect the free-ion ground state to have $J = \frac{7}{2}$. This eightfold degeneracy is partially lifted in a cubic crystalline field, yielding two Kramers doublets and a quartet (note that we are using the weak crystal-field scheme appropriate to the rare earths and discussed in Section 3–7). According to the calculations of Lea, Leask, and Wolf [68] one of the two doublets, labeled Γ_6 and Γ_7, should be lowest in energy.

The g value for isolated Tm^{2+} in CaF_2 is 3.453(3) and the g value for isolated Yb^{3+} in CaF_2 is 3.443(2) [69], both of which are very close to the value of $\frac{24}{7} = 3.4286$ predicted for the Γ_7 state and considerably different from the value of $\frac{8}{3} = 2.6667$ calculated for the Γ_6 state. Thus experimental evidence argues for a Γ_7 ground state. The calculated g value is obtained by requiring the same Zeeman splitting when expressed in terms of an effective spin of $\frac{1}{2}$ as when expressed in terms of the actual mixtures of eigenstates of $\mathbf{J}^2$ and J_z, that is,

$$g\beta H\langle S_z\rangle = g_L\beta H\langle J_z\rangle, \qquad (10\text{-}13)$$

where g_L is the Landé g factor for the lowest free-ion level ($g_L = \frac{8}{7}$ in this case), and the expectation values are taken using eigenfunctions of the effective and the actual Hamiltonian, respectively. Thus

$$g = 2g_L\langle J_z\rangle, \qquad (10\text{-}14)$$

and taking the actual wave function to be of the form (this ignores excited free-ion states)

$$|\rangle = \sum_{M_J} a_{M_J}|M_J\rangle, \qquad (10\text{-}15)$$

we obtain

$$g = 2g_L\sum_{M_J}|a_{M_J}|^2 M_J. \qquad (10\text{-}16)$$

Putting in the values of a_{M_J} given by Lea *et al.* [68] yields the results quoted above.

Isolated substitutional Yb^{3+} is charge-compensated remotely. Many types of associates result from local charge compensation. For example, in the alkaline-earth fluorides interstitial F^- ions can occur. They may occupy the cube body centers not normally occupied by alkaline-earth ions. A common neutral associate is formed by a substitutional trivalent rare-earth ion and an interstitial F^- in the nearest possible site. Such an imperfection has tetragonal symmetry (C_{4v}) and is described by the appropriate spin Hamiltonian (see Chapters 4 and 5). The structure of such a defect is shown in Fig. 10-11. The g factors for Yb^{3+} in CaF_2 are $g_\parallel = 2.420(4)$ and $g_\perp = 3.802(3)$, where the parallel or z axis is the particular one of the three cubic axes along which the association occurs [70]. In any sample all three directions of association are observed with equal likelihood, and the spectrum will look much like that in Fig. 5-2. The average g factor (the trace of $\mathbf{g}$ divided by 3) is $\bar{g} = 3.341$, a value close to that measured for cubic Yb^{3+} in CaF_2, 3.443, and also close to the value predicted for the Γ_7 state in cubic symmetry arising from the $J = \frac{7}{2}$ free-ion level. Lewis and Sabisky [71] have shown that $\bar{g}$ should approximately equal the cubic value if the deviation from cubic symmetry is an axial perturbation to the cubic crystal field. If this perturbation approach is employed, then $|g_\parallel - g_\perp|$ must be considerably less than $\bar{g}$, a rather poor approximation in this case. Rubins [72] has attempted to justify the near equality of $\bar{g}$ and the cubic g value for a wider range of conditions, but generally valid arguments seem lacking. Nevertheless this empirical rule is quite useful and is satisfied by most rare-earth ions in

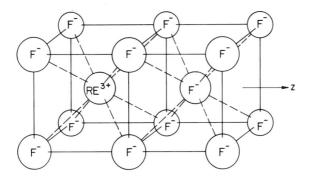

FIG. 10-11   Charge compensation of a trivalent rare-earth ion substituting for an alkaline-earth ion in an alkaline-earth fluoride crystal (such as CaF_2). Charge compensation is achieved by an interstitial F^- at a nearest body center. The resultant associate is tetragonal.

alkaline-earth halides having Γ_6 or Γ_7 ground states in cubic symmetry. Local charge compensation by H^- or D^- ions in the nearest interstitial site has also been observed for several rare-earth ions [73].

Spectra of Yb^{3+} ions are also observed in several sites having trigonal symmetry. One way which has been suggested for such an imperfection to be formed is the association of the positively charged substitutional Yb^{3+} ion with an O^{2-} impurity ion on a nearest-neighbor F^- site. Such a center is illustrated in Fig. 10-12. The Yb^{3+} center thought to have this

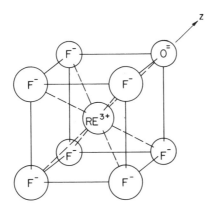

FIG. 10-12   A trigonal associated center in alkaline-earth fluorides resulting from local charge compensation of a trivalent rare-earth ion by an O^{2-} ion substituting for an F^- ion adjacent to the rare earth.

structure has $g_\parallel = 1.420(2)$ and $g_\perp = 4.389(5)$ [74]. If the spectrum is observed with the field along the axis of a given imperfection, the lines associated with that imperfection are split. This is believed to arise from the hyperfine interaction with the F^- ion opposite the O^{2-} ion. The particular fluorine site in question has also been occupied by H^- or D^- ions forming centers with slightly smaller anisotropies and smaller hyperfine splittings [74]. It has also been argued that rare-earth ions sometimes have an OH^- ion replacing one of the eight closest F^- ions. Similarly the possibility of an interstitial F^- in the next nearest interstitial site, which is along a $\langle 111 \rangle$ direction, is sometimes suggested to help explain the many trigonal centers observed for various rare earths.

Several orthorhombic Yb^{3+} centers have been observed in CaF_2. Three of these have been identified as associates of substitutional Yb^{+3} and substitutional Li^+, Na^+, or K^+ on the nearest possible Ca^{2+} site. Such an associated imperfection is pictured in Fig. 10-13. The principal

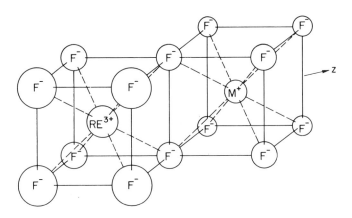

FIG. 10-13   An orthorhombic associate in CaF_2. The trivalent rare-earth ion is charge-compensated by an alkali ion (M^+) at a nearest Ca^{2+} site.

axes of **g** are [001], [110], and [1$\bar{1}$0] and all equivalent sets. If for the imperfection of Fig. 10-13 we regard these three axes as x, y, and z, then for the Yb^{3+} Na^+ center we have $g_x = 3.289(5)$, $g_y = 3.102(5)$, and $g_z = 3.926(5)$ [75]. We see that the g tensor is nearly axial, indicating that the noncubic crystal field is primarily the axial one arising from the effective negative charge at the Na^+ site. Similar results hold for the other two alkalies [75]. It has also been argued that the alkali can occupy the next nearest Ca site, forming a tetragonal center.

In the case of Nd^{3+}, orthorhombic spectra have been observed which can be explained on the basis of two substitutional Nd^{3+} ions as nearest neighbors. To obtain a neutral center, preserve the symmetry, and explain the association of two defects which should repel each other, it is postulated that two F^- ions occupy the two interstitial sites closest to the two Nd^{3+} ions. Such an imperfection is shown in Fig. 10-14. As we saw in Chapter 6, the spectrum of a pair of interacting paramagnets can be very complicated and may have little resemblance to the spectrum of the same paramagnet when isolated. In this case a relatively simple result occurs for Nd^{3+} pairs in SrF_2 [76]. The interaction is nearly the point dipole-dipole value, and the result is merely to double the number of lines. The resultant splitting is typically a few hundred gauss.

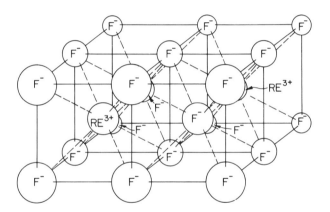

FIG. 10-14   An associate of two rare-earth ions and two interstitial F^- ions postulated to explain spectra observed in SrF_2 [76].

Anderson and Sabisky [77] have observed an associate of a trivalent rare-earth ion and a fluorine vacancy (an F center) with either one or two electrons trapped on it. For the positively charged state the electron occupies an orbital similar to that of an isolated F center. For the La^{3+} and Lu^{3+} cases the g values are very close to 2.00. The isolated F center [78] has $g = 1.9978(5)$.

Lanthanum behaves somewhat differently from the other rare-earth impurities in that La^{2+} has a single $5d$ electron rather than a $4f$ electron. In $SrCl_2$ [63] this leads to the dynamic Jahn-Teller effect discussed in Section 10–4. In other crystals the static Jahn-Teller effect may be observed [79].

The evidence available suggests that SrF_2 and BaF_2 produce for most rare-earth ions results similar to those of CaF_2. For $SrCl_2$ it does not appear that interstitial halogen ions are important in charge compensation. The most unusual of the fluorite structure halides is CdF_2. When heated in cadmium vapor rare-earth-doped CdF_2 frequently turns semiconducting [80, 81]. The interaction of conduction electrons and rare-earth ions has been observed in the electron paramagnetic resonance [81].

Anderson and Sabisky [82] have used combined optical and microwave techniques to extract a great deal more information about Tm^{2+} and Dy^{2+} centers than could be learned by electron paramagnetic resonance alone. For example, they have observed the EPR from an excited state of Dy^{2+}.

Positive identification of some of the associates discussed above has been made by observing $\Delta M_S = 0$ transitions between states split by the hyperfine interactions with the rare-earth nucleus and the host-crystal nuclei near the impurity. The technique for doing this, termed ENDOR or Electron Nuclear Double Resonance, was discussed in Section 5-4 and is described more fully in Section 11-4. Although the spin Hamiltonian terms necessary to describe the EPR spectra are usually few and very simple (for a Kramers doublet they consist of terms of the forms HS, SI, and I^2 where several different nuclear spins may enter), ENDOR spectra require the consideration of other more complicated terms. For all but the ions with a half-filled $4f$ shell (Eu^{2+} and Gd^{3+}) these additional terms arise because low-lying excited states give measurable contributions to the spin Hamiltonian in second or higher order. For a Kramers doublet terms in powers of S higher than 1 are not meaningful. However, if the value of I is large enough, the power of I can be greater than 1. Terms in the spin Hamiltonian of the forms HSI^2, SI^3, and I^4 have been detected in cubic and tetragonal symmetry [83].

In a similar fashion, if a Kramers doublet has an excited Γ_8 state rather close in energy, it may be necessary to include terms of the form H^3S in the spin Hamiltonian for the ground state. Such effects have been observed for Er^{3+} in ZnSe [84].

10-7 Diatomic Molecule-Ion Imperfections

A crystalline imperfection for which all electrons are in closed atomic shells or filled covalent bonds is not paramagnetic. It can become paramagnetic, however, by the addition of electrons or by the removal of electrons, that is, the addition of holes. In this section we will discuss hole centers in ionic crystals (called V centers in the parlance of color-center research). The alkali halides are the most extensively studied ionic crystals. Hole centers in alkali halides and many other ionic crystals containing halide ions are usually covalent molecule ions, in particular diatomic halogen-molecule negative ions. All molecule ions made up of the same two halogen atoms have approximately the same properties independently of the detailed structure of the imperfection or the particular host crystal. As evidence of this fact, the data for F_2^- molecule ions are listed in Table 10-7. The data are presented as if the spin Hamiltonian has axial symmetry, which is a very good approximation. The spin is $\frac{1}{2}$, and the principal hyperfine interaction is with the two ^{19}F nuclei in the molecule ion, each ^{19}F having $I = \frac{1}{2}$. Therefore the spin Hamiltonian is approximately

$$\mathcal{H} = g\beta H_z S_z + g_\perp \beta (H_x S_x + H_y S_y) + A S_z (I_{1z} + I_{2z})$$

$$+ B[S_x(I_{1x} + I_{2x}) + S_y(I_{1y} + I_{2y})]. \qquad (10\text{-}17)$$

Table 10-7
Spin Hamiltonian Parameters for F_2^-

Defect	Host Crystal	$g_{\parallel}$	$g_\perp$	A (G)	B (G)	Reference
V_K	LiF	2.0034	2.0239	883.7	57	85
V_K	NaF	2.0014	2.0220	897.1	47	"
V_K	KF	2.0020	2.0214	908.0	30	"
V_K	RbF	2.0034	2.0160	908.4		"
V_{KA}	NaF:Li	2.0020(1)	2.0219(2) 2.0231(2)	916.4(2)	<7	86
H	LiF:Na	2.0013(5)	2.012(2)	961.0(6)	75(25)	87
V_F	LiF	2.001(2)	2.023(2)	915	~ 0	88
$V_{\langle 111\rangle}$	LiF	2.0017	2.0105	1005.9	19.0	89
V_K	CaF_2	2.001(1)	2.020(1)	900(1)	48(2)	90
V_K	SrF_2	2.002(2)	2.022(2)	899(1)	44(1)	91
V_K	BaF_2	2.004(2)	2.024(2)	897(2)	42(1)	"
V_F	CaF_2	2.002(2)	2.019(2)	916(1)	45(10)	92
V_F	BaF_2	2.001(1)	2.017(1)	916(1)	40(10)	93
V_K	$KMgF_3$	2.0024(2)	2.025(1) 2.018(1)	884(2)	56(5)	94
	$NaHF_2$	2.0001(3)	2.016(1)	984.6(3)	64.0(1)	95
	KHF_2	2.002(1)	2.017(1)	955(1)	21(4)	96
	NH_4HF_2	1.9998(3)	2.015(1)	948.1(3)	15.9(1) 20.6(1)	95

With a few exceptions, an imperfection in an ionic halide-containing crystal which has trapped a hole is primarily a slightly modified X_2^- ion, where X is a halogen atom. Thus, if we can explain the paramagnetism of a free X_2^- molecule ion, we obtain considerable insight into most hole centers.

If we consider an hypothetical molecule consisting of two F$^-$ ions, we find that all molecular orbitals, both bonding and antibonding, are filled for the principal quantum numbers $n = 1$ and $n = 2$. The F$_2^-$ molecule ion results from removing an electron from the highest-energy antibonding orbital. In the simplest approximation this orbital would be formed from atomic $2p$ orbitals. If the $2p$ orbitals on the two atoms point toward each other, then maximum overlap occurs, resulting in the highest energy for the antibonding molecular orbital. Such an orbital is labeled σ_u in the free ion. The g factors and hyperfine parameters result from a slight elaboration of this description. The presence of additional ions near the F$_2^-$ does not significantly alter this description because the hole is so tightly bound in the molecule ion.

The several imperfections which are essentially homonuclear diatomic molecule ions can be distinguished by small quantitative differences in their spectra (both symmetry and parameter values), by differences in optical and thermal properties, and particularly by their ENDOR spectra.

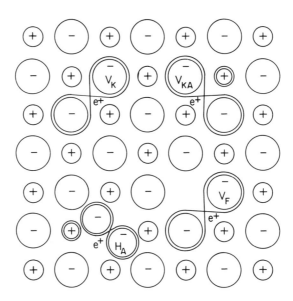

FIG. 10-15   Four trapped-hole centers which are essentially dihalide negative ions. These centers have been observed in alkali halides. A $\{100\}$ plane is shown. The V$_K$ center is a self-trapped hole. The V$_{KA}$ center is a hole trapped adjacent to an alkali impurity. The V$_F$ center is a hole trapped at an alkali vacancy, the antimorph of the F center. The H$_A$ center is a hole trapped on an interstitial halogen which is adjacent to an alkali impurity. This center was called the V$_1$ center before its structure was known. It occurs in sodium-doped KCl, for example. Another type of H$_A$ center is shown in Fig. 10-16.

The simplest such imperfection is called the V_K center (V for the color-center label denoting an excess hole center, and K for W. Känzig, who first observed it. This was the first hole center in alkali halides which was observed and identified by EPR [97]). The V_K center is a self-trapped hole, that is, at low temperatures ($\lesssim 100°K$) the hole becomes localized on a pair of adjacent substitutional halide ions (see Fig. 10-15). At somewhat higher temperatures the hole will diffuse about until it encounters an imperfection that will bind it. In this way other types of hole centers are formed, such as the V_{KA} center, a hole trapped adjacent to an alkali impurity [86] and again forming an X_2^- ion (see Fig. 10-15). Similarly the V_F center results when the hole is trapped at an alkali vacancy [88]. If halogen impurities are present, a heteronuclear diatomic molecule ion may result such as ICl^- or $BrCl^-$ with both halogens substitutional [98].

A rather different imperfection occurs when an interstitial halogen atom is created. This process accompanies the formation of F centers by the creation of negative-ion vacancies. The interstitial atom forms another of the ubiquitous molecule ions by bonding to a substitutional atomic ion. The resultant molecule ion occupies a substitutional site and is called an H center. The isolated interstitial appears to have either a $\langle 111 \rangle$ orientation [89] or a $\langle 110 \rangle$ orientation [100]. A variety of H centers can be formed by association of the interstitial halogen and one or two alkali impurity ions [99] (see Figs. 10-15 and 10-16). If fluorine is an impurity in an alkali halide, then FCl^-, FBr^-, and FI^- may be formed, depending on the crystal [101]. These heteronuclear diatomic molecular ions occupy

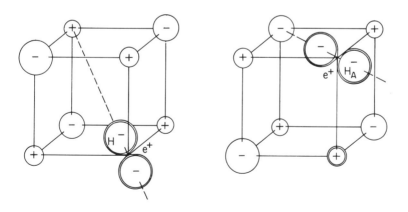

FIG. 10-16   One form of the H center is shown on the left as observed in LiF. An H center is a hole trapped at an interstitial halogen. On the right we show another type of H_A center, a hole trapped on an interstitial halogen near an alkali impurity. Figure 10-15 showed another form. The H_A center in this figure occurs in Na-doped LiF.

a single halogen site and are oriented with the internuclear axis along crystallographic $\langle 111 \rangle$ axes.

Other halide-containing crystals also have similar imperfections, particularly the alkaline-earth halides [90-93] having the fluorite crystal structure, and the ammonium halides [102] with the cesium chloride crystal structure. In both of these types of crystals the nearest halogen neighbors lie along $\langle 100 \rangle$ or cubic axes, unlike the $\langle 110 \rangle$ orientation of the sodium-chloride-structure alkali halides. However, not all ionic halides trap holes as X_2^- centers. For example, in AgCl the hole is trapped on a Ag^+ ion, forming paramagnetic Ag^{2+} [103].

In addition to halide diatomic molecule ions occupying single halide sites, many other molecular impurities can occur in alkali halides. We mentioned at the end of Section 7–2 the case of the O_2^- molecule ion, which substitutes at a halide-ion site and is oriented along $\langle 110 \rangle$ axes [104]. Since O_2^{3-} would be isoelectronic to F_2^-, we would need to remove two more antibonding electrons from the free molecule ion to arrive at the configuration for O_2^-. We would then find that the upper or σ_u orbital is not occupied at all and that a hole exists in the next highest orbital, the π_g orbital. This state has a twofold orbital degeneracy in the free molecule ion. Although this degeneracy is lifted in the crystal, the two levels are rather close together. Since these two states are mixed by the spin-orbit interaction, large shifts of the g factors from the spin-only value of 2 are observed (see Table 10-8). The characteristics of O_2^- in other hosts are rather similar [105]. Similar behavior is obtained for S_2^-, SSe^-, and Se_2^-

Table 10-8

Spin Hamiltonian Parameters for O_2^- in Alkali Halides

Host Crystal	g_x	g_y	g_z	A_x (MHz)	A_y (MHz)	A_z (MHz)
NaI	1.9996	2.0004	2.1859			
NaBr	1.9705	1.9663	2.3733			
NaCl	1.9483	1.9436	2.4529			
NaF	1.404	1.413	2.965	55	81	160
KI	1.9370	1.9420	2.4899	184.3	0	64.2
KBr	1.9268	1.9314	2.5203	181.3	0	71.1
KCl	1.9512	1.9551	2.4360	189.3	0	55.1
RbI	1.9674	1.9695	2.3774	193.7		
RbBr	1.9745	1.9763	2.3425			
RbCl	1.9836	1.9846	2.2947	201.6		

centers in alkali halides [106]. The larger spin-orbit interaction for sulfur or selenium yields still larger shifts in the g factors. The ground state is similar to that of O_2^- save for an increase in the principal quantum number.

Table 10-9

Spin Hamiltonian Parameters for N_2^- in Potassium Halides

Host Crystal	g_x	g_y	g_z	A_x (MHz)	A_y (MHz)	A_z (MHz)
KI	1.9937	1.984	1.8823	60.6	15	20
KBr	1.9956	2.000	1.8883	59.9	10	15
KCl	1.9978	2.000	1.9065	59.78	14.13	17.02

Continuing in this fashion, we expect N_2^- to be analogous to O_2^-. The π_g orbital is now singly occupied with consequences similar to O_2^- but with a negative g shift. The internuclear axis is still a $\langle 110 \rangle$ direction. Parameters for N_2^- in potassium halides are given in Table 10-9 [107].

References Cited in Chapter 10

[1] Chapter 2 of A. Carrington and A. D. McLachlan, *Introduction to Magnetic Resonance*, Harper and Row, New York, 1967, deals almost exclusively with the theory of atomic hydrogen electron paramagnetic resonance.

[2] *NMR Table*, 5th ed., Varian Associates, Palo Alto, Calif., 1965.

[3] P. Kusch, *Phys. Rev.* **100**, 1188 (1955).

[4] E. B. Nelson and J. E. Nafe, *Phys. Rev.* **75**, 1194 (1949).

[5] R. A. Weeks and M. Abraham, *J. Chem. Phys.* **42**, 68 (1965).

[6] R. G. Bessent, W. Hayes, J. W. Hodby, and P. A. S. Smith, *Proc. Roy. Soc. (London)* **A309**, 69 (1969).

[7] B. Welber, *Phys. Rev.* **136**, A1408 (1964).

[8] J. L. Hall and R. T. Schumacher, *Phys. Rev.* **127**, 1892 (1962).

[9] W. Burkersrode, *Z. Physik* **205**, 118 (1967).

[10] W. Hayes and J. W. Hodby, *Proc. Roy. Soc. (London)* **A294**, 359 (1966).

[11] F. Kerkhoff, W. Martienssen, and W. Sander, *Z. Physik* **173**, 184 (1963).

[12] G. Lehnert and J. M. Spaeth, *Phys. Stat. Solidi* **31**, 703 (1969).

[13] V. F. Koryagin and B. N. Grechushnikov, *Soviet Phys.-Sol. State* **7**, 2010 (1966).

[14] L. Shields, *J. Chem. Phys.* **45**, 2332 (1966).

[15] S. N. Foner, E. L. Cochran, V. A. Bowers, and C. K. Jen, *J. Chem. Phys.* **32**, 963 (1960).

[16] C. K. Jen, S. N. Foner, E. L. Cochran, and V. A. Bowers, *Phys. Rev.* **112**, 1169 (1958).

[17] M. Sharnoff and R. V. Pound, *Phys. Rev.* **132**, 1003 (1963).

[18] J. Lambe, *Phys. Rev.* **120**, 1208 (1960).

[19] S. A. Marshall, J. R. Gabriel, and R. A. Serway, *J. Chem. Phys.* **45**, 192 (1966).

[20] R. G. Bessent, W. Hayes, and J. W. Hodby, *Proc. Roy. Soc. (London)* **A297**, 376 (1967).

[21] J. M. Spaeth, *Z. Physik* **192**, 107 (1966).

[22] G. T. Trammell, H. Zeldes, and R. Livingston, *Phys. Rev.* **110**, 630 (1958).

[23] D. W. Feldman, J. G. Castle, Jr., and J. Murphy, *Phys. Rev.* **138**, A1208 (1965); D. W. Feldman, J. G. Castle, Jr., and G. R. Wagner, *Phys. Rev.* **145**, 237 (1966).

[24] S. Lee, V. P. Jacobsmeyer, and T. V. Hyncs, *Phys. Rev. Letters* **17**, 1245 (1966); W. Burkersrode, *Ann. Physik* **20**, 303 (1967).

[25] H. Blum, *Phys. Rev.* **161**, 213 (1967).

[26] C. K. Jen, V. A. Bowers, E. L. Cochran, and S. N. Foner, *Phys. Rev.* **126**, 1749 (1962).

[27] J. P. Goldsborough and T. R. Koehler, *Phys. Rev.* **133**, A135 (1964).

[28] R. A. Zhitnikov and N. V. Kolesnikov, *Soviet Phys.-Sol. State* **7**, 927 (1965).

[29] R. A. Zhitnikov, V. B. Koltsov, and N. I. Melnikov, *Phys. Stat. Solidi* **26**, 371 (1968).

[30] R. A. Zhitnikov and N. V. Kolesnikov, *Soviet Phys.-Solid State* **6**, 2645 (1965).

[31] P. G. Baranov, R. A. Zhitnikov, and N. I. Melnikov, *Phys. Stat. Solidi* **30**, 851 (1968).

[32] C. J. Delbecq, W. Hayes, M. C. M. O'Brien, and P. H. Yuster, *Proc. Roy. Soc. (London)* **A271**, 243 (1963).

[33] R. A. Zhitnikov and A. L. Oberli, *Soviet Phys.-Solid State* **7**, 1559 (1966).

[34] R. A. Zhitnikov, N. V. Kolesnikov, and V. I. Kosyakov, *Soviet Phys.-JETP* **17**, 815 (1963).

[35] R. A. Zhitnikov and N. V. Kolesnikov, *Soviet Phys.-Solid State* **7**, 1382 (1965).

[36] R. A. Zhitnikov and N. V. Kolesnikov, *Soviet Phys.-JETP* **19**, 65 (1964).

[37] P. H. Kasai, *Phys. Rev. Letters* **21**, 67 (1968).

[38] G. D. Watkins, in *Radiation Damage in Semiconductors*, Academic, New York, 1964, p. 97; see also J. W. Corbett, *Solid State Physics*, Suppl. 7 (F. Seitz and D. Turnbull, eds.), Academic, New York, 1966.

[39] A. Räuber and J. Schneider, *Phys. Stat. Solidi* **18**, 125 (1966).

[40] W. C. Holton and R. K. Watts, *J. Chem. Phys.* **51**, 1615 (1969).

[41] W. Dreybrodt and D. Silber, *Phys. Stat. Solidi* **20**, 337 (1967).

[42] K. Sugibuchi and Y. Mita, *Phys. Rev.* **147**, 355 (1966).

[43] R. Böttcher and J. Dziesiaty, *Phys. Stat. Solidi* **31**, K71 (1969).

[44] K. Suto and M. Aoki, *J. Phys. Soc. Japan* **24**, 955 (1968).

[45] J. H. Mackey, Jr., *J. Chem. Phys.* **39**, 74 (1963).

[46] K. Sugibuchi, *Phys. Rev.* **153**, 404 (1967).

[47] R. Röhrig and J. Schneider, *Phys. Letters* **30A**, 371 (1969).

[48] K. Suto and M. Aoki, *J. Phys. Soc. Japan* **22**, 1307 (1967).

[49] T. Iida and H. Watanabe, *Phys. Letters* **26A**, 541 (1968).

[50] R. Yokota and H. Imagawa, *J. Phys. Soc. Japan* **20**, 1537 (1965).

[51] L. Shields, *Trans. Faraday Soc.* **62**, 1042 (1966).

[52] A. R. Reinberg, *J. Chem. Phys.* **41**, 850 (1964); O. Schirmer, K. A. Müller, and J. Schneider, *Phys. Kond. Mat.* **3**, 323 (1965).

[53] W. V. Smith, P. P. Sorokin, I. L. Gelles, and G. J. Lasher, *Phys. Rev.* **115**, 1546 (1959); J. H. N. Loubser and L. DuPreez, *Brit. J. Appl. Phys.* **16**, 457 (1965).

[54] For a review of the properties of II-VI compounds refer to *Physics and Chemistry of II-VI Compounds* (M. Aven and J. S. Prener, eds.), North Holland, Amsterdam, 1967.

[55] A. Räuber and J. Schneider, *Phys. Letters* **3**, 230 (1963); J. Schneider, W. C. Holton, T. L. Estle, and A. Räuber, *Phys. Letters* **5**, 312 (1963).

[56] J. Schneider, A. Räuber, B. Dischler, T. L. Estle, and W. C. Holton, *J. Chem. Phys.* **42**, 1839 (1965).

[57] W. C. Holton, M. de Wit, and T. L. Estle, *International Symposium on Luminescence, The Physics and Chemistry of Scintillators* (N. Riehl and H. Kallmann, eds.), Karl Thiemig, Munich, 1966, p. 454.

[58] J. Schneider, B. Dischler, and A. Räuber, *J. Phys. Chem. Solids* **31**, 337 (1970).

[59] R. S. Title, G. Mandel, and F. F. Morehead, *Phys. Rev.* **136**, A300 (1964).

[60] Y. Otomo, H. Kusumoto, and P. H. Kasai, *Phys. Letters* **4**, 228 (1963).

[61] B. Dischler, A. Räuber, and J. Schneider, *Phys. Stat. Solidi* **6**, 507 (1964).

[62] F. S. Ham, *Phys. Rev.* **166**, 307 (1968); F. S. Ham, in *Electron Paramagnetic Resonance* (S. Geschwind, ed.), Plenum, New York, 1972.

[63] J. R. Herrington, T. L. Estle, and L. A. Boatner, *Phys. Rev.* **B3**, 2933 (1971).

[64] E. Fatuzzo and W. J. Merz, *Ferroelectricity*, North Holland, Amsterdam, 1967.

[65] A. W. Hornig, R. C. Rempel, and H. E. Weaver, *J. Phys. Chem. Solids* **10**, 1 (1959).

[66] L. Rimai and G. A. de Mars, *Phys. Rev.* **127**, 702 (1962).

[67] W. Low and E. L. Offenbacher, "Electron Spin Resonance of Magnetic Ions in Complex Oxides," in *Solid State Physics* (F. Seitz and D. Turnbull, eds.), Academic, New York, 1965, Vol. 17; for a recent study of interest, see K. A. Müller, W. Berlinger, and J. C. Slonczewski, *Phys. Rev. Letters* **25**, 734 (1970).

[68] K. R. Lea, M. J. M. Leask, and W. P. Wolf, *J. Phys. Chem. Solids* **23**, 1381 (1962). This reference gives the splitting of the free-ion levels for any of the rare-earth ions in cubic symmetry.

[69] W. Hayes and J. W. Twidell, *J. Chem. Phys.* **35**, 1521 (1961).

[70] U. Ranon and A. Yaniv, *Phys. Letters* **9**, 17 (1964).

[71] H. R. Lewis and E. S. Sabisky, *Phys, Rev.* **130**, 1370 (1963).

[72] R. S. Rubins, *Phys. Rev.* **B1**, 139 (1970).

[73] G. D. Jones, S. Peled, S. Rosenwaks, and S. Yatsiv, *Phys. Rev.* **183**, 353 (1969).

[74] S. D. McLaughlan and R. C. Newman, *Phys. Letters* **19**, 552 (1965).

[75] S. D. McLaughlan, *Phys. Rev.* **160**, 287 (1967).

[76] N. E. Kask and L. S. Kornienko, *Soviet Phys.-Solid State* **9**, 1795 (1968).

[77] C. H. Anderson and E. S. Sabisky, *Phys. Rev.* **B3**, 527 (1971).

[78] J. Arends, *Phys. Status Solidi* **7**, 805 (1964); W. Hayes and J. P. Scott, *Proc. Roy. Soc. (London)* **A301**, 313 (1967).

[79] W. Hayes and J. W. Twidell, *Proc. Phys. Soc.* **82**, 330 (1963).

[80] J. D. Kingsley and J. S. Prener, *Phys. Rev. Letters* **8**, 315 (1962).

[81] P. Eisenberger and P. S. Pershan, *Phys. Rev.* **167**, 292 (1968).

[82] E. S. Sabisky and C. H. Anderson, *Phys. Rev. Letters* **13**, 754 (1964); E. S. Sabisky and C. H. Anderson, *Appl. Phys. Letters* **13**, 214 (1968); C. H. Anderson and E. S. Sabisky, *Phys. Rev.* **178**, 547 (1969).

[83] J. M. Baker, W. B. J. Blake, and G. M. Copland, *Proc. Roy. Soc. (London)* **A309**, 119 (1969); J. M. Baker and W. B. J. Blake, *Proc. Roy. Soc. (London)* **A316**, 63 (1970).

[84] J. D. Kingsley and M. Aven, *Phys. Rev.* **155**, 235 (1967).

[85] C. E. Bailey, *Phys. Rev.* **136**, A1311 (1964).
[86] I. L. Bass and R. L. Mieher, *Phys. Rev.* **175**, 421 (1968).
[87] M. L. Dakss and R. L. Mieher, *Phys. Rev.* **187**, 1053 (1969).
[88] W. Känzig, *Phys. Rev. Letters* **4**, 117 (1960).
[89] Y. H. Chu and R. L. Mieher, *Phys. Rev.* **188**, 1311 (1969).
[90] W. Hayes and J. W. Twidell, *Proc. Phys. Soc.* **79**, 1295 (1962).
[91] W. Hayes, D. L. Kirk, and G. P. Summers, *Solid State Comm.* **7**, 1061 (1969).
[92] J. Sierro, *Phys. Rev.* **138**, A648 (1965).
[93] Y. Kazumata, *Phys. Stat. Solidi* **34**, 377 (1969).
[94] T. P. P. Hall, *Brit. J. Appl. Phys.* **17**, 1011 (1966).
[95] L. J. Vande Kieft and O. R. Gilliam, *Phys. Rev.* **B1**, 2015 (1970).
[96] F. B. Otto and O. R. Gilliam, *Phys. Rev.* **154**, 244 (1967).
[97] W. Känzig, *Phys. Rev.* **99**, 1890 (1955); T. G. Castner and W. Känzig, *J. Phys. Chem. Solids* **3**, 178 (1957); T. O. Woodruff and W. Känzig, *J. Phys. Chem. Solids* **5**, 268 (1958).
[98] W. Dreybrodt and D. Silber, *Phys. Stat. Solidi* **16**, 215 (1966); L. S. Goldberg and M. L. Meistrich, *Phys. Rev.* **172**, 877 (1968); C. J. Delbecq, D. Schoemaker, and P. H. Yuster, *Phys. Rev.* **B3**, 473 (1971).
[99] D. Schoemaker, *Phys. Rev.* **B3**, 3516 (1971).
[100] W. Känzig and T. O. Woodruff, *J. Phys. Chem. Solids* **9**, 70 (1958).
[101] J. W. Wilkins and J. R. Gabriel, *Phys. Rev.* **132**, 1950 (1963); D. Schoemaker, *Phys. Rev.* **149**, 693 (1966); W. Dreybrodt and D. Silber, *Phys. Stat. Solidi* **16**, 215 (1966).
[102] L. Vannotti, H. R. Zeller, K. Bachmann, and W. Känzig, *Phys. Kond. Mat.* **6**, 51 (1967).
[103] M. Höhne and M. Stasiw, *Phys. Stat. Solidi* **28**, 247 (1968).
[104] W. Känzig, *J. Phys. Chem. Solids* **23**, 479 (1962).
[105] J. E. Bennett, B. Mile, and A. Thomas, *Trans. Faraday Soc.* **64**, 3200 (1968).
[106] L. E. Vannotti and J. R. Morton, *Phys. Rev.* **161**, 282 (1967); L. E. Vannotti and J. R. Morton, *J. Chem. Phys.* **47**, 4210 (1967).
[107] J. R. Brailsford, J. R. Morton, and L. E. Vannotti, *J. Chem. Phys.* **50**, 1051 (1969).

CHAPTER 11

Double Resonance

We have devoted the greater part of this book to a discussion of simple electron paramagnetic resonance phenomena, that is, phenomena associated with the absorption of microwave power from a single, oscillating magnetic field by a paramagnetic sample in a quasi-static magnetic field. We also considered two related phenomena in Section 7–3, electrically stimulated transitions and ultrasonic paramagnetic resonance. In this chapter we will discuss double resonance phenomena, which are closely related to simple electron paramagnetic resonance except that two resonances are studied simultaneously. Examples of double resonance are masers, dynamic nuclear polarization, ENDOR, and some aspects of optical pumping. We will discuss each of these topics briefly after a simple illustration of the nature of double resonance.

11–1 General Characteristics of Double Resonance

In a double resonance experiment two oscillating fields are at or near resonance. Little is gained, however, by having the resonances uncoupled and performing thereby two uncorrelated but simultaneous magnetic resonance experiments. Hence in double resonance one of the two resonances influences the other. There are many variations of double resonance; it can be performed in a steady-state (CW) manner or by pulsed or other transient techniques. We will always assume that at least one of the two resonances occurs in the microwave-frequency range causing an EPR transition. The other frequency can be in the radio-frequency range (NMR), the microwave range (EPR), or as high as optical frequencies.

We will not attempt a general discussion but will limit ourselves to steady-state experiments, single-quantum transitions, and a description in terms of rate equations. Previously we employed rate equations in Section 2–4, especially Eq. (2-85), and briefly in Section 8–4, the latter in connection with a discussion of cross relaxation. By using rate equations we lose any ability to describe coherence effects arising from intense oscillating fields. The gain in simplicity, however, together with the ability to describe most of the observed effects, motivates this choice.

We are thus led to consider a system with three or more energy levels and to assume that one transition is saturated, at least partially. The saturation causes the populations of the levels to deviate from their thermal equilibrium values and results in a coupling between the two resonances.

For a system with several (≥ 4) energy levels, we illustrate in Fig. 11-1 the two cases which can arise. In (a) the saturated transition has a level in common with the other transition. In this case changing the population of the two levels between which the saturated transition occurs directly alters the population of one of the two levels between which the other transition occurs and thus generally causes a change in the other resonance signal. In (b) there is no direct influence of the saturation on the populations of the two levels involved in the other transition. However, spin-lattice relaxation may lead to changes in these populations, an indirect result of the saturation.

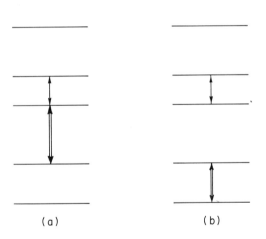

(a)   (b)

FIG. 11-1   Two types of possible double resonance experiments. **In (a) the** saturation of one transition (denoted by the double line joining the **two levels)** changes the population of one of the two terminal states of the **unsaturated** transition (single line) and thus changes the intensity of the unsaturated resonance. In (b) this direct effect does not exist. However, spin-lattice relaxation may lead to an indirect influence on the populations of other states and thus on the intensity of the unsaturated resonance.

Let us start by analyzing the simplest case, that of a system having three levels. The situation can be quite generally depicted as in Fig. 11-2. Aside from quantitative variations of the parameters, the only possible variation in this problem is in the relative positions of the levels, and this

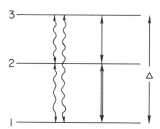

FIG. 11-2 Three-level system used in analyzing double resonance. The wavy lines denote relaxation transitions; the single straight line denotes the unsaturated transition whose intensity is influenced by saturating the transition shown by double straight lines. The energy difference between level 3 and level 1 is Δ.

can be easily allowed for. The rate equations can be written as a particular case of Eq. (2-85). Rather than attempt a general solution of this relatively uncomplicated problem, we will examine some of the simpler limiting behavior which can be deduced without solving the rate equations. We will take the magnetic dipole transition rate between levels 2 and 3 to be negligible compared to that from relaxation. The magnetic dipole transition rate between levels 1 and 2 will be taken as large enough to completely saturate the transition, resulting in equal populations, that is, $N_1 = N_2$. The results have their simplest form if we assume further that either relaxation between 1 and 3 or relaxation between 2 and 3 dominates. Choosing the former, we find

$$N_1 = N_2, \qquad \frac{N_3}{N_1} = e^{-\Delta/kT},$$ (11-1)

where Δ is $E_3 - E_1$. This result is independent of which of the three levels are involved as long as Δ and the three indices are appropriately chosen. Combining Eq. (11-1) with $N = N_1 + N_2 + N_3$ and using the fact that the unsaturated signal is proportional to $N_2 - N_3$, we obtain a signal proportional to

$$N_2 - N_3 = N \frac{1 - e^{-\Delta/kT}}{2 + e^{-\Delta/kT}}.$$ (11-2)

In the high-temperature limit this becomes

$$N_2 - N_3 = \frac{N}{3} \frac{\Delta}{kT}.$$ (11-3)

If we contrast this with the thermal-equilibrium population difference in the high-temperature limit,

$$N_2 - N_3 = \frac{N}{3} \frac{E_3 - E_2}{kT}, \tag{11-4}$$

we see that saturating transition $1 \rightleftharpoons 3$ will enhance the signal for transition $2 \rightleftharpoons 3$ if $\Delta > E_3 - E_2$, as depicted in Fig. 11-2. The signal is reduced if $0 < \Delta < E_3 - E_2$, and if Δ is negative we actually have an inverted population distribution (see Fig. 11-3). In the latter case the microwave magnetic field stimulates the paramagnet to emit more energy than it absorbs so that the signal is the negative of a standard absorption signal. The result is obtained by making Δ negative in Eqs. (11-2) and (11-3). No other permutation of the system brings in any significantly different behavior.

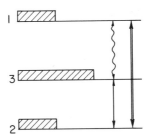

FIG. 11-3 Population inversion in a three-level system as a result of saturation of an EPR transition. The system is essentially the same as in Fig. 11-2 except that $\Delta < 0$. It is also assumed that the relaxation rate between states 1 and 3 is much faster than between 3 and 2. Observation of the $2 \rightleftharpoons 3$ EPR transition would result in an inverted (emission) signal.

A similar analysis can be carried out for a four-level system exemplifying case (b) of Fig. 11-1. To be specific we will consider the situation shown in Fig. 11-4. The two dominant relaxation processes and the two magnetic dipole transitions are shown. The unsaturated transition between levels 2 and 3 is inverted. Taking $\Delta_1 = E_2 - E_1$ and $\Delta_2 = E_4 - E_3$, we can show that the absorption signal (since it is negative it is actually emission) is proportional to

$$N_2 - N_3 = N \frac{e^{-\Delta_1/kT} - e^{\Delta_2/kT}}{2 + e^{-\Delta_1/kT} + e^{\Delta_2/kT}} \simeq -\frac{N}{4} \frac{\Delta_1 + \Delta_2}{kT}. \tag{11-5}$$

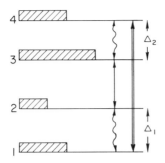

FIG. 11-4   Population inversion in a four-level system as a result of saturation of an EPR transition. Relaxation between states 3 and 4 and between states 1 and 2 is assumed to be much faster than between states 2 and 3. An emission signal would be observed for the $2 \rightleftharpoons 3$ transition.

11-2 Masers

Figures 11-3 and 11-4 illustrate the basic ideas of three- and four-level masers (acronym for microwave amplification by the stimulated emission of radiation) and, if extrapolated to optical frequencies, also for lasers. It would take an unusual paramagnet to have the simple properties we have assumed so far. However, even when all relaxation rates contribute or when complete saturation does not occur, inversion may still result. If a microwave field interacts with such a paramagnet, the field is amplified. If the gain is sufficiently high, oscillation can occur.

If we again consider the three-level paramagnet of Fig. 11-2 but saturate transition $1 \rightleftharpoons 3$ and observe transition $1 \rightleftharpoons 2$, we find a signal proportional to

$$N_1 - N_2 = N \frac{(W_{21} - W_{12}) - (W_{32} - W_{23})}{2W_{21} + 2W_{23} + W_{12} + W_{32}}, \qquad (11\text{-}6)$$

where the W_{ij} are the relaxation rates for transitions from level i to level j (see Section 2–4). Equation (11-6) results from solving the following three equations: $\Sigma_i N_i = N$, $N_1 = N_3$, $dN_2/dt = 0$. The ratios of the phonon emission rates to the phonon absorption rates are given by

$$\frac{W_{21}}{W_{12}} = \exp\left(\frac{E_2 - E_1}{kT}\right),$$

$$\frac{W_{32}}{W_{23}} = \exp\left(\frac{E_3 - E_2}{kT}\right), \qquad (11\text{-}7)$$

which, using the high-temperature approximation, allows us to write Eq. (11-6) as

$$N_1 - N_2 = \frac{N}{3kT} \frac{W_{12}(E_2 - E_1) - W_{23}(E_3 - E_2)}{W_{12} + W_{23}}. \qquad (11\text{-}8)$$

Thus in the high-temperature limit, if inversion is to occur, that is, $N_1 - N_2 < 0$, we must have

$$W_{23}(E_3 - E_2) > W_{12}(E_2 - E_1). \qquad (11\text{-}9)$$

The corresponding result for partial saturation would be still more complicated but would be straightforward, in principle, to calculate.

The major advantage of a maser preamplifier is the possibility of having the paramagnetic material near absolute zero with a corresponding reduction in the noise temperature as compared with conventional microwave preamplification techniques involving hot cathodes.

The first proposal along the lines of the foregoing argument was made by Bloembergen [1], and the first experimental demonstration of such a device operating in the microwave range was given by Scovil, Feher, and Seidel [2]. A lanthanum ethyl sulfate crystal containing 0.5% gadolinium was used as the working substance. For a more detailed discussion of solid-state masers, some of the standard references on the subject should be consulted [3].

It is of considerable scientific interest that the three-level maser preamplifier has been used quite successfully in radio-telescope applications. The 1421 MHz emission line from galactic hydrogen (arising from relative reorientation of the nuclear and electronic magnetic moments that are in hyperfine interaction) is at a frequency which lends itself extremely well to maser amplification, using common microwave sources for the saturating power. Since there is no opportunity to increase the power available from a galactic source, optimum signal-to-noise ratio in the preamplification is the only possible approach to weak source regions of the galaxy.

11-3 Dynamic Nuclear Polarization [4]

Masers involve two transitions in or near the microwave-frequency range. In this section we discuss double resonance phenomena in which one transition is normally in the microwave-frequency range but the other is in the radio-frequency range. The former is an electron paramagnetic resonance transition, whereas the latter is a nuclear magnetic resonance transition.

The simplest system we can study is one having $S = I = \frac{1}{2}$, a four-level system. If we also assume cubic or spherical symmetry, the resultant paramagnet will generally be described by the spin Hamiltonian

$$\mathcal{H} = g\beta\mathbf{H}\cdot\mathbf{S} + A\mathbf{S}\cdot\mathbf{I} - g_n\beta_n\mathbf{H}\cdot\mathbf{I}, \qquad (11\text{-}10)$$

whose solution in first order is [see Eq. (5-75)]

$$E = g\beta H M_S + A M_S M_I - g_n\beta_n H M_I. \qquad (11\text{-}11)$$

We show the four resultant energy levels in Fig. 11-5. We also indicate the dominant transitions resulting from a simple assumption concerning the relaxation. If we assume that modulation of the electronic Zeeman interaction dominates relaxation, that is, that relaxation results from terms of the type THS [see Eqs. (7-6) and (7-9)], then the $\Delta M_S = \pm 1$, $\Delta M_I = 0$ transitions, shown by the vertical lines in Fig. 11-5, would be the most rapid. The "flip-flop" transition $(1 \rightleftharpoons 3)$ corresponding to $\Delta M_S = \pm 1$, $\Delta M_I = \mp 1$ also results from this relaxation mechanism because the two states involved (1 and 3) are not eigenstates of S_3 and I_3 (the components of $\mathbf{S}$ and $\mathbf{I}$ along $\mathbf{H}$). The term proportional to $S_+I_- + S_-I_+$ in the spin Hamiltonian (written in the 123-coordinate system) causes the high-field states with quantum numbers $M_S = -\frac{1}{2}$, $M_I = \frac{1}{2}$ and $M_S = \frac{1}{2}$, $M_I = -\frac{1}{2}$ to be mixed in moderate magnetic fields. This admixture allows matrix elements of THS-type operators between states 1 and 3, causing this relaxation to occur.

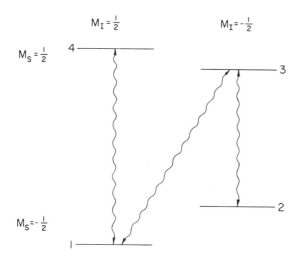

FIG. 11-5   The energy levels for a system with $S = I = \frac{1}{2}$, assuming $g > 0$, $A > 0$, and $g_n > 0$. The relaxation transitions which dominate are shown by wavy lines. The Hamiltonian of the system is given in Eq. (11-10).

If for the present argument we assume that all possible transitions are resolved, we can attempt to influence the nuclear level populations and hence enhance or invert the NMR transitions or simply polarize the nuclei by saturating any of three EPR transitions. The two transitions allowed in high field ($1 \rightleftharpoons 4$ and $2 \rightleftharpoons 3$ or $\Delta M_S = \pm 1$, $\Delta M_I = 0$) result from components of H_1 normal to H, whereas the transition allowed only if A is not negligible compared to $g\beta H$ ($1 \rightleftharpoons 3$ or $\Delta M_S = \pm 1$, $\Delta M_I = \mp 1$) arises only if components of H_1 parallel to H are present. As in Sections 11–1 and 11–2, we obtain simple results easily if we consider complete saturation. Neglecting the effect of all energy splittings on the populations except $g\beta H \equiv \Delta$, and making the high-temperature approximation, we obtain the results given in Table 11-1. Actually the population differences in thermal equilibrium are not zero, as implied by Table 11-1, but rather the small values given by

$$N_1 - N_2 = N_3 - N_4 = \frac{N}{4}\frac{A}{2kT},$$

$$N_1 + N_4 - N_2 - N_3 = \frac{N}{2}\frac{\delta}{kT},$$

(11-12)

Table 11-1

Effect of Saturating EPR Transitions on Nuclear Populations for the System Shown in Fig. 11-5

Transition Saturated	$N_1 - N_2$	$N_3 - N_4$	$N_1 + N_4 - N_2 - N_3$
$1 \rightleftharpoons 4$	0	$-\dfrac{N}{4}\dfrac{\Delta}{kT}$	$\dfrac{N}{4}\dfrac{\Delta}{kT}$
$2 \rightleftharpoons 3$	$\dfrac{N}{4}\dfrac{\Delta}{kT}$	0	$\dfrac{N}{4}\dfrac{\Delta}{kT}$
$1 \rightleftharpoons 3$	$-\dfrac{N}{4}\dfrac{\Delta}{kT}$	$\dfrac{N}{4}\dfrac{\Delta}{kT}$	$-\dfrac{N}{2}\dfrac{\Delta}{kT}$

where $\delta \equiv g_n \beta_n H$, and we have assumed for simplicity that $\Delta \gg A \gg \delta \gg A^2/\Delta$. Thus we find that the observation of either NMR transition ($1 \rightleftharpoons 2$ or $3 \rightleftharpoons 4$) may result in a considerable enhancement of the signal strength. For example, observation of transition $1 \rightleftharpoons 2$ while completely saturating the EPR transition $2 \rightleftharpoons 3$ will increase the signal by the ratio $2\Delta/A$. If, however, the EPR transition between levels 1 and 3 is saturated, then the magnitude of the signal is again increased by the same ratio but the signal is inverted, that is, power is extracted from the sample by the radio-frequency field. The result of observing the two NMR transitions by sweeping the r-f frequency is shown in Fig. 11-6.

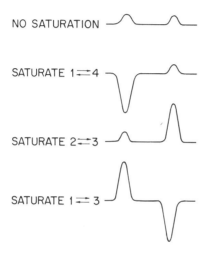

FIG. 11-6 Observation of the NMR transitions by sweeping the frequency for the system depicted in Fig. 11-5. The results are shown for no saturation and for the saturation of the three possible EPR transitions. The ratio of the enhanced to the unenhanced signals is about $2\Delta/A$, where $\Delta = g\beta H$.

If the experiment is not concerned with measuring an NMR signal but monitors nuclear polarization by some other means, then the last column in Table 11-1 is the appropriate population difference, that is, the difference in population for $M_I = \frac{1}{2}$ and $M_I = -\frac{1}{2}$ ("spin up" and "spin down"). Saturation of the weak $1 \rightleftharpoons 3$ EPR transition causes the greatest nuclear polarization. The nuclear polarization of radioactive nuclei can be detected by the anisotropy of the radiation emitted. It is also possible to observe the nuclear polarization if the nuclei in question participate in nuclear scattering [5].

The situation would be somewhat different if the hyperfine splitting made a negligible contribution to the energy and as a result the two allowed EPR transitions ($\Delta M_I = 0$) were not resolved. If we make the same assumption about which relaxation transitions dominate as we did for Fig. 11-5, then we are dealing with the situation shown in Fig. 11-7. If we now saturate the EPR transitions (we must saturate both since they are unresolved), we find that $N_1 = N_3$ and $N_2 = N_4$, but, ignoring $\delta \equiv g_n \beta_n H$ with respect to $\Delta \equiv g\beta H$, we find that $N_4/N_1 = \exp(-\Delta/kT)$. Thus the two coincident NMR transitions have an intensity proportional to $N_1 + N_3 - N_2 - N_4 = (N/2)(\Delta/kT)$ in the high-temperature limit. Hence the NMR signal is enhanced by the ratio Δ/δ. This case is the closest analog in non-metals to the method of polarization first proposed by Overhauser [6] for metals. As a result this polarization technique and other closely related ones are often referred to as the Overhauser effect.

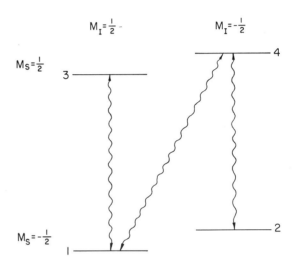

FIG. 11-7   The energy levels for a system with $S = I = \frac{1}{2}$ and negligible hyperfine interaction. The quantities g and g_n are assumed positive. Note that the levels are labeled differently from those in the somewhat similar system in Fig. 11-5, that is, they are labeled from 1 to 4 in order of increasing energy. The dominant relaxation rates are shown by wavy lines.

If we saturate either of the EPR transitions which are forbidden in the absence of electron-nuclear interactions ($1 \rightleftharpoons 4$ or $2 \rightleftharpoons 3$), we have what is referred to as the solid effect [7]. As long as the $\Delta M_I = 0$ relaxation transitions dominate, an enhancement of the NMR signal is obtained. If the $1 \rightleftharpoons 4$ transition is saturated, the NMR signal is proportional to $N_1 + N_3 - N_2 - N_4 = -(N/2)(\Delta/kT)$ and the signal is inverted and enhanced by a factor of Δ/δ. Saturation of the $2 \rightleftharpoons 3$ transition gives the same enhancement but no inversion. For a recent discussion of the solid effect and other competing possibilities see the second reference in citation 4.

In Fig. 11-7, if the relaxation transition between levels 2 and 3 dominates all others for which $\Delta M_I = \pm 1$, then saturation of the normally allowed EPR transitions will cause the NMR signal to be inverted but enhanced by the usual factor of Δ/δ. This is colloquially called the Underhauser effect.

The principal result of all of the dynamic nuclear polarization schemes which we have discussed in this section is the production of nuclear population differences comparable to electronic ones. This means enhancements of nuclear signals which can in principle be of the order of 1000 (the figure is 657 for protons and is larger for most other nuclei). In real situations this ratio is not achieved, a consequence of many complications which we chose to ignore in our simple discussion [8].

11-4 ENDOR [9]

In Section 11-3 we considered the effect on NMR intensities of saturating EPR transitions. In this section we will discuss a technique which employs the saturation of NMR transitions in order to change the intensity of EPR transitions. This phenomenon, which is called ENDOR, an acronym for Electron Nuclear Double Resonance, was first described by Feher [9]. The usual objective in ENDOR experiments is to study NMR transitions of nuclei having significant hyperfine coupling with some paramagnet under circumstances in which the direct observation of an NMR signal, even if enhanced by one of the polarization schemes of Section 11-3, would be difficult or impossible. The result is an increase in the sensitivity to NMR transitions, which measure the hyperfine interaction with a greater accuracy than can be obtained strictly by EPR. In particular it is possible to study hyperfine structure which is unresolved in the EPR spectrum because each hyperfine line is so broad that adjacent lines overlap. The resultant bell-shaped EPR "line" is inhomogeneously broadened.

To illustrate how ENDOR works let us return to the system ($S = \frac{1}{2}$, $I = \frac{1}{2}$) of Fig. 11-5. Making the same assumptions about the dominant relaxation rates and also assuming that all transitions are resolved, we have the situations shown in Fig. 11-8. We show the populations in the high-temperature limit of the four levels, first for complete saturation of the $1 \rightleftharpoons 4$ EPR transition and then for the application of an additional saturating r-f field corresponding to the $3 \rightleftharpoons 4$ NMR transition. As before, we neglect all energy splittings except $\Delta \equiv g\beta H$. Examination of the populations of levels 1 and 4 shows a significant change, $(N/8)(\Delta/kT)$, as a result of saturation of the NMR transition. This suggests that changes may be produced in the EPR signal even though they would not occur here because we have assumed complete saturation of the EPR transition. The result is no signal, because of the equality of the populations. Partial saturation of the EPR transition would lead to a nonzero EPR signal which

would then be changed upon saturation of the NMR signal. We will
analyze this case below.

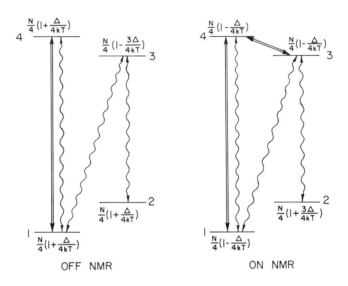

FIG. 11-8 Illustration of how ENDOR works, using the system shown in
Fig. 11-5. Saturation of the $1 \rightleftharpoons 4$ EPR transition yields the population shown
on the left. If in addition the $3 \rightleftharpoons 4$ NMR transition is saturated, the populations
change as shown on the right. If the EPR transition had been only partially
saturated, this effect would have led to a change in the EPR signal which would
occur at nuclear magnetic resonance. This use of an EPR signal to detect an
NMR transition is termed ENDOR (<u>E</u>lectron <u>N</u>uclear <u>D</u>ouble <u>R</u>esonance).

We can see from examining Fig. 11-8 that, had we chosen to saturate
the other NMR transition ($3 \rightleftharpoons 4$), we would observe no change in populations and thus we would not detect this transition by ENDOR (at least
for the simple situation considered here). However, if we were to partially
saturate the other EPR transition ($2 \rightleftharpoons 3$), then we could observe the
$1 \rightleftharpoons 2$ NMR transition but not the one between levels 3 and 4.

To examine this description of ENDOR somewhat more quantitatively,
in fact to actually show that the EPR intensity will respond to the NMR,
let us consider the system of Fig. 11-8 in more detail. Using the simple
assumption concerning the relaxation rates that was made in Section 11-3
after Eq. (11-11), we find the fastest relaxation between levels 1 and 4 and
between levels 2 and 3. The next fastest relaxation is between levels 1 and 3,
the "flip-flop" transition. If we partially saturate the $1 \rightleftharpoons 4$ EPR transition,

that is to say, if an oscillating electromagnetic field stimulates transitions between 1 and 4 at a rate comparable to the relaxation rates, then the rate equation for the population of level 1 is

$$\frac{dN_1}{dt} = -N_1(w + W_{14}) + N_4(w + W_{41}) = 0, \tag{11-13}$$

yielding

$$\frac{N_4}{N_1} = \frac{w + W_{14}}{w + W_{41}} \equiv e^{-\Delta'/kT}, \tag{11-14}$$

where we have considered only the fastest rates in the rate equation: w is the magnetic dipole transition rate, W_{14} is the phonon absorption rate, and W_{41} is the relaxation rate for phonon emission. In Eq. (11-14) we define a quantity Δ' which expresses the extent of saturation. The parameter Δ' is zero for complete saturation and is equal to $\Delta = g\beta H$ for no saturation since $W_{14}/W_{41} = e^{-\Delta/kT}$. The EPR signal in the absence of saturation of the NMR transition is given by the solution of Eq. (11-14) together with

$$\frac{N_3}{N_1} = \frac{N_3}{N_2} = e^{-\Delta/kT}, \tag{11-15}$$

$$N_1 + N_2 + N_3 + N_4 = N.$$

The EPR signal is then proportional to

$$N_1 - N_4 = \frac{N}{4} \frac{\Delta_1}{kT} \left(1 + \frac{\Delta_1}{4kT} + \frac{\Delta}{4kT}\right) \tag{11-16}$$

in the high-temperature limit. If the NMR transition between levels 3 and 4 is saturated, we must solve Eq. (11-14) together with

$$N_3 = N_4, \qquad \frac{N_3}{N_4} = e^{-\Delta/kT}, \tag{11-17}$$

$$N_1 + N_2 + N_3 + N_4 = N,$$

which yields

$$N_1 - N_4 = \frac{N}{4} \frac{\Delta_1}{kT} \left(1 - \frac{3\Delta_1}{4kT} + \frac{\Delta}{4kT}\right). \tag{11-18}$$

The ENDOR signal is proportional to the difference between the EPR signal with NMR saturation and that without, that is,

$$-\frac{N}{8} \frac{\Delta_1}{kT} \frac{\Delta - \Delta_1}{kT}. \tag{11-19}$$

In this case the nuclear saturation produces a decrease in the EPR intensity or a negative ENDOR signal. Had we chosen to partially saturate the $2 \rightleftharpoons 3$ EPR transition, saturation of the $1 \rightleftharpoons 2$ NMR transition would have produced a positive ENDOR signal. If we compare the ENDOR signal intensity to the EPR signal intensity [proportional to Eqs. (11-19) and (11-16), respectively], we find their ratio to be $(\varDelta - \varDelta_1)/2kT$. Since $\varDelta - \varDelta_1$ is comparable to $\varDelta$, we would expect this ratio to vary from about $1/10$ in the liquid-helium temperature range to about $1/1000$ at liquid-nitrogen temperatures. The ENDOR signal is thus somewhat weaker than the EPR signal but more intense than the NMR signal that could be observed directly; the latter could be less intense by six or more orders of magnitude than the EPR signal.

We have chosen a simple model for the ENDOR process and perhaps one that does not correspond to common physical situations. In more realistic situations ENDOR occurs because of transient effects, changes in the effective relaxation time, and nuclear spin diffusion. However, the consequences are roughly the same no matter what the mechanism, that is, NMR transitions can be observed for nuclei which are coupled to the paramagnet directly or indirectly. As a result we observe the hyperfine splittings more directly and usually with much greater precision. The resultant ENDOR spectra were alluded to briefly in the last two paragraphs of Chapter 5.

11-5 Optical Pumping

If a frequency in the optical region is chosen to produce the transition complementary to the microwave EPR transition, the subject of double resonance greatly increases in its variety and complexity. Most studies of electron paramagnetic resonance are concerned with the ground manifold of states, usually those with energies within a few reciprocal centimeters of the lowest level. Combined optical-EPR experiments can extend EPR to excited states. The study of several states is of considerable value in understanding complicated paramagnets, such as defects in solids. Another feature of such combined experiments is the possibility of uniquely and unambiguously relating EPR and optical spectra. In a complicated system several EPR spectra and several optical spectra may be observed. The relationship, if any, to each other can often be difficult to establish in the absence of combined optical-EPR experiments.

A simple model [10] will illustrate most of the possibilities. We will discuss this model with reference to some of the corresponding observations in real and more complicated systems. Consider a paramagnet consisting of four levels, two being the Zeeman levels of a spin-$\frac{1}{2}$ ground-state manifold and the other two being the Zeeman levels for an excited-state manifold with spin of $\frac{1}{2}$. This energy level diagram is shown in Fig. 11-9.

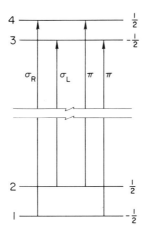

FIG. 11-9 Simple four-level system used to explain optical-EPR double resonance. The system consists of a ground Kramers doublet, levels 1 and 2, and an excited Kramers doublet, levels 3 and 4. The difference in energy between the ground-state manifold and the excited-state manifold lies in the optical frequency region (note the break in the energy scale). The polarization for absorption is shown, under the assumption of electric dipole selection rules between two $J = \frac{1}{2}$ states. The π-polarized transitions occur if the light is polarized parallel to the magnetic field. The σ-polarized components result for polarizations perpendicular to the field. The transition labeled σ_R occurs if right circularly polarized radiation is used, and σ_L occurs for left circular polarization (some authors use the reverse convention on circular polarization).

Normally levels 1 and 2 are within 1 cm^{-1} or less of each other, and both are populated at the temperatures typical of EPR experiments. However, levels 3 and 4 are usually thousands of reciprocal centimeters from 1 and 2. They are never populated thermally, therefore, and one cannot see EPR in the excited state without exciting the system nonthermally.

If we assume that optical transitions between the lower doublet and the upper doublet occur with selection rules characteristic of electric dipole transitions between states with $J = \frac{1}{2}$, we obtain the results for absorption shown in Fig. 11-9. The transitions labeled π are polarized with the electric field parallel to the magnetic field. The transitions labeled σ occur for polarizations in which the electric field is perpendicular to the magnetic field. The two σ transitions correspond to opposite senses of circularly polarized light. Linearly polarized or unpolarized light in which the direction of propagation is along the magnetic field will cause both σ transitions. The role of σ_R and σ_L radiation is reversed for emission. In all cases the frequency of the light must be in resonance with the frequency of the transition, $\Delta E/h$. In addition to the optical resonance transitions, an optical-EPR experiment involves the EPR transitions at microwave frequencies and spin-lattice relaxation.

Two main categories of optical-EPR double resonance experiments exist, those associated with EPR in the excited-state manifold and those involving EPR in the ground-state manifold. Since the excited states cannot be studied without optical excitation, there is potentially more to be learned from studying the excited-state EPR. An important feature of such experiments is that one can replace detection of microwave quanta by detection of optical quanta. The much greater sensitivity possible in detection of the higher-energy optical quanta can be exploited for either ground or excited states. It is also possible to relate either kind of EPR observation to the optical properties of the sample.

Possibly the most straightforward optical-EPR double resonance experiment is one in which the EPR of the ground-state manifold is detected directly by the usual microwave techniques. Resonance optical radiation is then allowed to cause transitions, and the resultant changes in the ground-state EPR are studied. If the four optical transitions among the Zeeman levels are resolved, they can be excited individually. If this is not the case, transitions can be selected on the basis of their polarization selection rules (see Fig. 11-9). As an example consider the use of right circularly polarized light to cause transition $1 \rightarrow 4$. If radiative decay from the excited state is more probable than relaxation between the excited Zeeman levels, then state 4 will decay to states 1 and 2 by emission of photons of the appropriate polarization. Decays which repopulate level 1 may again lead to optical absorption and a transition to state 4. In this way, if ground-state spin-lattice relaxation did not intervene, all of the paramagnets would eventually be pumped into state 2. The attendant EPR would then be an emission signal of large intensity. The actual alteration in population would be determined by the competition between the optical pumping rate and the spin-lattice relaxation (or conceivably the EPR transition rate). Clearly relaxation within the excited-state manifold also reduces the effect.

If a sufficient overpopulation of state 2 is achieved, one can obtain maser action (see Section 11–2). Optically pumped microwave masers have been operated in a number of materials [11]. In addition changes in ground-state EPR intensities, frequently including changes from absorption to emission, have been observed in many materials [12]. Not all of these observations can be explained by the simple arguments just given. A closely related observation is that of nuclear spin polarization by optical pumping [13].

A simple variation of the experiment discussed above leads to optical detection of the ground-state EPR. Consider again the excitation of transition $1 \rightarrow 4$ by circularly polarized resonance radiation. If the optical pumping of the paramagnets proceeded until virtually all were in state 2, the absorption of the circularly polarized radiation would decrease to a negligible value. Absorption will recur, however, if transitions between states 1 and 2 are induced by a microwave field. In this way the ground-state EPR can be observed by the change in absorption of the resonance radiation; this constitutes a commonly used technique for optical pumping in gases [14]. We will not discuss this subject although it is very similar in many ways to the solid-state aspects, which we do treat. Changes in optical absorption caused by EPR transitions have been observed in several materials [15]. Somewhat similar experiments in which changes in the optical Faraday rotation were used to detect EPR have been reported [16].

Again using the simple system of Fig. 11-9, we can detect the ground-state EPR by observation of the emitted light. Consider the case in which either σ- or π-polarized light causes transitions to states 3 and 4. Since the thermal equilibrium populations of levels 1 and 2 will be different, we would expect that the populations of levels 3 and 4 would likewise differ (again assuming that radiative decay occurs before spin-lattice relaxation). Thus, if we were to examine any of the four optical emission lines, assuming that they are resolvable, the effect of saturating the ground-state EPR could be seen. This would be possible because equalizing the population of levels 1 and 2 will cause levels 3 and 4 to have equal populations, thereby changing the intensity of the emission lines. This type of effect has been seen in $Al_2O_3 : Cr^{3+}$, although the system is considerably more complicated [17]. Several variations of this scheme could be imagined, such as observing the change in the intensity of the circularly polarized emission coming out parallel to the magnetic field. It is possible also to conceive of a variety of pumping schemes, such as pumping a single resolved transition or using only one circularly polarized σ component.

The experiments discussed so far in this section involved the EPR of the ground-state manifold. It is also possible to study the excited-state EPR. The most straightforward way in principle, although not necessarily in practice, is to generate a sufficient excited-state population to observe the EPR directly as a microwave absorption. This can occur for the simple system of Fig. 11-9 if we use light to produce transitions to the excited state. If the radiative lifetime is long enough, this population may be sufficient for the detection of microwave absorption. The required population difference between levels 3 and 4 may result from thermalization in the excited state or from the use of polarized light to preferentially populate the levels. In practice such experiments are usually performed on long-lived metastable states, which must be populated indirectly. The direct transitions to such states are too weak to permit the generation of significant excited-state populations with available light sources. A number of excited states have been studied by direct detection of the EPR [18].

Direct detection of the excited-state EPR does not take advantage of the gain in sensitivity that can be obtained by detecting optical quanta.

There are many ways of doing this, but a change in the nature of the luminescent emission is probably the most obvious. Referring again to Fig. 11-9, consider the case in which the four optical absorption or emission lines are resolvable. If we were to excite the $1 \to 4$ transition and observe the emission from the $3 \to 1$ transition, we would expect to see nothing if spin-lattice relaxation in the excited state is much slower than the radiative decay. However, if EPR transitions between states 3 and 4 are excited, then the $3 \to 1$ emission will occur and can be used to monitor the excited-state EPR. Such an experiment has been performed for Cr^{3+} in Al_2O_3 [19], although the system is more complicated than our simple example.

If the optical Zeeman spectrum was not resolved, it would still be possible to observe the EPR in the excited state by observing the effect on the circularly polarized components of the emission. If we assume thermalization in the excited state, then level 3 will have a greater population than level 4 and the emission will have a right circularly polarized component which is larger than the left circularly polarized component. Saturation of the $3 \rightleftharpoons 4$ EPR transition will reduce the right circularly polarized component and increase the left circularly polarized component. The excited state of Mn^{4+} in Al_2O_3 has been observed in essentially this way [20], and the excited states of Cr^{3+} and V^{2+} in MgO and of Eu^{2+} in CaF_2 and SrF_2 have also been studied [21]. In these latter systems the excited states are ^2E_g states; hence the observed EPR spectra are characteristic of the dynamic Jahn-Teller effect discussed in Section 10–4. For Eu^{2+} in CaF_2 a microwave modulation of the emission is observed to result from the excited-state EPR [22]. This coherence effect cannot be explained by our simple model using population arguments alone. The effect is similar to the existence of a transverse magnetization precessing about a static magnetic field at the Larmor frequency (see Chapter 2).

Another method of optically detecting the excited-state EPR involves observing changes in the emission intensity which arise from selective reabsorption of the emitted light. If for Fig. 11-9 the two σ transitions are resolved, then σ light emitted in the fluorescence of this system will be more strongly reabsorbed by the $1 \to 4$ transition of other similar paramagnets in the crystal than it will be by the $2 \to 3$ transition. This is so because of the greater population of level 1 in thermal equilibrium. Thus, if we monitor the total intensity of the σ-polarized light normal to the magnetic field, we would expect to see a change in the intensity if the relative populations of levels 3 and 4 were disturbed by EPR in the excited state. This approach has been used to study Cr^{3+} in Al_2O_3 [23].

Just as the ground-state EPR could be observed by changes in the optical emission, so it is possible to observe the effect of excited-state EPR on the absorption. This has been done for F centers (an electron trapped at a negative-ion vacancy) in alkali halides [24] by observing the change in the absorption of circularly polarized light resulting from EPR in the excited state. This technique has been elaborated so that ENDOR is observed in the excited state of F centers in KI [25], a microwave–optical–radio-frequency triple resonance experiment (see also reference 13).

Although we will not discuss optical pumping for electrons in the energy bands of solids, several recent papers have considered this topic[26]. Finally we note that some of the advantages of optical-EPR double resonance experiments also result from the use of light to change the charge states of paramagnetic defects in crystals [27].

References Cited in Chapter 11

[1] N. Bloembergen, *Phys. Rev.* **104**, 324 (1956).

[2] H. E. D. Scovil, G. Feher, and H. Seidel, *Phys. Rev.* **105**, 762 (1957).

[3] J. R. Singer, *Masers*, Wiley, New York, 1959; A. A. Vuylsteke, *Elements of Maser Theory*, Van Nostrand, Princeton, N.J., 1960; A. E. Siegman, *Microwave Solid State Masers*, McGraw-Hill, New York, 1963. Also consult H. W. Moos, *Am. J. Phys.* **32**, 589 (1964) for additional references.

[4] For more information see C. D. Jeffries, *Dynamic Nuclear Orientation*, Interscience, New York, 1963. A brief indication of recent developments is given in M. Borghini and K. Scheffer, *Phys. Rev. Letters* **26**, 1362 (1971).

[5] See *Polarization Phenomena in Nuclear Reactions* (H. H. Barschall and W. Haeberli, eds.), University of Wisconsin Press, Madison, Wisc., 1971, and the proceedings of earlier symposia in the series.

[6] A. W. Overhauser, *Phys. Rev.* **89**, 689 (1953); *Phys. Rev.* **92**, 411 (1953).

[7] A. Abragam and W. G. Proctor, *Compt. Rend.* **246**, 2253 (1958).

[8] See reference 4 and M. Borghini, *Phys. Rev. Letters* **16**, 318 (1966); T. B. J. Swanenburg, G. M. Van den Heuvel, and N. J. Poulis, *Physica* **35**, 369 (1967); J. J. Hill, *Phys. Rev.* **157**, 204 (1967).

[9] G. Feher, *Phys. Rev.* **103**, 834 (1956). For an extensive discussion of the subject see Chapter 4 of A. Abragam and B. Bleaney, *Electron Paramagnetic Resonance of Transition Ions*, Oxford, New York, 1970.

[10] S. Geschwind, G. E. Devlin, R. L. Cohen, and S. R. Chinn, *Phys. Rev.* **137**, A1087 (1965); S. Geschwind, "Special Topics in Hyperfine Structure in EPR," in *Hyperfine Interactions* (A. J. Freeman and R. B. Frankel, eds.), Academic, New York, 1967.

[11] D. P. Devor, I. J. D'Haenens, and C. K. Asawa, *Phys. Rev. Letters* **8**, 432 (1962); E. S. Sabisky and C. H. Anderson, *Appl. Phys. Letters* **8**, 298 (1966); E. S. Sabisky and C. H. Anderson, *IEEE J. Quantum Electronics* **QE-3**, 287 (1967).

[12] B. R. McAvoy, D. W. Feldman, J. G. Castle, Jr., and R. W. Warren, *Phys. Rev. Letters* **6**, 618 (1961); N. V. Karlov, J. Margerie, and Y. Merle D'Aubigne, *J. Phys. Radium (France)* **24**, 717 (1963); D. H. Tanimoto, W. M. Ziniker, and J. O. Kemp, *Phys. Rev. Letters* **14**, 645 (1965); C. H. Anderson, H. A. Weakliem, and E. S. Sabisky, *Phys. Rev.* **143**, 223 (1966).

[13] W. B. Grant, L. F. Mollenauer, and C. D. Jeffries, *Phys. Rev.* **B4**, 1428 (1971).

[14] T. R. Carver, *Science* **141**, 599 (1963).

[15] I. Wieder, *Phys. Rev. Letters* **3**, 468 (1959); C. K. Asawa and R. A. Satten, *Phys. Rev.* **127**, 1542 (1962); H. Panepucci and L. F. Mollenauer, *Phys. Rev.* **178**, 589 (1969).

[16] J. M. Daniels and H. Wesemeyer, *Can. J. Phys.* **36**, 405 (1958); K. E. Rieckhoff and D. J. Griffiths, *Can. J. Phys.* **41**, 33 (1963); Y. Hayashi, M. Fukui, and H. Yoshioka, *J. Phys. Soc. Japan* **23**, 312 (1967).

[17] G. F. Imbusch and S. Geschwind, *Phys. Rev. Letters* **17**, 238 (1966).

[18] C. A. Hutchison, Jr., and B. W. Mangum, *J. Chem. Phys.* **34**, 908 (1961); H. Seidel, *Phys. Letters* **7**, 27 (1963); R. W. Brandon, R. E. Gerkin, and C. A. Hutchison, Jr., *J. Chem. Phys.* **41**, 3717 (1964); E. S. Sabisky and C. H. Anderson, *Phys. Rev. Letters* **13**, 754 (1964); E. S. Sabisky and C. H. Anderson, *Phys. Rev.* **148**, 194 (1966); R. H. Clarke and C. A. Hutchison, Jr., *J. Chem. Phys.* **54**, 2962 (1971); R. H. Clarke and C. A. Hutchison, Jr., *Phys. Rev. Letters* **27**, 638 (1971).

[19] S. Geschwind, G. E. Devlin, R. L. Cohen, and S. R. Chinn, *Phys. Rev.* **137**, A1087 (1965).

[20] G. F. Imbusch, S. R. Chinn, and S. Geschwind, *Phys. Rev.* **161**, 295 (1967).

[21] L. L. Chase, *Phys. Rev.* **168**, 341 (1968); L. L. Chase, *Phys. Rev.* **B2**, 2308 (1970).

[22] L. L. Chase, *Phys. Rev. Letters* **21**, 888 (1968).

[23] S. Geschwind, R. J. Collins, and A. L. Schawlow, *Phys. Rev. Letters* **3**, 545 (1959); W. H. Culver, R. A. Satten, and C. R. Viswanathan, *J. Chem. Phys.* **38**, 775 (1963).

[24] L. F. Mollenauer, S. Pan, and S. Yngvesson, *Phys. Rev. Letters* **23**, 683 (1969).

[25] L. F. Mollenauer, S. Pan, and A. Winnacker, *Phys. Rev. Letters* **26**, 1643 (1971).

[26] G. Lampel, *Phys. Rev. Letters* **20**, 491 (1968); R. R. Parsons, *Phys. Rev. Letters* **23**, 1152 (1969); C. Hermann and G. Lampel, *Phys. Rev. Letters* **27**, 373 (1971).

[27] W. C. Holton, J. Schneider, and T. L. Estle, *Phys. Rev.* **133**, A1638 (1964).

APPENDIX A

Quantum-Mechanical Properties of Angular Momenta

We list below a number of the more useful properties of angular momenta (in units of $\hbar$). Everything will be given in terms of **J**, but one can equally well consider any of the standard angular momenta— **J, L, S, I, F, l, s, j**, etc.—to be involved.

1. Commutators

$$[J_a, J_b] \equiv J_a J_b - J_b J_a = iJ_c$$

Here a, b, c are x, y, z or a cyclic permutation (all other commutators are zero).

2. Raising and Lowering Operators

$$J_+ \equiv J_x + iJ_y \qquad\qquad J_x = \tfrac{1}{2}(J_+ + J_-)$$

$$J_- \equiv J_x - iJ_y \qquad\qquad J_y = \frac{1}{2i}(J_+ - J_-)$$

3. Commutators Again

$$[J_z, J_\pm] = \pm J_\pm$$

$$[J_+, J_-] = 2J_z$$

4. The Operations

$$J_z |M_J\rangle = M_J |M_J\rangle \qquad\qquad \mathbf{J}^2 |M_J\rangle = J(J+1)|M_J\rangle$$

$$J_\pm |M_J\rangle = \sqrt{J(J+1) - M_J(M_J \pm 1)}\,|M_J \pm 1\rangle$$

5. Orbital Angular Momentum

$$l_x = -i\left(y\frac{\partial}{\partial z} - z\frac{\partial}{\partial y}\right) \text{ and cyclic permutations of } x, y, z.$$

6.   Irreducible Tensor Operators

$$[J_z, T_{lm}] = m T_{lm}$$

$$[J_\pm, T_{lm}] = \sqrt{l(l+1) - m(m \pm 1)} \, T_{lm \pm 1}$$

Hence $T_{11} = -J_+$, $T_{10} = \sqrt{2} J_z$, $T_{1-1} = J_-$ are components of an irreducible tensor operator.

7.   Coupling of Two Angular Momenta

$$\mathbf{J} = \mathbf{j}_1 + \mathbf{j}_2$$

$$|J, M\rangle = \sum_{\substack{m_1, m_2 \\ m_1 + m_2 = M}} \langle j_1 m_1 j_2 m_2 | j_1 j_2 J M \rangle |j_1 m_1\rangle |j_2 m_2\rangle$$

where $\langle j_1 m_1 j_2 m_2 | j_1 j_2 J M \rangle$ are Clebsch-Gordan coefficients (see, for example, M. Tinkham, *Group Theory and Quantum Mechanics*, McGraw-Hill, New York, 1964).

Solutions of the Spin Hamiltonian Eigenvalue Problem to Second Order

In Chapter 5 we confined our attention almost exclusively to first-order calculations. Although this restriction is simple and convenient when discussing qualitative features, such treatment is frequently inadequate when making precise quantitative comparisons with experiment. In this appendix we illustrate only one of a large number of possible second-order calculations, namely, the solution of the eigenvalue problem for Eq. (5-57):

$$\mathcal{H} = \beta \mathbf{H} \cdot \mathbf{g} \cdot \mathbf{S} + \mathbf{S} \cdot \mathbf{A} \cdot \mathbf{I}, \tag{B-1}$$

where we assume that the second term (the hyperfine interaction) is small in relation to the first term. Following Section 5-3, we write the Hamiltonian in terms of ζ and ζ' so that $\hat{\zeta} = \mathbf{H} \cdot \mathbf{g}/gH$ and $\hat{\zeta}' = \mathbf{H} \cdot \mathbf{g} \cdot \mathbf{A}/gHK$. For this choice of axes there are no terms in the Hamiltonian involving S_ξ or S_η alone and no terms involving $S_\zeta I_{\xi'}$ or $S_\zeta I_{\eta'}$. There are, however, terms in the hyperfine interaction involving S_ξ and S_η, and these produce the higher-order effects.

To write these terms let us develop convenient expressions for the several coordinate systems involved. We show these in Fig. B-1. The η and η' axes are chosen to be in the xy plane. From this we see that

$$\hat{\zeta} = \frac{\mathbf{H} \cdot \mathbf{g}}{gH}, \qquad \hat{\zeta}' = \frac{\mathbf{H} \cdot \mathbf{g} \cdot \mathbf{A}}{gHK},$$

$$\hat{\eta} = \frac{\hat{\zeta} \times \hat{\mathbf{z}}}{|\hat{\zeta} \times \hat{\mathbf{z}}|}, \qquad \hat{\eta}' = \frac{\hat{\zeta}' \times \hat{\mathbf{z}}}{|\hat{\zeta}' \times \hat{\mathbf{z}}|}, \tag{B-2}$$

$$\hat{\xi} = \hat{\eta} \times \hat{\zeta}, \qquad \hat{\xi}' = \hat{\eta}' \times \hat{\zeta}'.$$

We may now write Eq. (B-1) in terms of these coordinates, with the result

$$\mathcal{H} = g\beta H S_\zeta + K S_\zeta I_{\zeta'} + \hat{\eta} \cdot \mathbf{A} \cdot \hat{\zeta}' S_\eta I_{\zeta'} + \hat{\xi} \cdot \mathbf{A} \cdot \hat{\zeta}' S_\xi I_{\zeta'}$$

$$+ \hat{\eta} \cdot \mathbf{A} \cdot \hat{\eta}' S_\eta I_{\eta'} + \hat{\eta} \cdot \mathbf{A} \cdot \hat{\xi}' S_\eta I_{\xi'} + \hat{\xi} \cdot \mathbf{A} \cdot \hat{\eta}' S_\xi I_{\eta'} + \hat{\xi} \cdot \mathbf{A} \cdot \hat{\xi}' S_\xi I_{\xi'}. \tag{B-3}$$

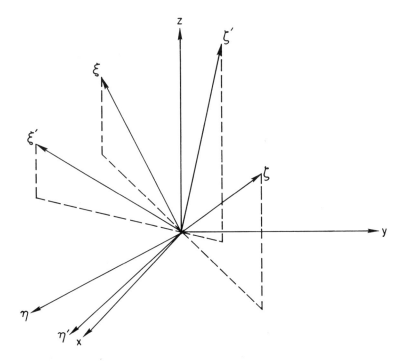

FIG. B-1   Coordinate systems used in the second-order solutions of the eigen-value problem arising from the Hamiltonian of Eq. (B-1). The Cartesian coor-dinate system xyz is determined by the principal axes or symmetry axes of the paramagnet. The Cartesian coordinate system $\xi\eta\zeta$ is determined by taking the ζ axis to be along $\mathbf{H}\cdot\mathbf{g}$ and η to be in the xy plane. Using this coordinate system the only spin operator in the Hamiltonian for the Zeeman interaction is S_ζ and the electronic spin is quantized along the ζ axis. Similarly the coordinate system $\xi'\eta'\zeta'$ is determined by choosing ζ' to be parallel to $\mathbf{H}\cdot\mathbf{g}\cdot\mathbf{A}$ and requiring that η' be in the xy plane. The first-order solutions result from diagonal nuclear spin operators ($I_{\zeta'}$ only) if the nuclear spin is quantized along ζ'.

It is more convenient to work with the raising and lowering operators (see Appendix A):

$$S_\xi = \tfrac{1}{2}(S_+ + S_-), \qquad S_\eta = \frac{1}{2i}(S_+ - S_-),$$

$$I_{\xi'} = \tfrac{1}{2}(I_+ + I_-), \qquad I_{\eta'} = \frac{1}{2i}(I_+ - I_-).$$

$$(B\text{-}4)$$

Note that $S_\pm$ and $I_\pm$ are referred to different coordinate systems, neither of which is a principal axis system in general. Thus we have

$$\mathcal{H} = g\beta H S_\zeta + K S_\zeta I_{\zeta'} + \left(\frac{1}{2i}\hat{\mathbf{\eta}}\cdot\mathbf{A}\cdot\hat{\mathbf{\zeta}}' + \tfrac{1}{2}\hat{\mathbf{\xi}}\cdot\mathbf{A}\cdot\hat{\mathbf{\zeta}}'\right)S_+ I_{\zeta'}$$

$$+\left(-\frac{1}{2i}\hat{\mathbf{\eta}}\cdot\mathbf{A}\cdot\hat{\mathbf{\zeta}}' + \tfrac{1}{2}\hat{\mathbf{\xi}}\cdot\mathbf{A}\cdot\hat{\mathbf{\zeta}}'\right)S_- I_{\zeta'}$$

$$+\left(-\tfrac{1}{4}\hat{\mathbf{\eta}}\cdot\mathbf{A}\cdot\hat{\mathbf{\eta}}' + \frac{1}{4i}\hat{\mathbf{\eta}}\cdot\mathbf{A}\cdot\hat{\mathbf{\xi}}' + \frac{1}{4i}\hat{\mathbf{\xi}}\cdot\mathbf{A}\cdot\hat{\mathbf{\eta}}' \quad \tfrac{1}{4}\hat{\mathbf{\xi}}\cdot\mathbf{A}\cdot\hat{\mathbf{\xi}}'\right)S_+ I_+$$

$$\text{(B-5)}$$

$$+\left(-\tfrac{1}{4}\hat{\mathbf{\eta}}\cdot\mathbf{A}\cdot\hat{\mathbf{\eta}}' - \frac{1}{4i}\hat{\mathbf{\eta}}\cdot\mathbf{A}\cdot\hat{\mathbf{\xi}}' - \frac{1}{4i}\hat{\mathbf{\xi}}\cdot\mathbf{A}\cdot\hat{\mathbf{\eta}}' + \tfrac{1}{4}\hat{\mathbf{\xi}}\cdot\mathbf{A}\cdot\hat{\mathbf{\xi}}'\right)S_- I_-$$

$$+\left(\tfrac{1}{4}\hat{\mathbf{\eta}}\cdot\mathbf{A}\cdot\hat{\mathbf{\eta}}' + \frac{1}{4i}\hat{\mathbf{\eta}}\cdot\mathbf{A}\cdot\hat{\mathbf{\xi}}' - \frac{1}{4i}\hat{\mathbf{\xi}}\cdot\mathbf{A}\cdot\hat{\mathbf{\eta}}' + \tfrac{1}{4}\hat{\mathbf{\xi}}\cdot\mathbf{A}\cdot\hat{\mathbf{\xi}}'\right)S_+ I_-$$

$$+\left(\tfrac{1}{4}\hat{\mathbf{\eta}}\cdot\mathbf{A}\cdot\hat{\mathbf{\eta}}' - \frac{1}{4i}\hat{\mathbf{\eta}}\cdot\mathbf{A}\cdot\hat{\mathbf{\xi}}' + \frac{1}{4i}\hat{\mathbf{\xi}}\cdot\mathbf{A}\cdot\hat{\mathbf{\eta}}' + \tfrac{1}{4}\hat{\mathbf{\xi}}\cdot\mathbf{A}\cdot\hat{\mathbf{\xi}}'\right)S_- I_+ \,.$$

Before analyzing the general case let us specialize to the well-studied case of axial, hexagonal, trigonal, or tetragonal symmetry and symmetric tensors. Writing all vector and tensor components in terms of the principal axis coordinate system, x, y, z, we have

$$\mathbf{H} = H(l, m, n),$$

$$\mathbf{g} = \begin{pmatrix} g_\perp & 0 & 0 \\ 0 & g_\perp & 0 \\ 0 & 0 & g_\parallel \end{pmatrix},$$

$$\text{(B-6)}$$

$$\mathbf{A} = \begin{pmatrix} B & 0 & 0 \\ 0 & B & 0 \\ 0 & 0 & A \end{pmatrix}.$$

From these we can now calculate the required unit vectors:

$$\hat{\mathbf{\zeta}} = \frac{1}{g}(lg_\perp, mg_\perp, ng_\parallel), \qquad g = \sqrt{g_\perp^2(l^2+m^2)+g_\parallel^2 n^2},$$

$$\zeta' = \frac{1}{gK}(lg_\perp B, \, mg_\perp B, \, ng_\parallel A), \qquad gK = \sqrt{g_\perp^2 B^2(l^2+m^2)+g_\parallel^2 A^2 n^2},$$

$$\hat{\eta} = \hat{\eta}' = \frac{1}{\sqrt{l^2+m^2}}(m, \, -l, \, 0), \tag{B-7}$$

$$\hat{\xi} = \frac{1}{g\sqrt{l^2+m^2}}[-nlg_\parallel, \, -mng_\parallel, \, (l^2+m^2)g_\perp],$$

$$\hat{\xi}' = \frac{1}{gK\sqrt{l^2+m^2}}[-nlg_\parallel A, \, -mng_\parallel A, \, (l^2+m^2)g_\perp B].$$

Calculating now the proper mixed components of **A**, we obtain

$$\hat{\eta} \cdot \mathbf{A} \cdot \hat{\zeta}' = 0,$$

$$\hat{\xi} \cdot \mathbf{A} \cdot \hat{\zeta}' = n\sqrt{l^2+m^2}\,\frac{g_\parallel g_\perp}{g^2}\frac{A^2-B^2}{K},$$

$$\hat{\eta} \cdot \mathbf{A} \cdot \hat{\eta}' = B,$$

$$\hat{\eta} \cdot \mathbf{A} \cdot \hat{\xi}' = 0, \tag{B-8}$$

$$\hat{\xi} \cdot \mathbf{A} \cdot \hat{\eta}' = 0,$$

$$\hat{\xi} \cdot \mathbf{A} \cdot \hat{\xi}' = \frac{AB}{K}.$$

Substituting in Eq. (B-5), we obtain

$$\mathcal{H} = g\beta H S_\zeta + K S_\zeta I_{\zeta'} + \tfrac{1}{2}n\sqrt{l^2+m^2}\,\frac{g_\parallel g_\perp}{g^2}\frac{A^2-B^2}{K}(S_+I_{\zeta'}+S_-I_{\zeta'})$$

$$+ \frac{1}{4}\frac{B(A-K)}{K}(S_+I_+ + S_-I_-) + \frac{1}{4}\frac{B(A+K)}{K}(S_+I_- + S_-I_+).$$

$$\tag{B-9}$$

To solve for the energy we will use perturbation theory [Eq. (5-99)]. We will take the first two terms in Eq. (B-9) as the unperturbed Hamiltonian; the remainder is the perturbation. In this way all diagonal matrix elements belong to the unperturbed Hamiltonian and all off-diagonal matrix elements represent perturbations. Thus to second order we obtain

$$E = g\beta H_{\perp s} + KM_S M_I + \tfrac{1}{2}n^2(l^2 + m^2)\frac{g_{\parallel}^2 g_{\perp}^2}{g^4}\frac{(A^2 - B^2)^2}{K^2}\frac{_s M_I^2}{g\beta H}$$

$$+ \frac{1}{4}\frac{B^2(A^2 + K^2)}{K^2 g\beta H}M_S[I(I+1) - M_I^2] - \frac{1}{2}\frac{AB^2}{Kg\beta H}M_S[S(S+1) - M_S^2].$$

$$\text{(B-10)}$$

Calculating the energy difference for the strong $\Delta M_S = \pm 1$, $\Delta M_I = 0$ transitions, we obtain

$$h\nu = E(M_S) - E(M_S - 1) = g\beta H + KM_I + \tfrac{1}{2}n^2(1 - n^2)\frac{g_{\parallel}^2 g_{\perp}^2}{g^4}\frac{(A^2 - B^2)^2}{K^2}\frac{M_I^2}{g\beta H}$$

$$+ \frac{1}{4}\frac{B^2(A^2 + K^2)}{K^2 g\beta H}[I(I+1) - M_I^2] + \frac{1}{2}\frac{AB^2}{Kg\beta H}M_I(2M_S - 1). \quad \text{(B-11)}$$

The magnetic field can then be obtained as

$$H = \frac{h\nu}{g\beta} - \frac{K}{g\beta}M_I - \tfrac{1}{2}n^2(1 - n^2)\frac{g_{\parallel}^2 g_{\perp}^2}{g^4}\frac{(A^2 - B^2)^2}{g\beta K^2 h\nu}M_I^2$$

$$- \frac{1}{4}\frac{B^2(A^2 + K^2)}{g\beta K^2 h\nu}[I(I+1) - M_I^2] - \frac{1}{2}\frac{AB^2}{g\beta Kh\nu}M_I(2M_S - 1). \quad \text{(B-12)}$$

Returning now to the general case and Eq. (B-5), let us define three quantities as follows:

$$K_1 \equiv \tfrac{1}{2}\hat{\xi}\cdot \mathbf{A}\cdot \hat{\zeta}' + \frac{1}{2i}\hat{\eta}\cdot \mathbf{A}\cdot \hat{\zeta}',$$

$$K_2 \equiv \tfrac{1}{4}\hat{\xi}\cdot \mathbf{A}\cdot \hat{\xi}' - \tfrac{1}{4}\hat{\eta}\cdot \mathbf{A}\cdot \hat{\eta}' + \frac{1}{4i}\hat{\xi}\cdot \mathbf{A}\cdot \hat{\eta}' + \frac{1}{4i}\hat{\eta}\cdot \mathbf{A}\cdot \hat{\xi}', \quad \text{(B-13)}$$

$$K_3 \equiv \tfrac{1}{4}\hat{\xi}\cdot \mathbf{A}\cdot \hat{\xi}' + \tfrac{1}{4}\hat{\eta}\cdot \mathbf{A}\cdot \hat{\eta}' - \frac{1}{4i}\hat{\xi}\cdot \mathbf{A}\cdot \hat{\eta}' + \frac{1}{4i}\hat{\eta}\cdot \mathbf{A}\cdot \hat{\xi}'.$$

In terms of these quantities our Hamiltonian [Eq. (B-5)] has the form

$$\mathcal{H} = g\beta H S_{\zeta} + KS_{\zeta}I_{\zeta'} + K_1 S_+ I_{\zeta'} + K_1^* S_- I_{\zeta'} + K_2 S_+ I_+ + K_2^* S_- I_-$$

$$+ K_3 S_+ I_- + K_3^* S_- I_+. \quad \text{(B-14)}$$

Using perturbation theory taken to second order to solve Eq. (B-14) just as we did for Eq. (B-9), we obtain

$$E = g\beta HM_S + KM_SM_I$$

$$+ \frac{2}{g\beta H}\{|K_1|^2 M_S M_I^2 + (|K_2|^2 - |K_3|^2)[S(S+1) - M_S^2]M_I$$

$$+ (|K_2|^2 + |K_3|^2)M_S[I(I+1) - M_I^2]\}. \tag{B-15}$$

This result is a generalization of Eq. (B-10). The solution for a given symmetry involves the calculation of $|K_1|^2$, $|K_2|^2$, and $|K_3|^2$, as well as g and K required for the first-order description.

To illustrate the use of Eq. (B-15) we consider the case of orthorhombic symmetry (D_{2h}, D_2, C_{2v}), described in first order by Eqs. (5-10), (5-60), and (5-64). Using Eqs. (5-10), (5-62), (5-64), and (B-2), we have

$$\hat{\zeta} = g^{-1}(g_x l, g_y m, g_z n),$$

$$\hat{\eta} = (g_x^2 l^2 + g_y^2 m^2)^{-1/2}(g_y m, -g_x l, 0),$$

$$\hat{\xi} = g^{-1}(g_x^2 l^2 + g_y^2 m^2)^{-1/2}(-g_z g_x nl, -g_y g_z mn, g_x^2 l^2 + g_y^2 m^2),$$

$$\hat{\zeta}' = (gK)^{-1}(A_x g_x l, A_y g_y m, A_z g_z n), \tag{B-16}$$

$$\hat{\eta}' = (A_x^2 g_x^2 l^2 + A_y^2 g_y^2 m^2)^{-1/2}(A_y g_y m, -A_x g_x l, 0),$$

$$\hat{\xi}' = (gK)^{-1}(A_x^2 g_x^2 l^2 + A_y^2 g_y^2 m^2)^{-1/2}(-A_z A_x g_z g_x nl,$$

$$- A_y A_z g_y g_z mn, A_x^2 g_x^2 l^2 + A_y^2 g_y^2 m^2).$$

We obtain the required coefficients, given in Eq. (B-13), as

$$|K_1|^2 = \frac{1}{4g^2 K^2}(A_x^4 g_x^2 l^2 + A_y^4 g_y^2 m^2 + A_z^4 g_z^2 n^2 - g^2 K^4),$$

$$|K_2|^2 - |K_3|^2 = -\frac{A_x A_y A_z}{4K},$$
$$\tag{B-17}$$

$$|K_2|^2 + |K_3|^2 = \frac{1}{8g^2 K^2}[A_y^2 A_z^2(g_y^2 m^2 + g_z^2 n^2) + A_z^2 A_x^2(g_z^2 n^2 + g_x^2 l^2)$$

$$+ A_x^2 A_y^2(g_x^2 l^2 + g_y^2 m^2)],$$

which together with Eq. (B-15) gives the energy correct to second order.

If these results are particularized to axial symmetry ($A_x = A_y$ and $g_x = g_y$), then Eq. (B-10) is obtained.

To extend these calculations to third order it is necessary to insert more accurate energy denominators and to employ some terms resulting from fourth-order perturbation theory, which give results whose magnitudes are of third order. There are no contributions from third-order perturbation theory as such.

APPENDIX C

Relative Intensity to First Order in Perturbation Theory of Hyperfine Lines from N Nuclei of Spin I with Identical Hyperfine Interactions [see Eq. (5-90)]

I	N	M_I												
		0	1	2	3	4	5	6	7	8	9	10	11	12
0	Any	1												
$\frac{1}{2}$	2	2	1											
	4	6	4	1										
	6	20	15	6	1									
	8	70	56	28	8	1								
	12	924	792	495	220	66	12	1						
1	1	1	1											
	2	3	2	1										
	3	7	6	3	1									
	4	19	16	10	4	1								
	6	141	126	90	50	21	6	1						
	8	1107	1016	784	504	266	112	36	8	1				
$\frac{3}{2}$	2	4	3	2	1									
	4	44	40	31	20	10	4	1						
	6	580	546	456	336	216	120	56	21	6	1			
	8	8092	7728	6728	5328	3823	2472	1428	728	322	120	36	8	1

I	N	\multicolumn{16}{c}{M_I}
		0	1	2	3	4	5	6	7	8	9	10	11	12	13	14	15
$\frac{5}{2}$	2	6	5	4	3	2	1										
	4	146	140	125	104	80	56	35	20	10	4	1					
	6	4332	4221	3906	3431	2856	2247	1666	1161	756	456	252	126	56	21	6	1
$\frac{7}{2}$	2	8	7	6	5	4	3	2	1								
	4	344	336	315	284	246	204	161	120	84	56	35	20	10	4	1	
$\frac{9}{2}$	2	10	9	8	7	6	5	4	3	2	1						

I	N	\multicolumn{14}{c}{M_I}
		1/2	3/2	5/2	7/2	9/2	11/2	13/2	15/2	17/2	19/2	21/2	23/2	25/2	27/2
$\frac{1}{2}$	1	1													
	3	3	1												
$\frac{3}{2}$	1	1													
	3	12	10	6	3	1									
$\frac{5}{2}$	1	1													
	3	27	25	21	15	10	6	3	1						
$\frac{7}{2}$	1	1													
	3	48	46	42	36	28	21	15	10	6	3	1			
$\frac{9}{2}$	1	1													
	3	75	73	69	63	55	45	36	28	21	15	10	6	3	1

The spectra are all symmetric about the center ($M_I = 0$).

Index